Men's Fitness magazine

Workout Manual 2013

Editor Jon Lipsey

Additional words Ben Ince, Sam Rider, Joel Snape, Joe Warner
Design Fanni Williams
Managing Editor Chris Miller
Subeditor Gareth Beach
Art Director Donovan Walker

Photography Tom Miles, Duncan Nicholls, packshotfactory.co.uk, Danny Bird, Getty, Shutterstock
Models Mark Hughes, Kirk Miller, Toby Rowland, Richard Scrivener@WAthletic, David Peters, Peter Sheath@MOT

MAGBOOK

Group Publisher **Russell Blackman**
Group Managing Director **Ian Westwood**
Digital Production Manager **Nicky Baker**
International Business Development Director **Dharmesh Mistry**
Operations Director **Robin Ryan**
Managing Director of Advertising **Julian Lloyd-Evans**
Newstrade Director **David Barker**
Commercial & Retail Director **Martin Belson**
Chief Operating Officer/ Chief Financial Officer **Brett Reynolds**
Group Finance Director **Ian Leggett**
Chief Executive Officer **James Tye**
Chairman **Felix Dennis**

WORKOUT MANUAL 2013 ISBN **1-78106-049-5**
To license this product please contact Nicole Adams on +44 (0) 20 7907 6134 or nicole_adams@dennis.co.uk

Advertising
Katie Wood katie_wood@dennis.co.uk
Matt Wakefield matt_wakefield@dennis.co.uk

The health and fitness information presented in this book is an educational resource and is not intended as a substitute for medical advice. Consult your doctor or healthcare professional before performing any of the exercises described in this book or any other exercise programme, particularly if you are pregnant, or if you are elderly or have chronic or recurring medical conditions. Do not attempt any of the exercises while under the influence of alcohol or drugs. Discontinue any exercise that causes you pain or severe discomfort and consult a medical expert. Neither the author of the information nor the producer nor distributors of such information make any warranty of any kind in regard to the content of the information presented in this book.

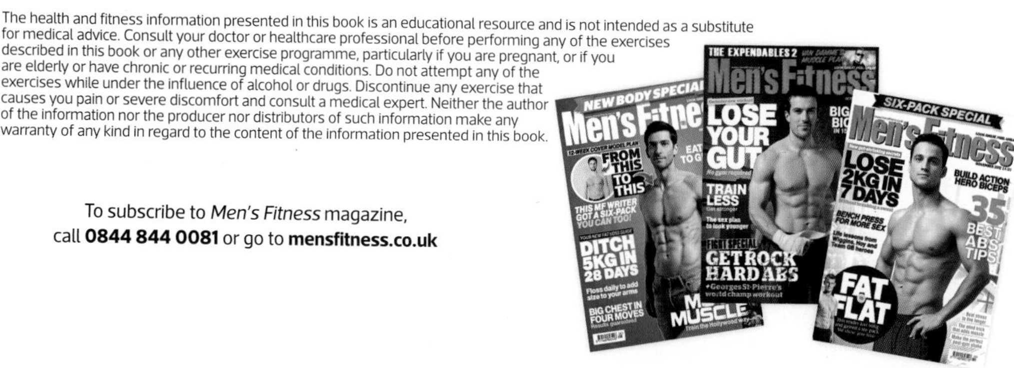

Introduction

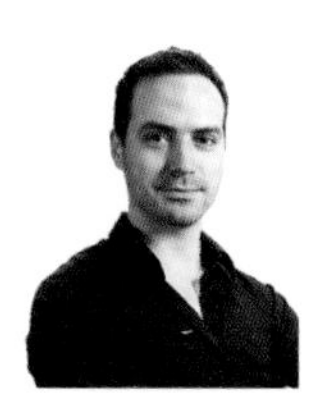

Welcome to the *Men's Fitness* Workout Manual, the ultimate collection of workouts and advice from the pages of Britain's finest fitness magazine.

Whatever your goals, you'll find something to help in these pages, from the big moves that should form the fundamentals of any workout to tailored plans for putting the finishing touches to your new body. There's also a nutrition section packed with advice on how to shop, cook and eat better, including tips on how to eat healthily wherever you are. We've also picked some of the most inspiring sports workouts from the mag, including advice from Olympians and former UFC champions. Finally, for those whose ultimate target is to have an impressive six-pack, we've got the latest and best abs moves – to be used in combination with our series of home workouts to burn away unwanted body fat.

Jon Lipsey, Editor, *Men's Fitness*

Contents

8-37
Must-Do Moves
Key muscle-building exercises

38-87
12-Week Plan
Your best ever body plan

88-95
Nutrition
Eat right to fuel your training

96-117
Sports Drills
Pro performance tips

119-128
Abs Training
New moves that carve six-packs

130-145
Home Workouts
Circuits that burn off your belly

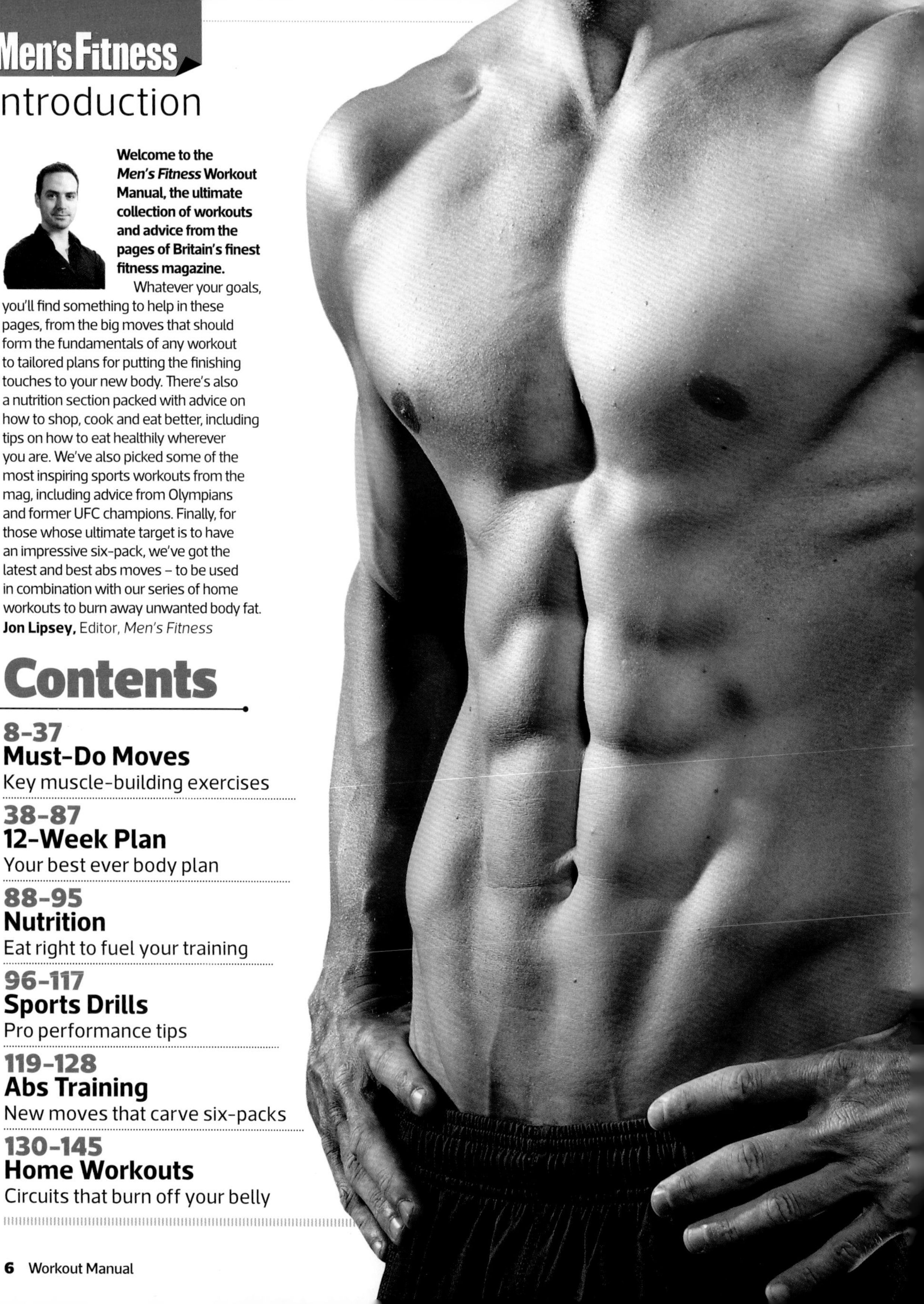

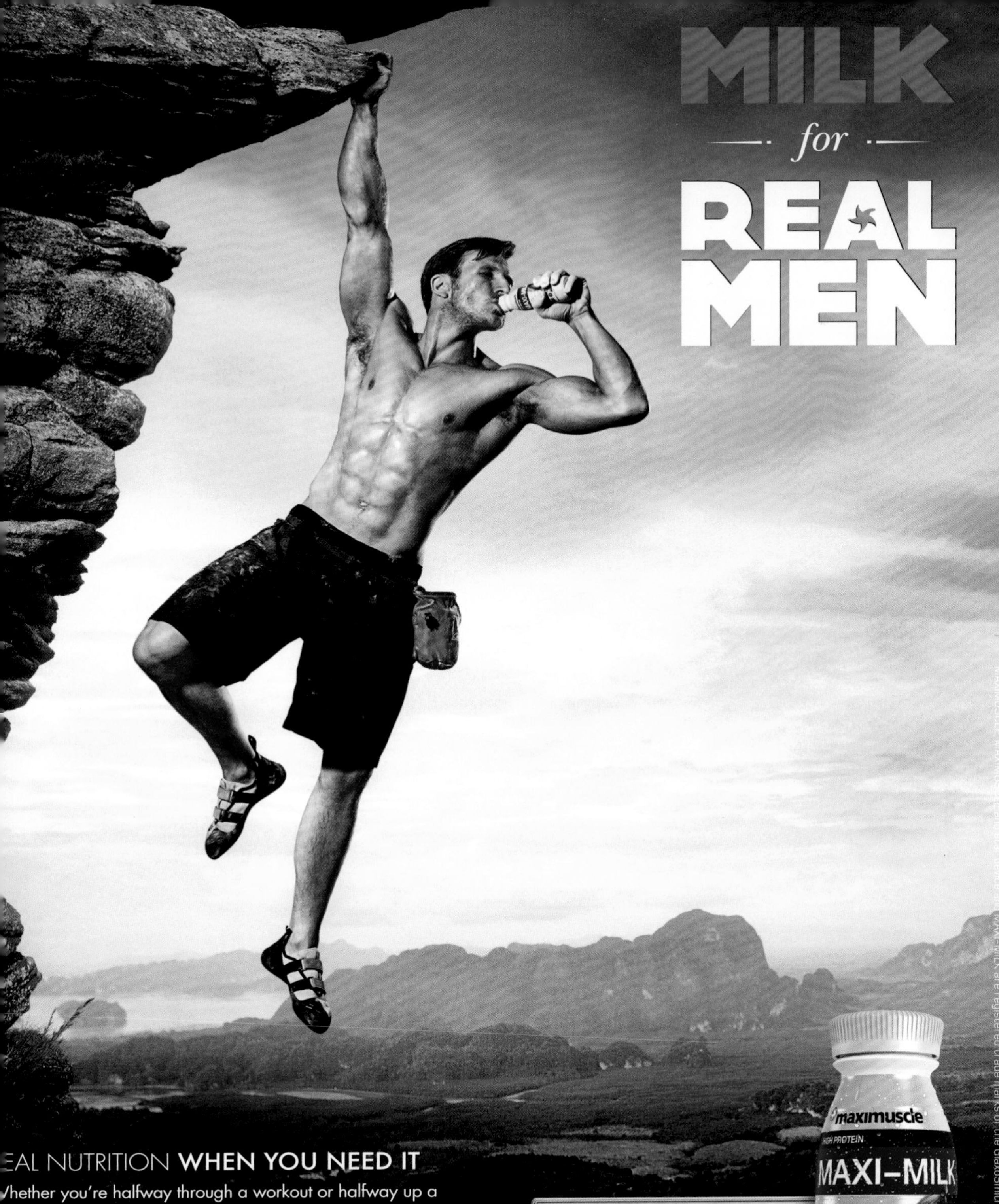
MILK
for
REAL
MEN
MAXIMUSCLE, MAXIMUSCLE and star device and MAXI-MILK are registered trade marks of the GlaxoSmithKline group of companies.

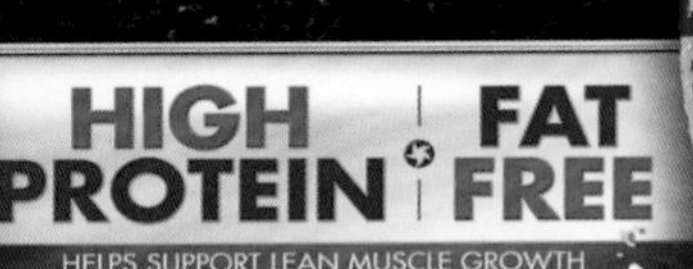
HIGH PROTEIN
FAT FREE
HELPS SUPPORT LEAN MUSCLE GROWTH

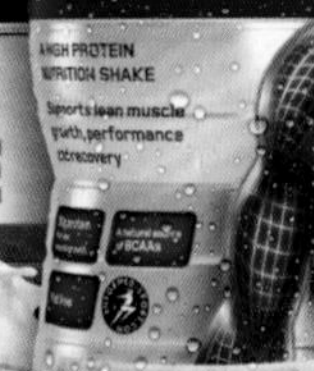
maximuscle
HIGH PROTEIN
MAXI-MILK

EAL NUTRITION **WHEN YOU NEED IT**
Vhether you're halfway through a workout or halfway up a
ountain, if you need a quick hit on the go, grab yourself a Maxi-
ilk. It's got 30g of high quality protein, it's rich in BCAAs and it's
so fat free. So, basically it's great at building lean muscles and
elping you do manly things.
acebook.com/maximuscle

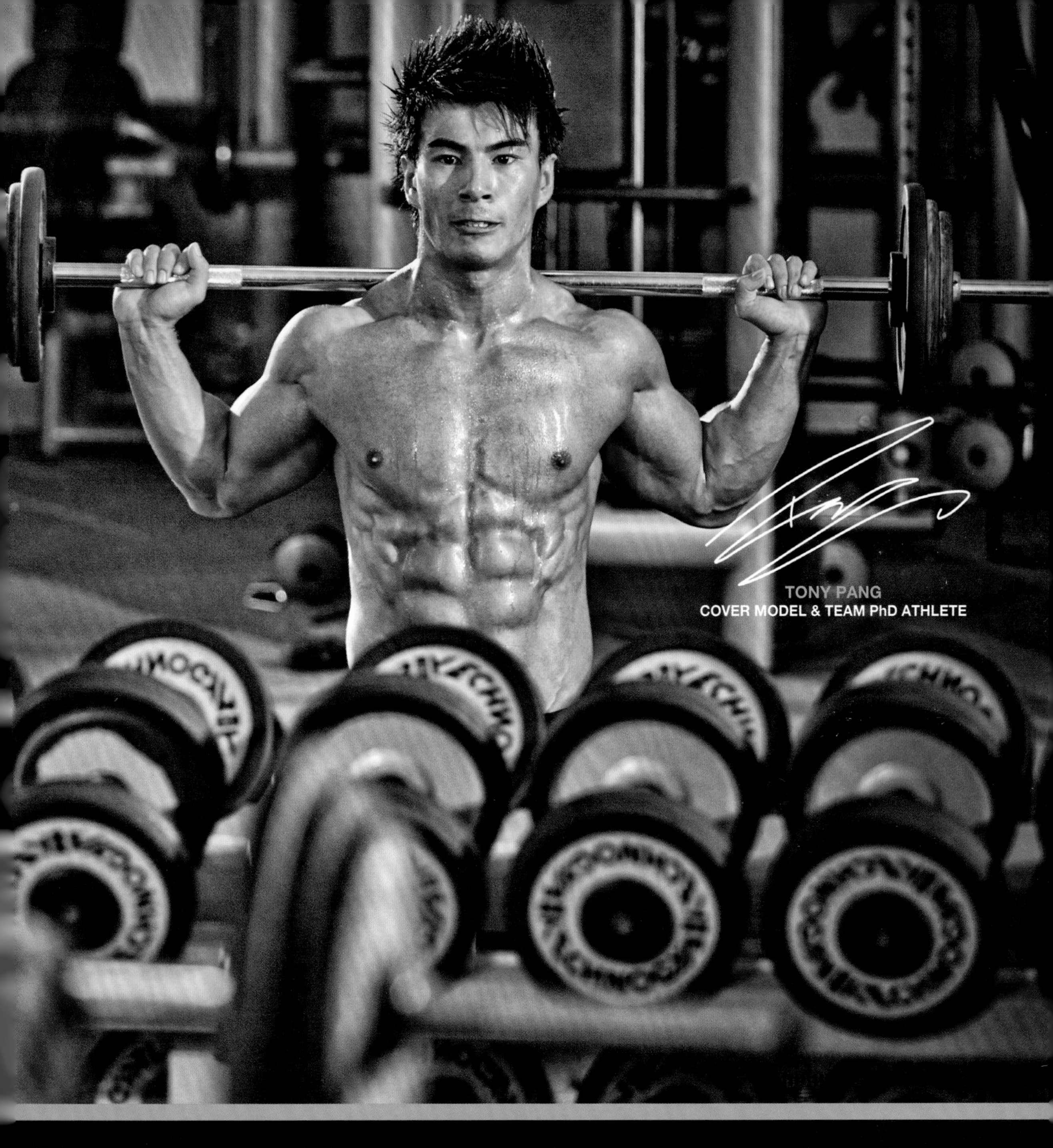
TONY PANG
COVER MODEL & TEAM PhD ATHLETE

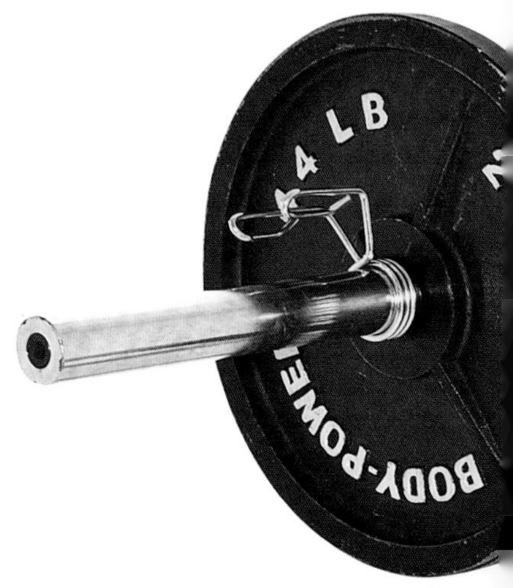

Must-do moves

Get a body part blitz with the best moves for each main muscle group

It's not true that all men want to look the same. But every man in the gym has one or more muscle groups that he'd like to develop. You might want to add size to your biceps, make your back a bit thicker or bring out your abs. Whatever your target body part, this chapter contains the key moves you'll need to develop it.

The key to making real progress with a particular muscle group is to hit it with a variety of exercises that emphasise different areas of the muscle group while also working in slightly different movement patterns. Doing multiple exercises for the same muscle group will also help you stress the maximum amount of muscle fibres, which means you get maximum repair and increased muscle growth.

BODY PART WORKOUTS IN THIS SECTION

Chest	p12
Quads	p14
Biceps	p16
Hamstrings	p18
Triceps	p20
Glutes	p22
Upper back	p24
Abs	p26
Shoulders	p28
Lats	p31

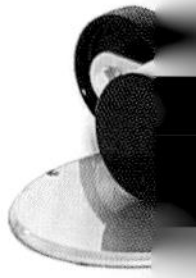

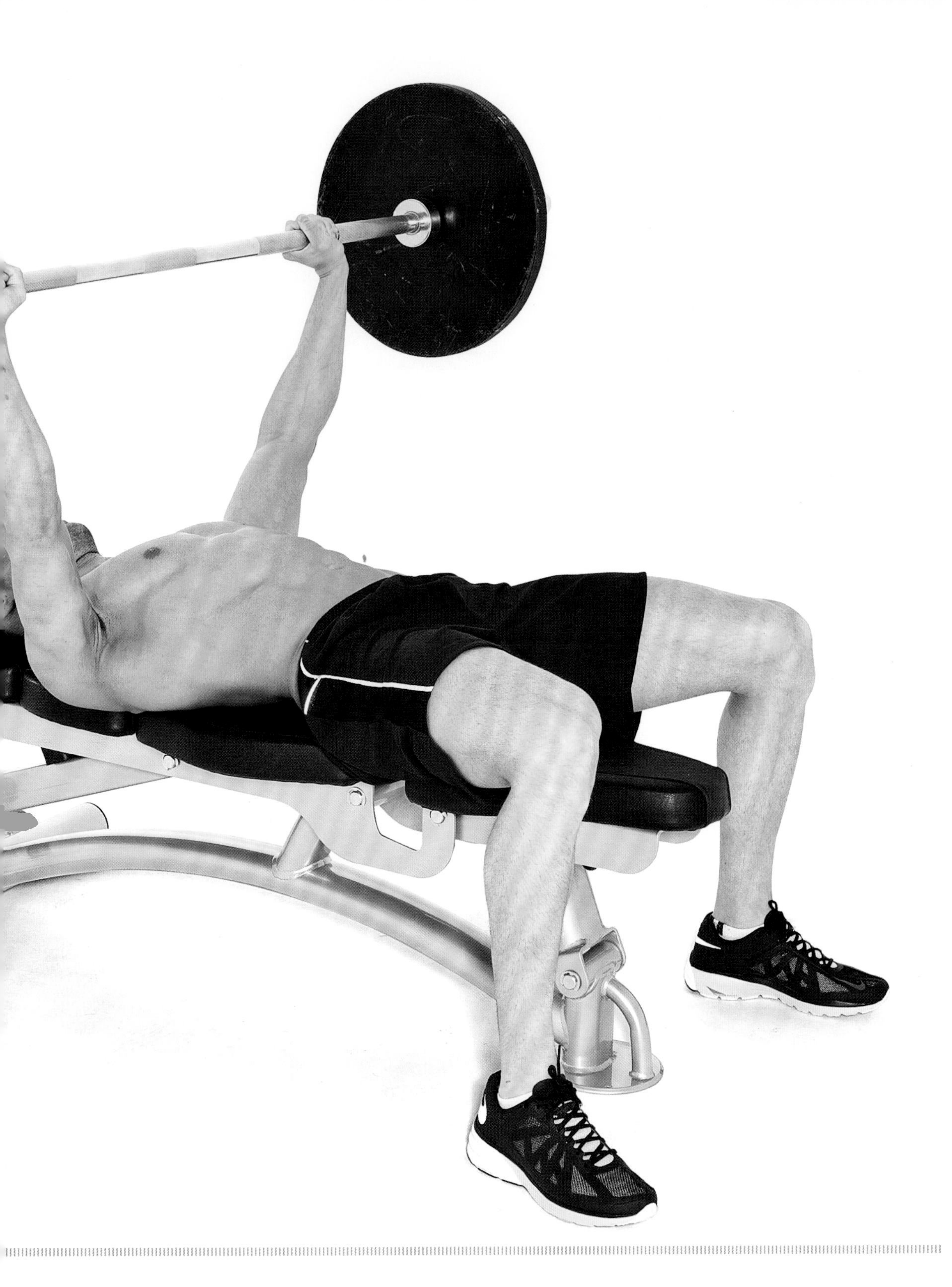

Must-Do Moves

Chest

Build big pecs by starting with this classic gym move

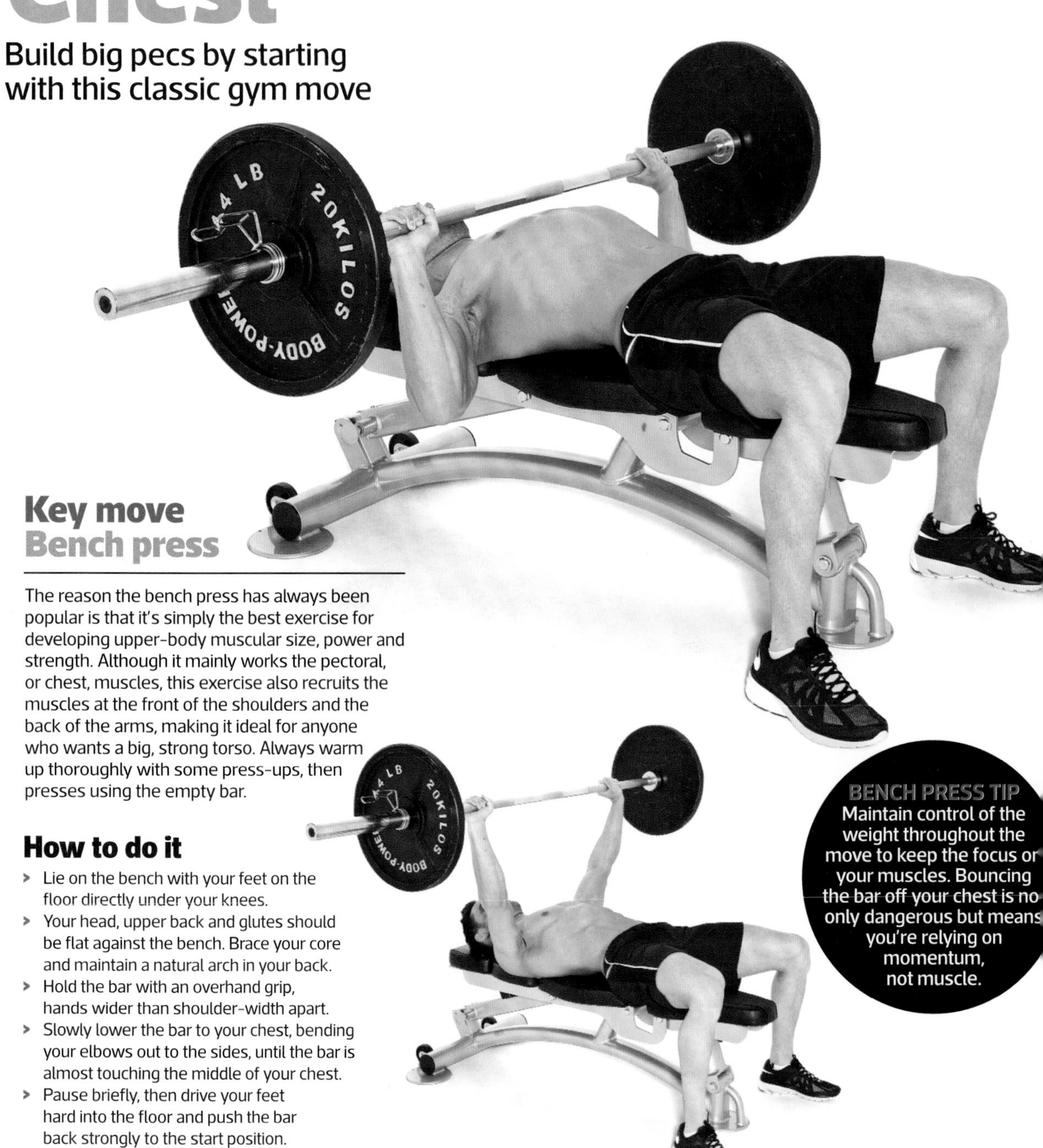

Key move
Bench press

The reason the bench press has always been popular is that it's simply the best exercise for developing upper-body muscular size, power and strength. Although it mainly works the pectoral, or chest, muscles, this exercise also recruits the muscles at the front of the shoulders and the back of the arms, making it ideal for anyone who wants a big, strong torso. Always warm up thoroughly with some press-ups, then presses using the empty bar.

How to do it

- Lie on the bench with your feet on the floor directly under your knees.
- Your head, upper back and glutes should be flat against the bench. Brace your core and maintain a natural arch in your back.
- Hold the bar with an overhand grip, hands wider than shoulder-width apart.
- Slowly lower the bar to your chest, bending your elbows out to the sides, until the bar is almost touching the middle of your chest.
- Pause briefly, then drive your feet hard into the floor and push the bar back strongly to the start position.

BENCH PRESS TIP
Maintain control of the weight throughout the move to keep the focus on your muscles. Bouncing the bar off your chest is no only dangerous but means you're relying on momentum, not muscle.

Dumbbell flye

This move isolates your chest muscles, taking your arms out of the equation so all the work has to be done by your chest.

How to do it

- Lie on an incline bench holding a dumbbell in each hand directly above your chest, arms straight and palms facing each other.
- Make sure your head and shoulders are supported on the bench and your feet are flat on the floor.
- With a slight bend in your elbows, slowly lower the weights out to the side as far as is comfortable.
- Don't arch your back.
- Use your pecs to reverse the movement and raise the weights back to the top.

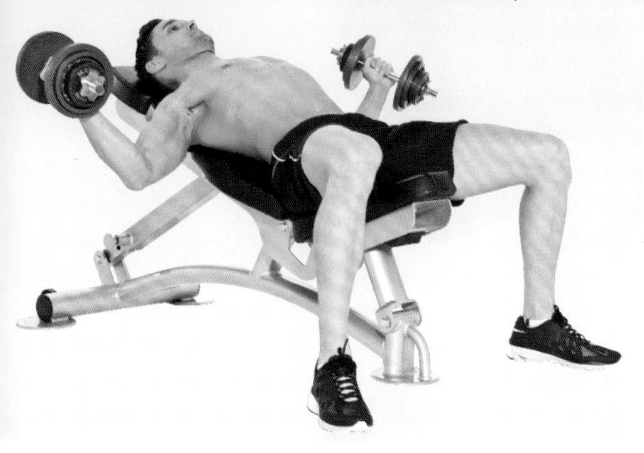

Cable crossover

It's hard to truly isolate your powerful chest muscles – the arms and shoulders nearly always get in on the act because of the way your upper body muscles move together. But this move is a great way to work the chest because using cables, rather than dumbbells, for resistance ensures that there is constant tension throughout the move, which forces your chest to work hard to control the weight.

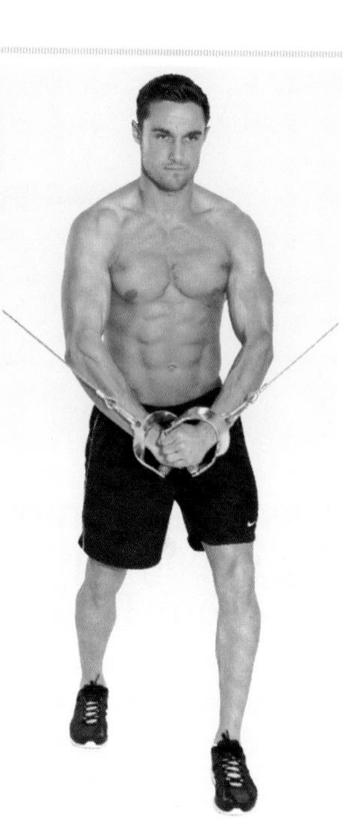

How to do it

- Stand in the middle of a cable machine with a split stance, holding a D-handle attachment in each hand and with the cable set above shoulder height.
- Keeping a natural arch in your back, your core braced and your upper body still, bring your hands down in an arc to meet in front of your torso.
- Pause briefly and squeeze your chest muscles, then return to the start slowly and with the weight under full control.

Incline dumbbell press

Tilting the bench places the focus on the upper part of your chest, as well as your triceps and the front of your shoulders. Using dumbbells allows for a greater range of motion.

How to do it

- Lie on a bench set at a 30-45° angle holding a dumbbell in each hand at shoulder-height.
- Keep your feet flat on the floor and your back against the bench.
- Press the weight directly above your head, but don't lock out your elbows at the top.
- Slowly lower the weight back down to your chest, flaring your elbows out to the side.

Clap press-up

Having to clap between press-ups means you have to push up from the floor very quickly, turning a humble bodyweight exercise into an explosive muscle-building move.

How to do it

- Start in a press-up position and lower until your chest is just above the ground, keeping your elbows close to your sides.
- Press back up powerfully so that your hands leave the floor. Quickly clap them together.
- Land on your hands and descend into the next rep.

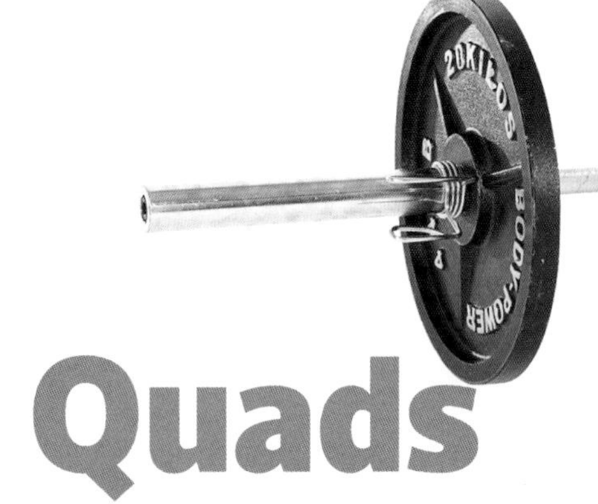

Quads

Master these moves to build big, strong legs that give you a platform for all-over muscle

Key move Squat

There's a reason the squat is called 'king of the lifts' – it targets not only the quads but also the glutes, hamstrings, core and back, making it the single most important exercise in your muscle-building arsenal. Although your legs are the obvious target, squats create an overall anabolic environment that triggers the release of extra testosterone and growth hormone. This means that mastering the squat will give you bigger, stronger leg muscles and have a similarly galvanising effect on your upper body and abs.

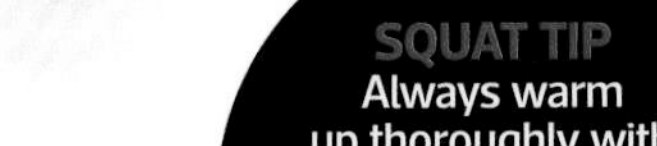

SQUAT TIP
Always warm up thoroughly with some bodyweight squats, then using the empty bar before adding serious weight.

How to do it

- Rest the bar against the back of your shoulders – not on your neck – and hold it with an overhand grip slightly wider than shoulder width.
- Your feet should be just wider than shoulder-width apart with your toes pointing outwards slightly.
- Slowly lower yourself, keeping your chest and chin up while maintaining a natural arch in your back. Keep the weight on your heels and your body upright, and don't let your knees roll inwards or forwards.
- Bring your body down until your thighs are at least parallel to the floor. The deeper you can squat, the better.
- Drive back up through your heels.

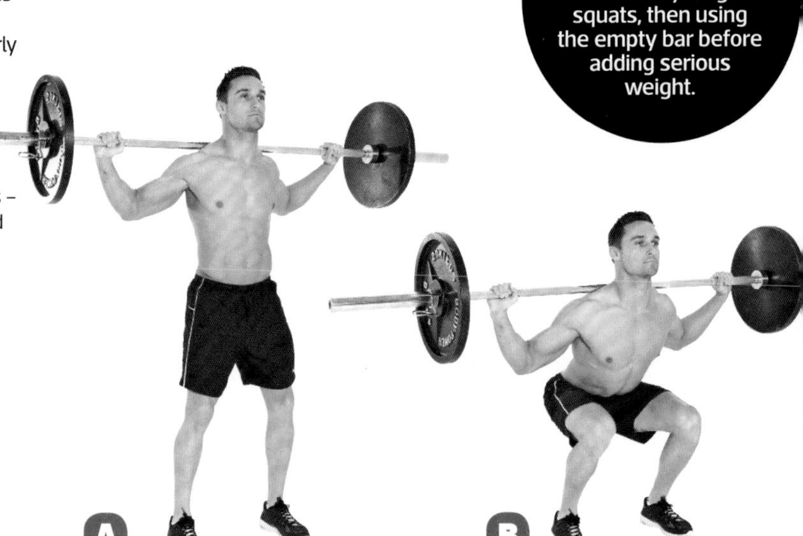

ront squat

Resting the bar on the front of your shoulders targets your quads while aking emphasis off your lower back. n this position you can't lean forward, o you get a bigger range of motion.

low to do it

- Rest the bar on the front of your shoulders, gripping it with your hands crossed in front of you, your elbows pointing forward and your feet shoulder-width apart.
- Maintain a natural arch in your back and keep your core braced throughout the move.
- Squat down until your thighs are at least parallel to the floor.
- Push back up through your heels.

Sumo squat

This stance puts the emphasis on your hard-to-hit inner thighs. Make sure your feet point out to the sides more than in a normal squat to avoid placing excessive strain on your knees.

How to do it

- Stand with a bar resting across your shoulders with a wide stance, so that your feet are wider than shoulder-width apart. Keep your feet pointing out to the sides.
- Maintain a natural arch in your back and keep your core braced throughout the move.
- Squat down until your thighs are at least parallel to the floor.
- Push back up through your heels.

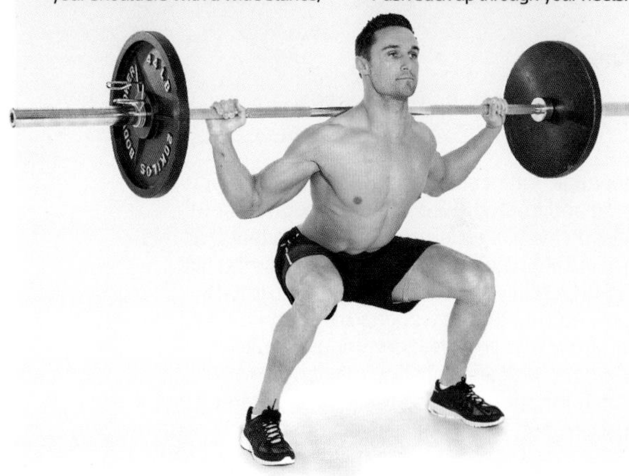

ateral lunge

.ike the sumo squat, this move argets the often-forgotten inner nigh muscles. Ignoring them can ead to muscular imbalances and njury, while strengthening them nproves all your lower-body lifts s well as sports performance.

low to do it

- Stand tall with feet close together, holding a dumbbell in each hand.
- Keeping your core braced and head looking forward, take a big step to one side and lower your body down towards the leading leg. Your knee should stay in line with your toes.
- Push back off the leading leg and repeat on the other side.

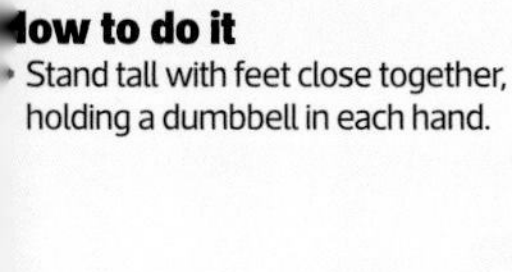

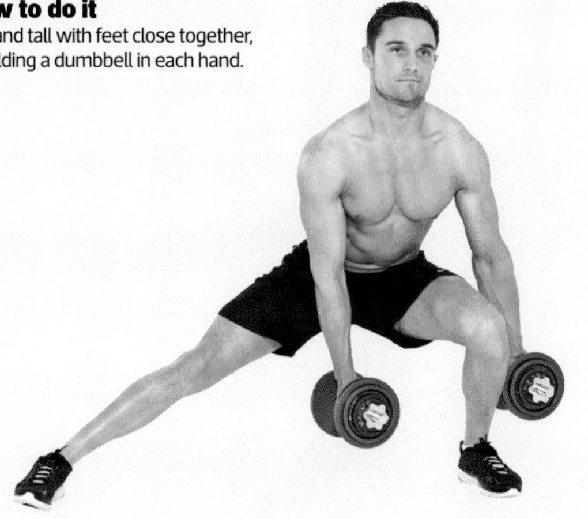

Hack squat

Holding the bar behind your body forces you to keep your torso upright to manage the weight, and so improves your ability to perform normal squats correctly and safely. This variation places less strain on your back but greater emphasis on your powerful quad muscles.

How to do it

- Stand in front of a barbell with your feet shoulder-width apart.
- Squat down and hold the bar with an overhand grip.
- Keeping your feet flat on the floor, knees in line with your toes, head up and core braced and a neutral arch in your back, push through your heels until you're fully upright.
- Lower again until your thighs are at least parallel to the floor.

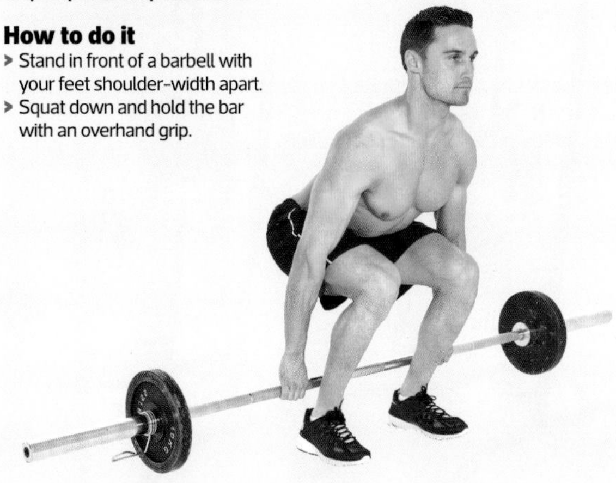

Biceps

The five moves that can lead to big upper-arm gains

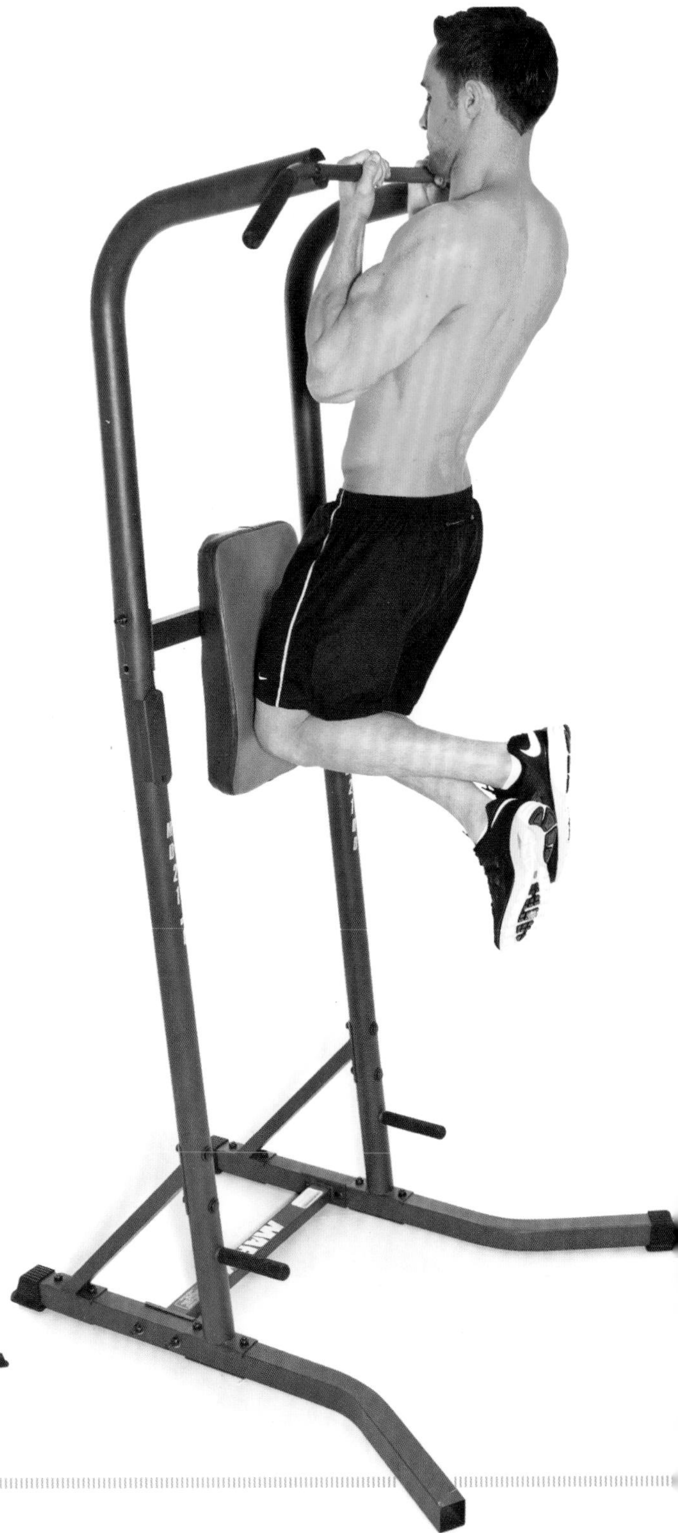

Key move Chin-up

Many people intent on building big arms stick with the tried and trusted biceps curl. Although a useful muscle-building exercise, the curl isn't as tough as this compound lift, which is arguably the most effective way of targeting your biceps muscles for growth. Not only do your biceps work hard throughout the move, you also recruit the powerhouse muscles of the upper back and consequently ensure a big growth-hormone response, resulting in greater gains not just on your biceps but all over your body.

How to do it

- Hold the bar with an underhand grip with your hands shoulder-width apart.
- Start from a dead hang with your arms fully extended.
- Pull yourself up by squeezing your lats together.
- Once your chin is higher than your hands, pause briefly, then slowly lower yourself back to the start.

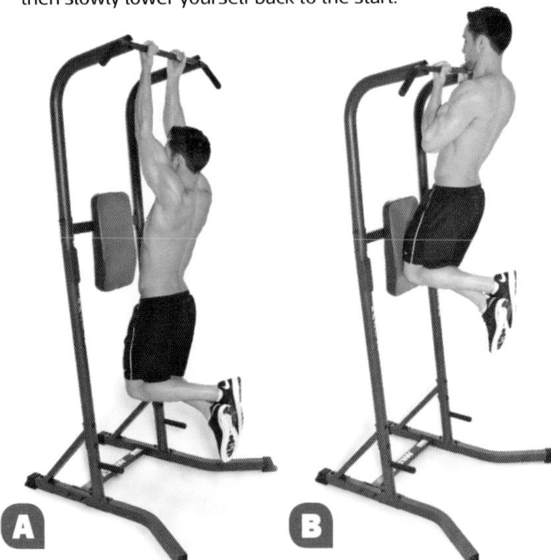

ıcline dumbbell curl

ʒy doing biceps curls on an incline ɟench, you move through a greater ange of motion than when standing ɪp, so your biceps work harder.

ɬow to do it

- Sit on a bench set on an incline between 30° and 45° holding a dumbbell in each hand.
- Keeping your back flat against the bench and your elbows close to your sides, slowly curl the dumbbells up to shoulder height.
- Squeeze your biceps at the top of the move and then slowly return to the start.

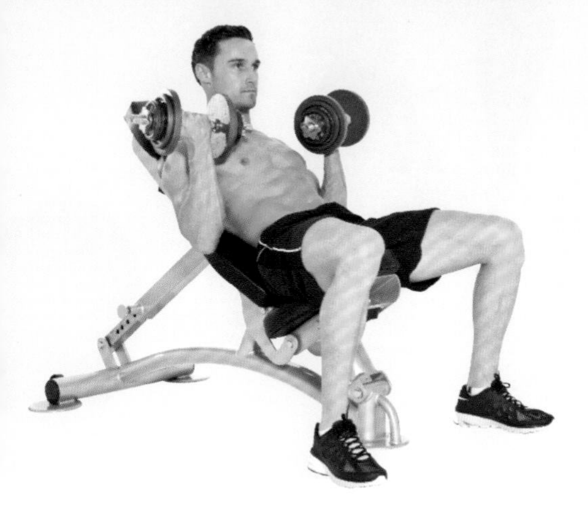

One-arm preacher curl

Resting your upper arm on an upright bench stabilises it, taking momentum out of the equation and forcing your biceps to do all the work. Training each arm individually also removes the risk of your dominant arm doing more of the work, resulting in balanced growth. Straighten your arm fully at the bottom of the move and squeeze your biceps at the top for maximum muscle gains.

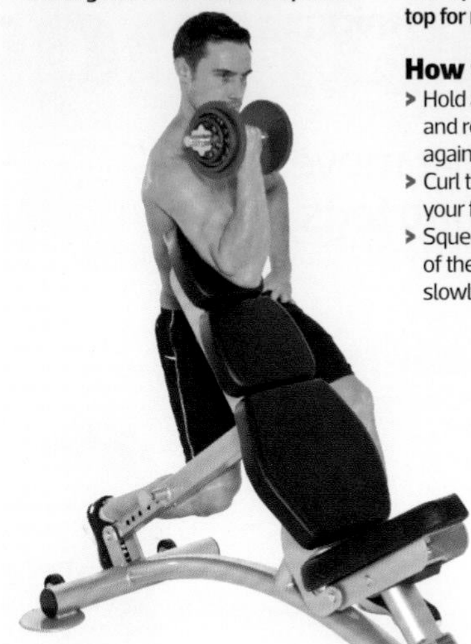

How to do it

- Hold a dumbbell in one hand and rest that upper arm against an upright bench.
- Curl the weight up until your forearm is vertical.
- Squeeze your biceps at the top of the move and then lower slowly back to the start.

Z-bar biceps curl

ɬsing an EZ-bar, which has a zigzagged niddle, allows you turn your hands ıwards slightly, unlike a barbell. This akes some of the strain off your wrists ınd allows the focus of the weight to ɪe solely on your biceps, forcing them ɔ work harder throughout the move.

ɬow to do it

- Stand tall with your shoulders back and feet close together, holding an EZ-bar with an underhand grip with hands just outside your hips.
- Keeping your elbows tucked in to your sides, curl the bar up towards your chest, stopping just before your forearms reach vertical.
- Lower the bar back slowly to the start. Avoid rocking back and forth to generate momentum, because this takes the emphasis away from the biceps.

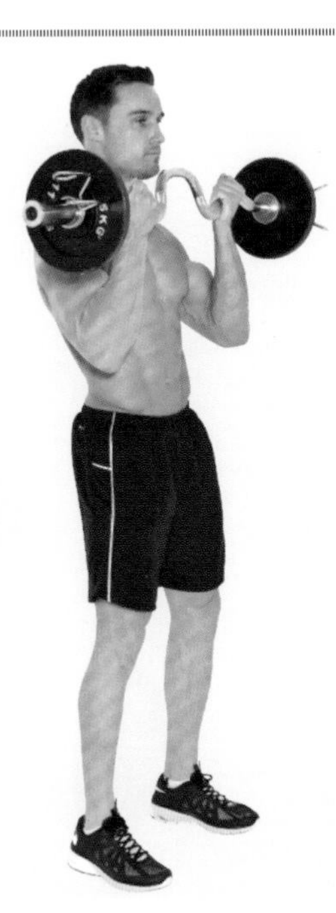

Hammer curl

This move shifts some of the emphasis towards the forearms, making it a good exercise for working the muscles responsible for grip strength. A stronger grip will reward you with better performance in a host of other lifts, not just those focusing on the biceps.

How to do it

- Stand tall with your shoulders back and feet close together, holding a dumbbell in each hand.
- Turn your wrists so that your palms face each other. Maintain this grip throughout the move.
- Keeping your elbows close to your side, slowly raise the dumbbells to shoulder height, squeezing your biceps at the top of the move.
- Slowly return the weights to the start position and repeat.

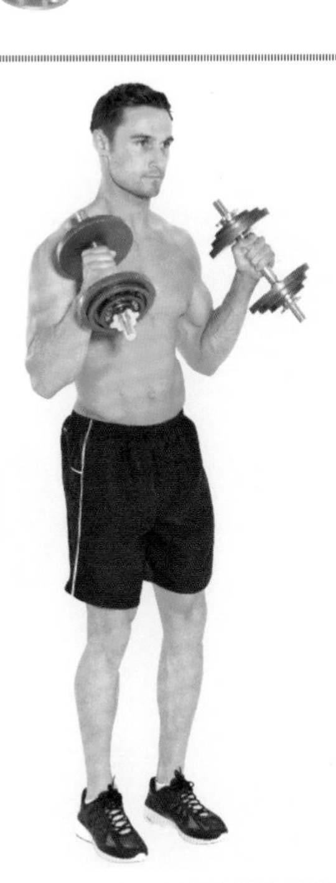

Hamstrings

Perfect these five moves to build big, strong legs

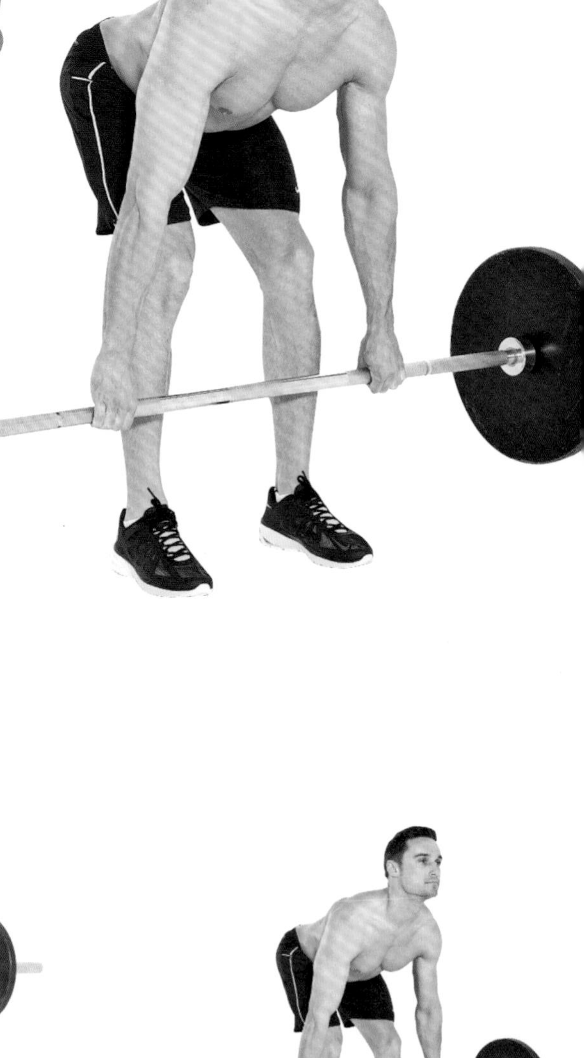

Key move
Romanian deadlift

This is one of the best moves for building muscle mass on the backs of your legs. Perfect form is vital to protect your lower back from injury.

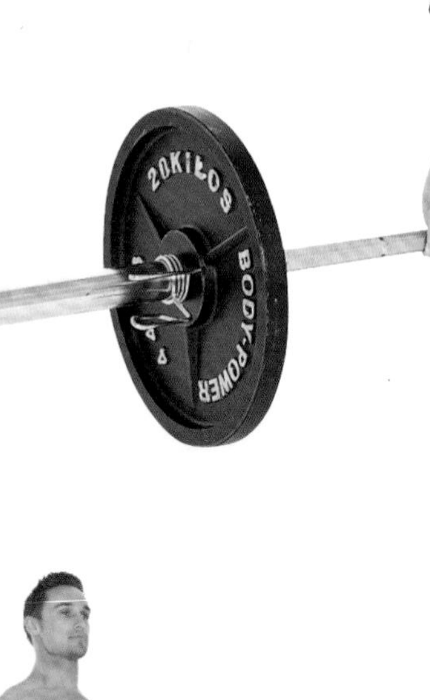

How to do it

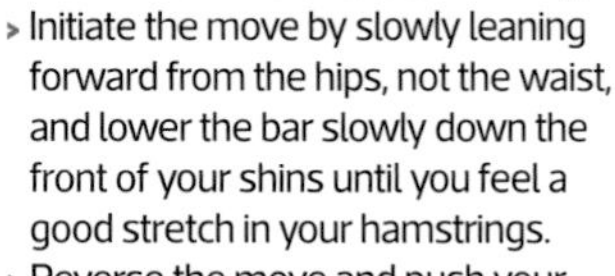

- Stand tall with your feet shoulder-width apart, holding a barbell with an overhand grip just outside your hips. Keep your shoulder blades retracted, torso upright, core braced and a natural arch in your back.
- Initiate the move by slowly leaning forward from the hips, not the waist, and lower the bar slowly down the front of your shins until you feel a good stretch in your hamstrings.
- Reverse the move and push your hips forward to return to the start.

A

B

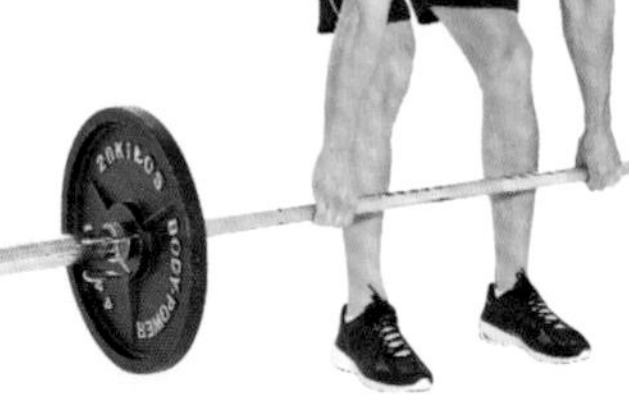

unge

As well as the hamstrings and glutes, unges also involve stabilising muscles such as adductors and hip flexors that need to be strong for you to move with speed, power and co-ordination.

How to do it

- Stand tall with a barbell resting on the back of your shoulders. Point your elbows down to retract your shoulder blades and keep your back upright and core braced throughout.
- Take a big step forward, keeping your knee over your front foot and not letting it go beyond it.
- Lower until both knees are bent at 90°, then push back off your front foot to return to the start position.

Gym ball leg curl

Even though you are only using your own bodyweight, this is still a surprisingly tough move that hits your hamstrings hard.

How to do it

- Lie with your head, shoulders and upper back on a gym mat and with your feet together on top of a gym ball. Your body should form a straight line from head to heels.
- Keeping your back straight, raise your hips and drag the ball towards your backside with your heels.
- Pause briefly at the top of the move, then slowly return to the start.

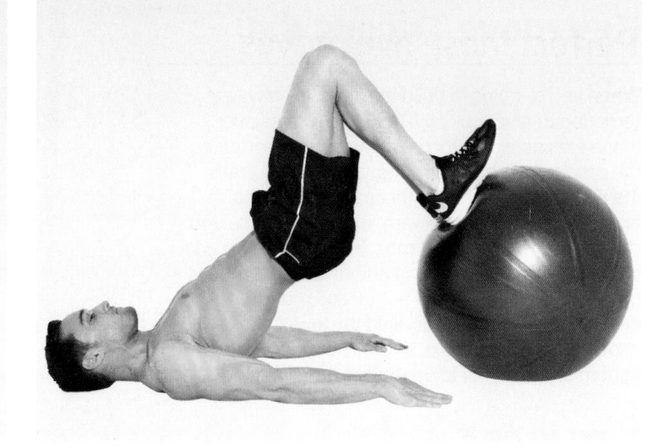

umbbell lateral lunge and touch

This move targets the often-forgotten inner-thigh muscles. Ignoring them can lead to muscular imbalances and injury, while strengthening them will improve all lower-body lifts and sports performance.

How to do it

- Stand tall with your feet close together, holding a dumbbell in each hand.
- Keeping your core braced and head looking forward, take a big step to one side and lower your body towards the leading leg, with your knee in line with your toes.
- Reach down with the dumbbells, keeping your back straight, and touch them to the floor, or as far as you can comfortably reach.
- Push back off the leading leg and repeat on the other side.

Jump lunge

The explosive power required to jump high enough to switch legs and land in another lunge leads to rapid muscle growth and has huge transferable value to many sports.

How to do it

- Start in a lunge position, then jump straight up.
- Switch legs in mid-air to land with your other foot forward.
- Descend straight into a lunge and repeat.

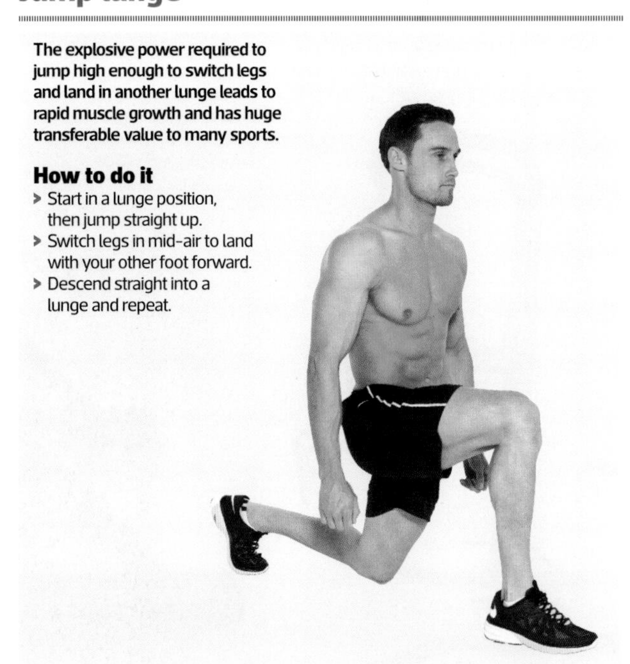

Triceps

Do these five moves to add size and strength to your arms

Key move Triceps dip

When you're trying to build big arms, it's always tempting to favour biceps-boosting moves over those exercises that focus on the triceps because the results are so visually impressive – but that's the wrong approach. The triceps make up about two-thirds of your upper-arm musculature, so you can't afford to ignore this muscle if you want to add size and strength. The dip is one of the best moves to target all three parts of the triceps muscle, as well as being great for working the lower chest, shoulders and your core, which you must keep tight to prevent your lower body from swinging.

How to do it

- Grip parallel bars, keeping your body upright.
- With your elbows pointing straight back, lower your body as far down as you can comfortably go without stressing your shoulders.
- Keep your core braced and don't swing your legs for momentum.

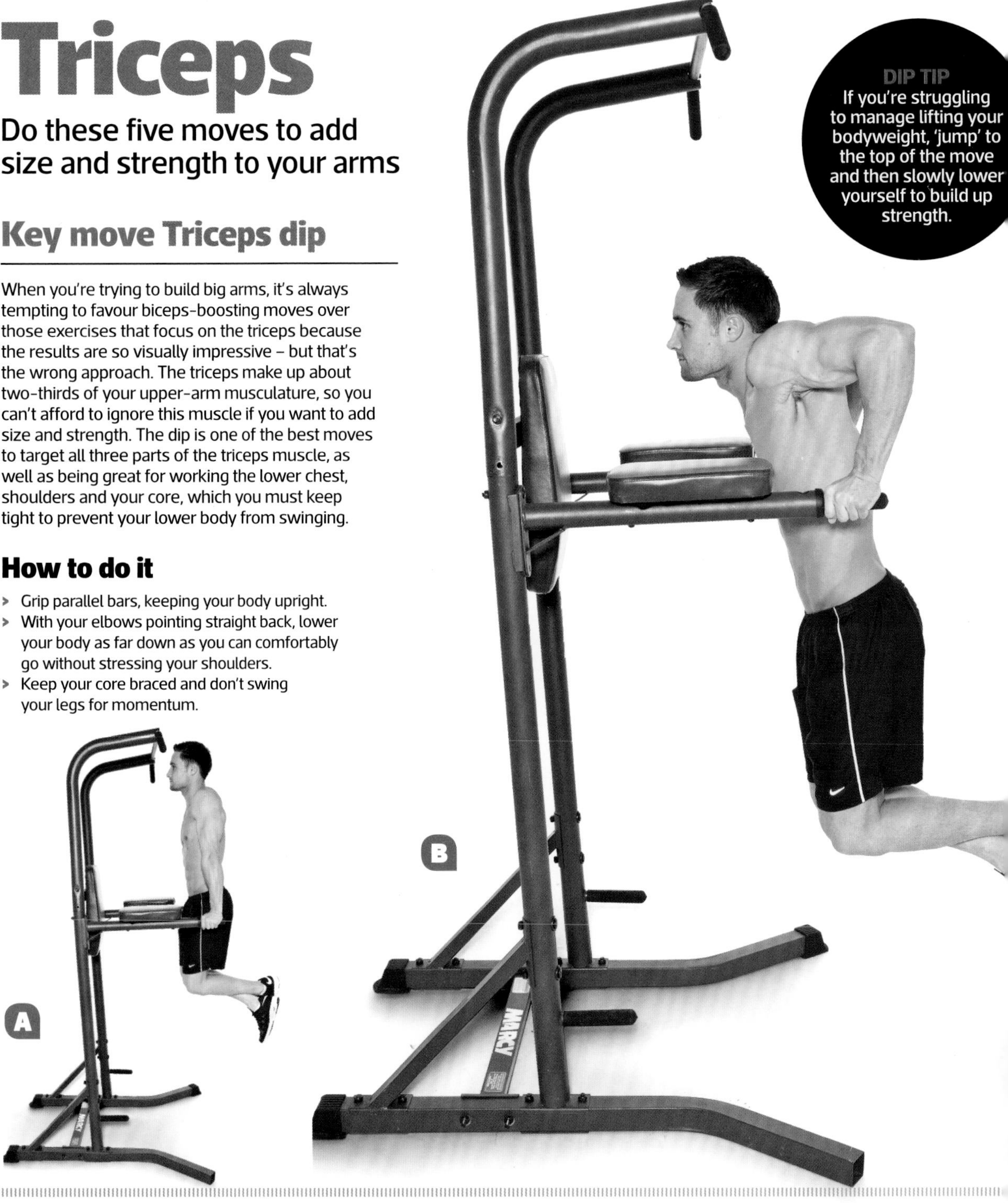

DIP TIP
If you're struggling to manage lifting your bodyweight, 'jump' to the top of the move and then slowly lower yourself to build up strength.

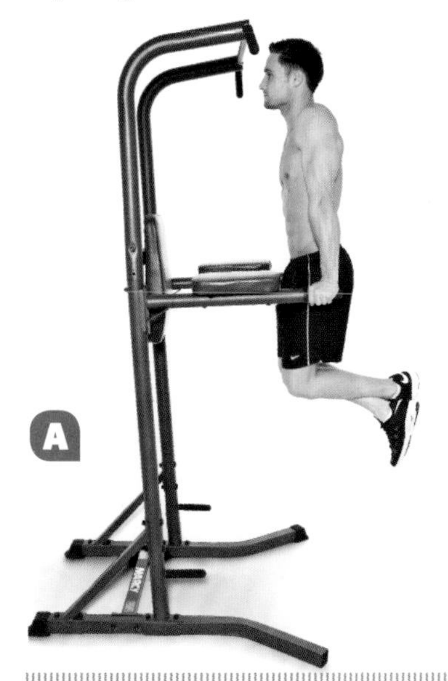

lose-grip bench press

Bringing your hands closer together transfers the focus of this move away from the chest and to the triceps.

How to do it

- Lie flat on a bench holding a barbell with a close, overhand grip. Aim for a fist-sized gap between your hands.
- Keep your head, shoulders and back supported by the bench, your core braced and your feet flat on the floor.
- Lower the bar slowly to your chest, keeping your elbows close in to your sides to keep the emphasis on your triceps.
- Push back up powerfully, but don't lock out your elbows.

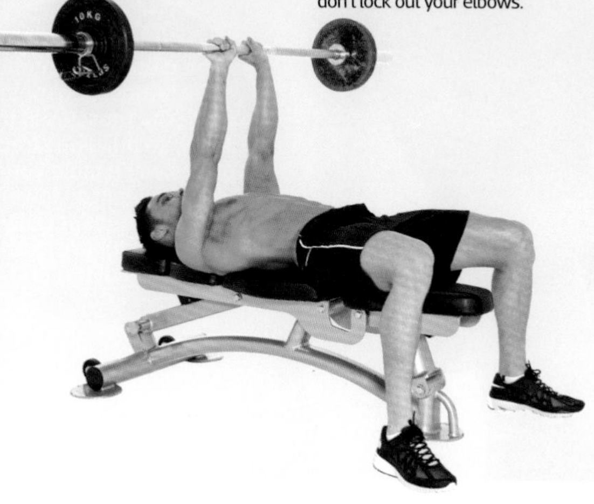

Lying EZ-bar triceps extension

This move works to isolate your triceps, forcing the muscle to work hard throughout as you control the weight on the way down before raising it again. Start by using a light weight because you need to manage the weight safely as you lower it towards your head.

How to do it

- Lie flat on a bench, holding an EZ-bar above you with straight arms.
- Slowly lower the bar towards the top of your head by bending your elbows, which should point upwards throughout the move.
- Without arching your back, return the bar to the start position.

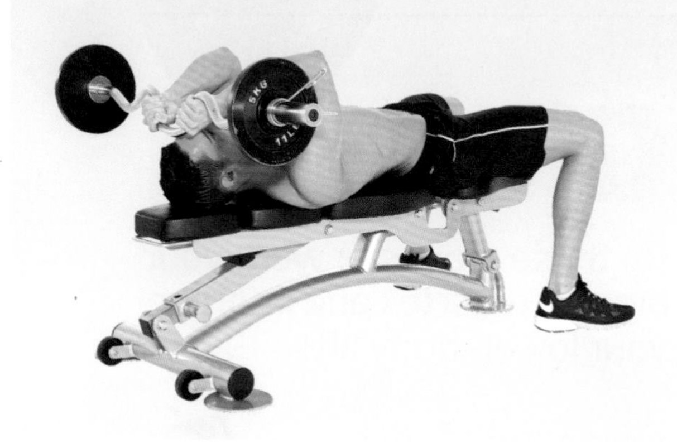

able press-down

The advantage of using a cable machine is that it provides resistance throughout the whole move, forcing your triceps to work hard to manage the weight on the way up as well as on the way down. Keep your elbows close to your sides so that the emphasis stays on your triceps.

How to do it

- Stand tall at a cable machine with a double rope handle or straight bar handle attached at head height.
- Keeping your elbows tucked in, press the handle down without leaning forwards.
- Squeeze your triceps at the bottom of the move, then slowly return to the start.

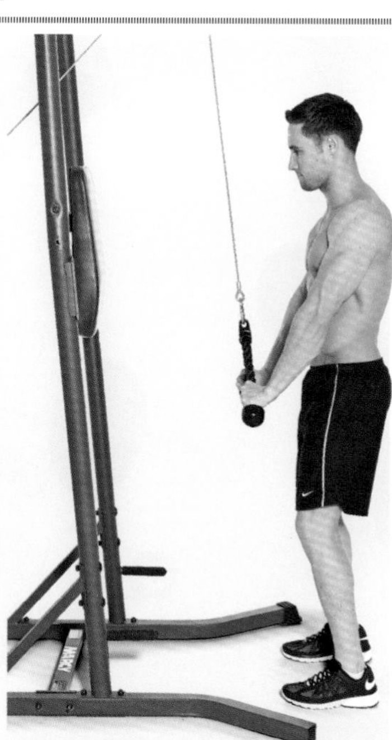

Cable kickback

Using a cable provides greater resistance to your muscles throughout the move, making this a harder and more worthwhile exercise than the dumbbell version.

How to do it

- Rest one hand and one knee on a bench, maintaining a natural curve in your back.
- Hold a cable rope in your free hand, ensuring that there's tension.
- Press the handle straight back, moving only at the elbow.
- Squeeze your triceps at the top of the move, then return to start.

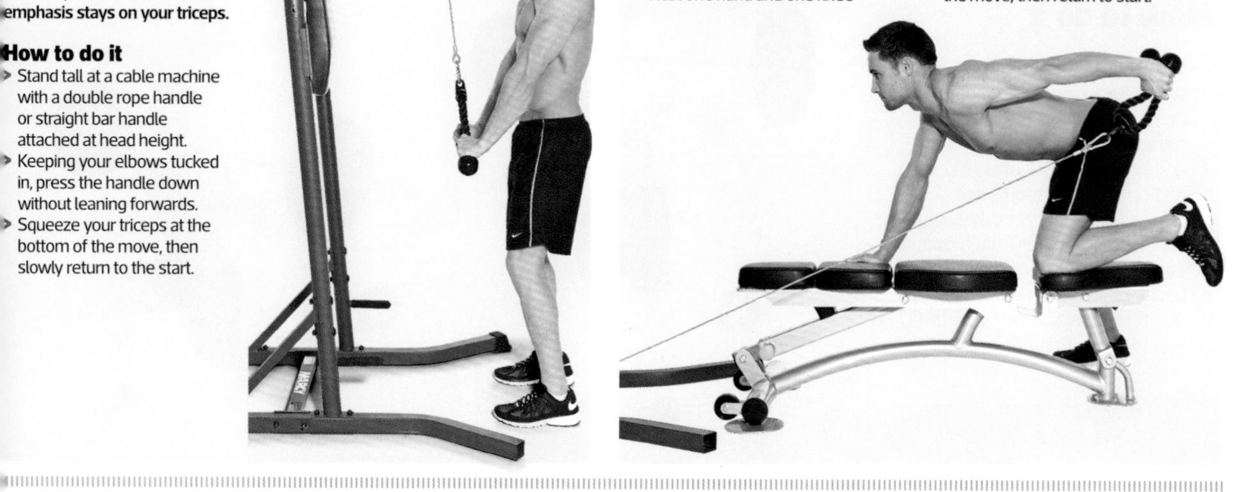

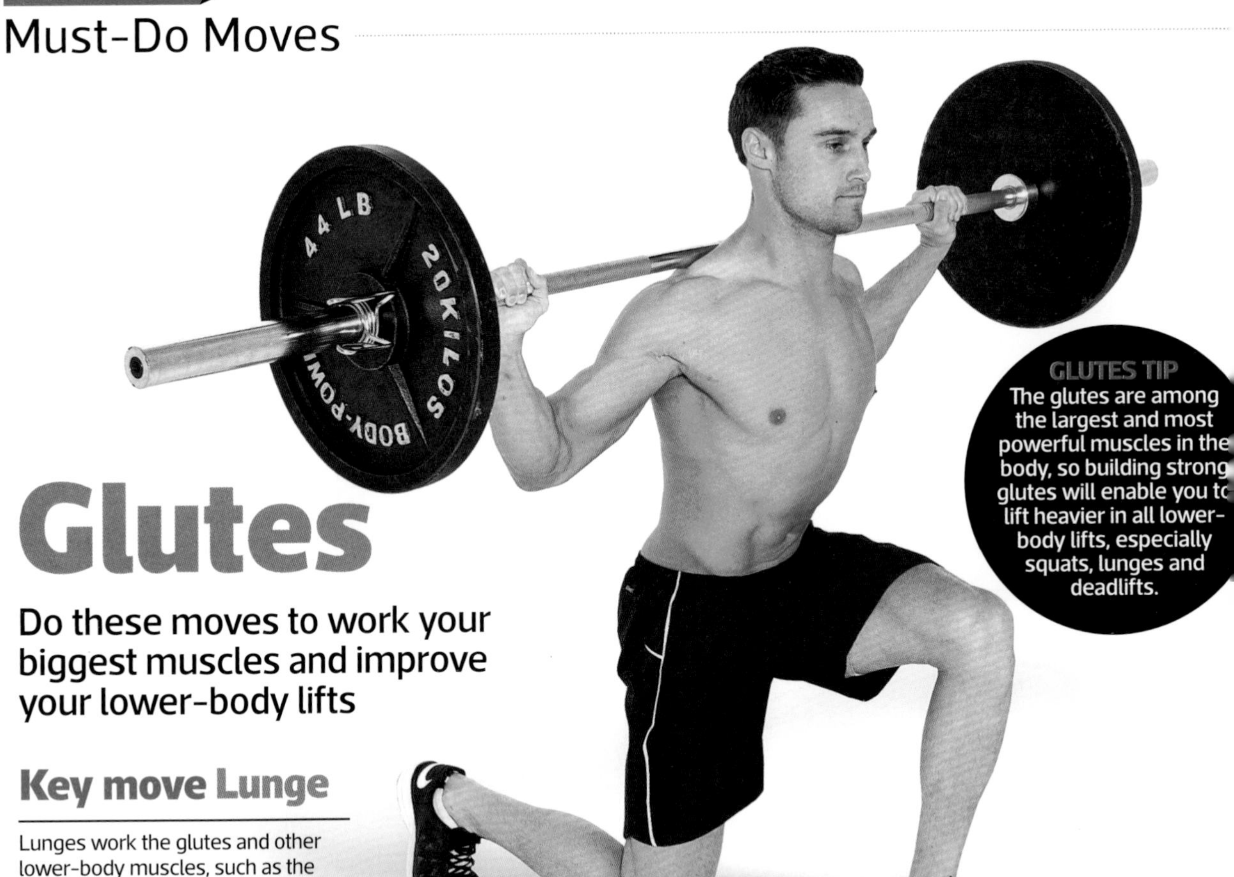

GLUTES TIP
The glutes are among the largest and most powerful muscles in the body, so building strong glutes will enable you to lift heavier in all lower-body lifts, especially squats, lunges and deadlifts.

Glutes

Do these moves to work your biggest muscles and improve your lower-body lifts

Key move Lunge

Lunges work the glutes and other lower-body muscles, such as the quads, hamstrings and calves, as well as many stabilising muscles – including your core – to allow you to move with speed and power.

How to do it

- Stand tall with a barbell resting on the back of your shoulders. Point your elbows down to retract your shoulder blades, and keep your back upright and core braced throughout.
- Take a big step forward, keeping your knee over your front foot and ensuring it doesn't go beyond it.
- Lower until both knees are bent at 90°, then push back off your front foot to return to the start position.

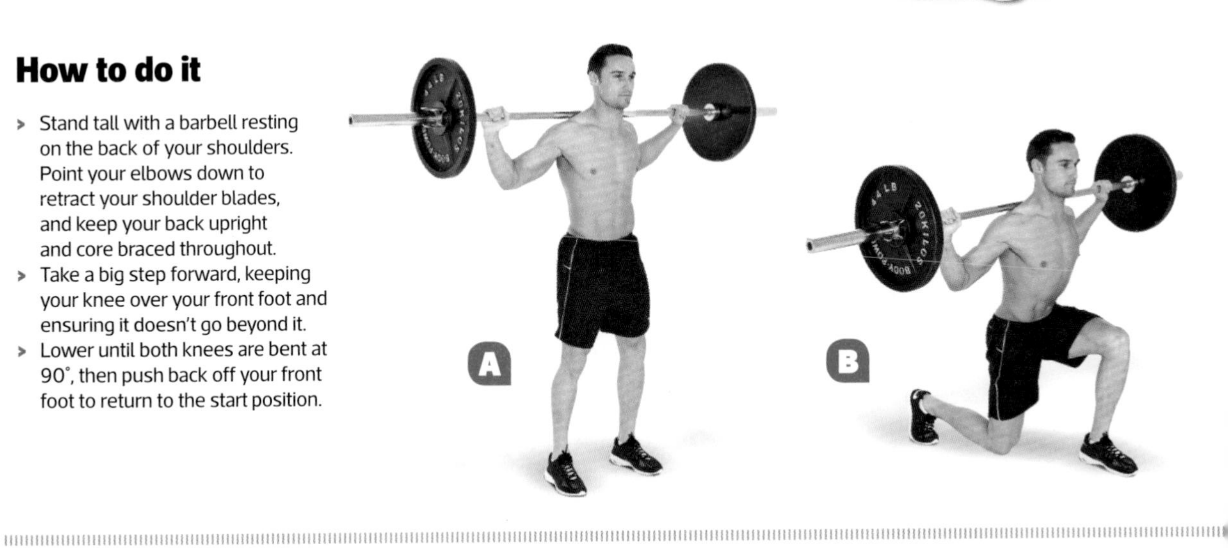

umbbell step-up

t's a move you do countless times each day when climbing stairs, but adding extra weight with dumbbells will craft powerful glutes.

How to do it

- Stand in front of a bench set no higher than knee height, holding a dumbbell in each hand.
- Keeping your back straight and your core braced, place one foot on the bench, then the other.
- Step back down, leading with the same leg. Alternate leading legs with every rep.

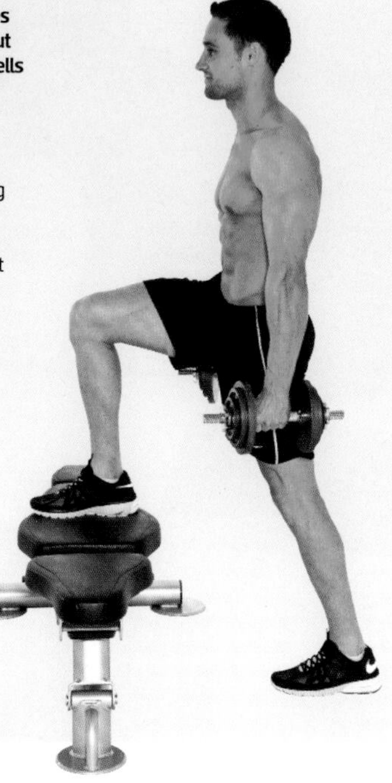

One-leg squat

This tough unilateral move forces all the work on to one leg, while your core has to work hard to stabilise your upper body.

How to do it

- Stand on one leg.
- Keeping your knee in line with your toes, squat down as far as you can go.
- Stand back up and complete a set on the same leg, swapping legs for the next set.

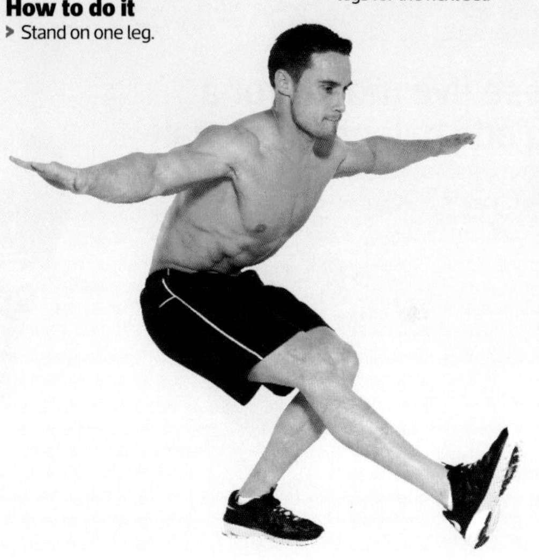

ulgarian split squat

Placing your back foot on a bench behind you takes that leg out of the equation, forcing your front leg and the glutes muscles on that side to handle the entire workload.

How to do it

- Rest a barbell across the back of your shoulders and rest your back foot on a bench. Your front leg should be about a metre in front of the bench with toes pointing ahead.
- Keeping your torso upright, bend your front leg until your thigh is parallel to the floor.
- Keep your knee in line with your toes and don't let it travel beyond your toes.

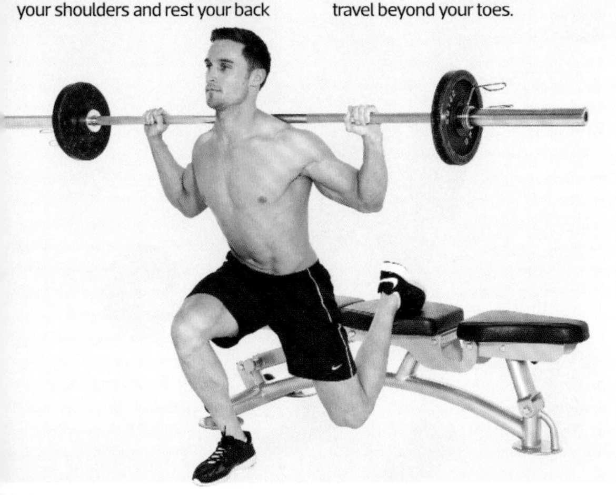

Glute raise

This is one of the best moves for isolating your glute muscles.

How to do it

- Lie flat on the floor with your knees bent at right angles and your feet apart.
- Keeping your core braced, raise your lower back off the floor by squeezing your glutes.
- Pause at the top of the move for one second, then slowly lower back to the start position.

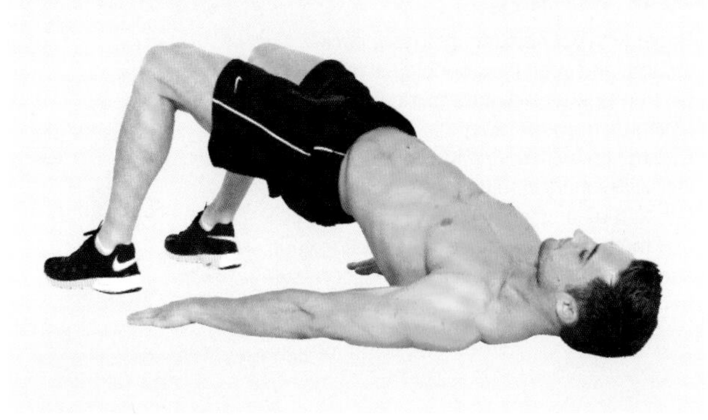

Upper back

Do these five moves for a strong and balanced top half

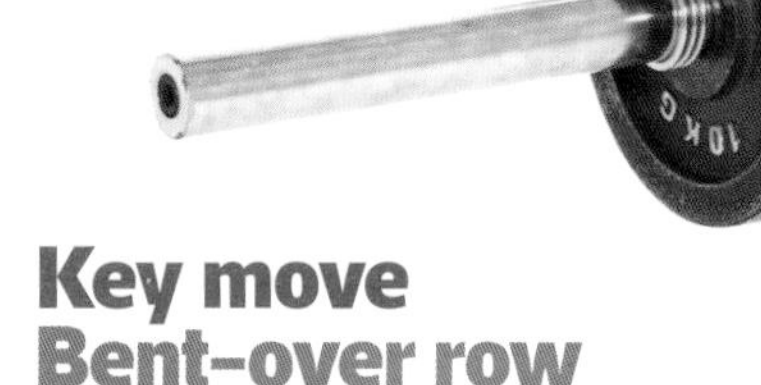

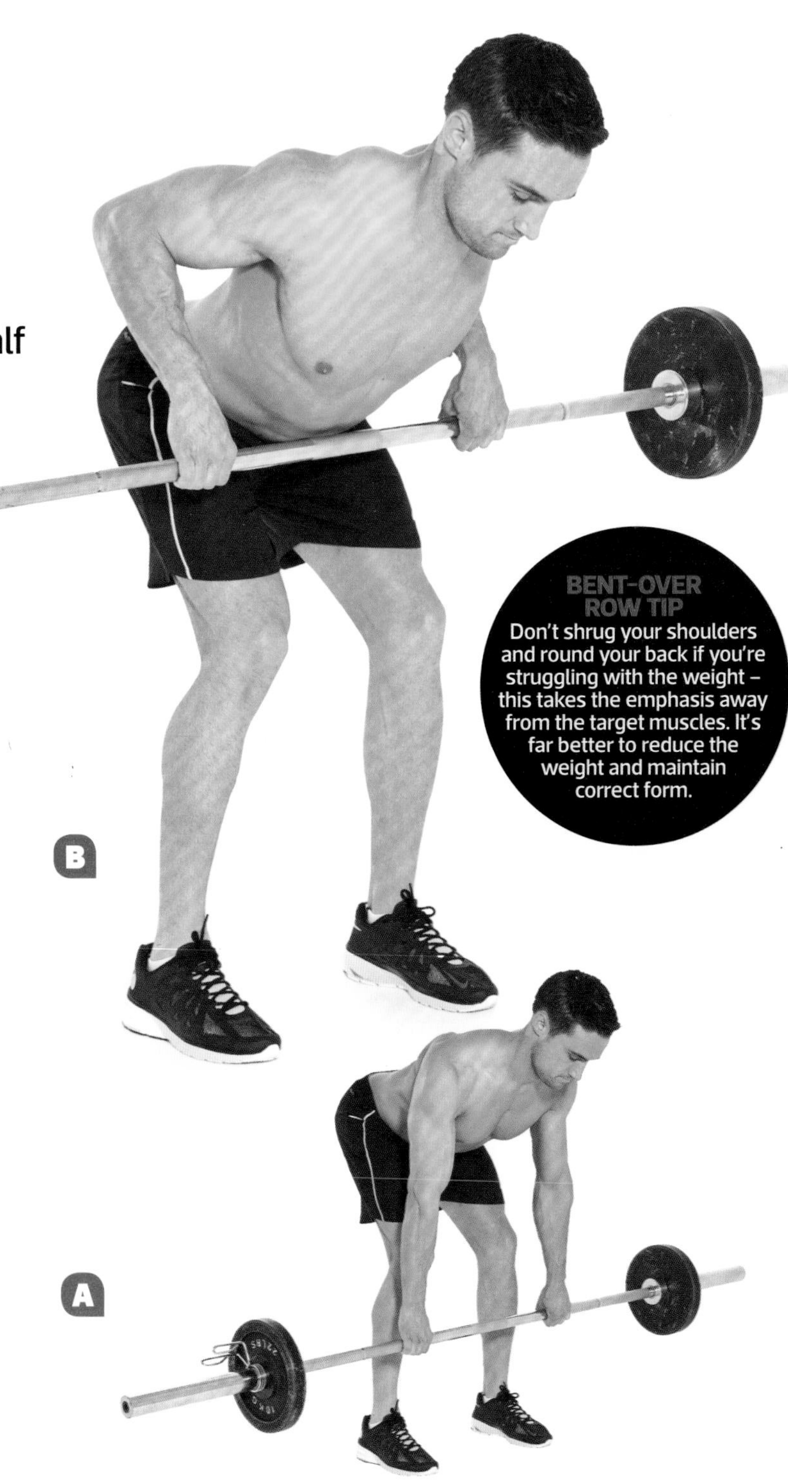

Key move
Bent-over row

It may be tempting to let the bench press dominate your workout, but concentrating on your pecs at the expense of your back can lead to a muscle imbalance that not only looks rubbish but also increases your risk of injury. This move works the opposite muscle group, the upper back (traps, lats, rhomboids and rear deltoids), as well as your biceps and abs, helping to keep your torso stable. The move is overlooked by many, but should be a key weapon in your muscle-building arsenal.

How to do it

- Begin with your core braced, your back straight and your shoulder blades retracted.
- Bend your knees slightly and lean forwards from the hips.
- Grip the bar with your hands placed just wider than shoulder-width apart, letting the bar hang at knee level.
- Pull the bar to your sternum, retracting your shoulder blades to allow the bar to come up to your chest, then lower slowly to the start.

BENT-OVER ROW TIP

Don't shrug your shoulders and round your back if you're struggling with the weight – this takes the emphasis away from the target muscles. It's far better to reduce the weight and maintain correct form.

hrug

hrugs have a limited range of motion compared with many other lifts, which means that you can use really heavy weights to help build big and strong traps and create wide shoulders.

How to do it

- Stand in front of two heavy dumbbells.
- Squat down and securely grip a weight in each hand with a neutral grip.
- Stand up, keeping your core braced and a natural arch in your back.
- Shrug your shoulders up towards your ears, keeping your arms straight.
- Hold for a second at the top position before slowly lowering the weights back down.
- You can also perform shrugs with a heavy barbell using an overhand grip just outside your hips.

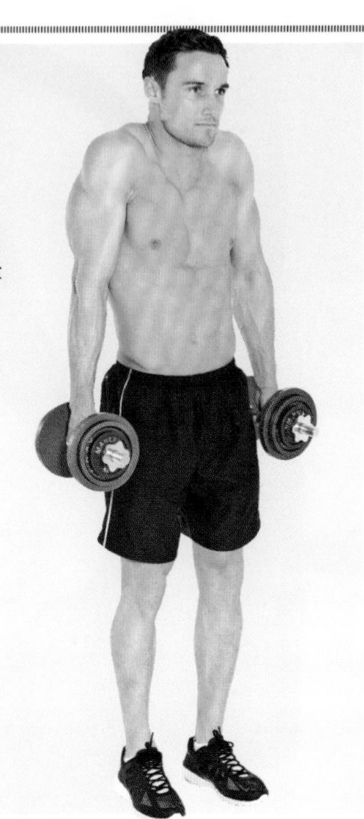

Seated cable row

Hitting your back muscles while seated allows you to go heavy and focus all your efforts on the target muscle groups, resulting in big muscle-mass gains.

How to do it

- Sit with a flat back and a slight bend in your knees, using a neutral grip to hold a double D-handle attached to the bottom pulley of a cable machine.
- Ensure that there is tension in the cable before you begin.
- Pull the handle to your sternum, keeping upper-body movement to a minimum, and squeeze your shoulder blades together.
- Return slowly to the start.

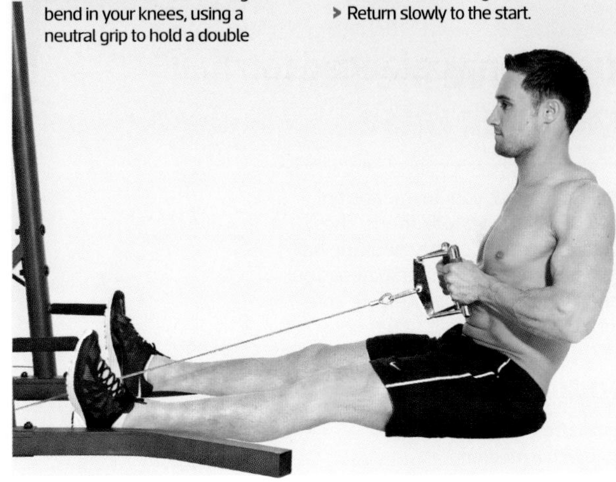

pright row

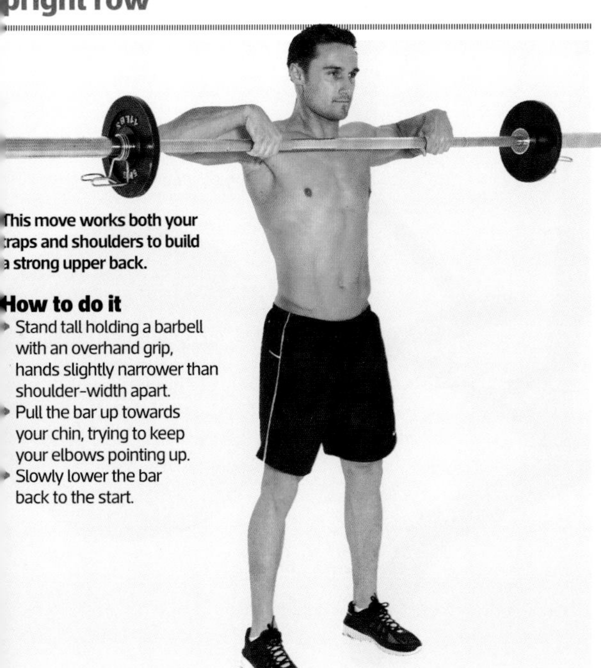

This move works both your traps and shoulders to build a strong upper back.

How to do it

- Stand tall holding a barbell with an overhand grip, hands slightly narrower than shoulder-width apart.
- Pull the bar up towards your chin, trying to keep your elbows pointing up.
- Slowly lower the bar back to the start.

One-arm row

Working one arm at a time helps encourage balanced growth, lessening the risk of injury.

How to do it

- Rest your left knee and left hand on a bench, holding a dumbbell in your right hand close to the floor.
- Keeping your back straight, use your back muscles and biceps to row the weight up to your side, leading with your elbow.
- Repeat on the other side.

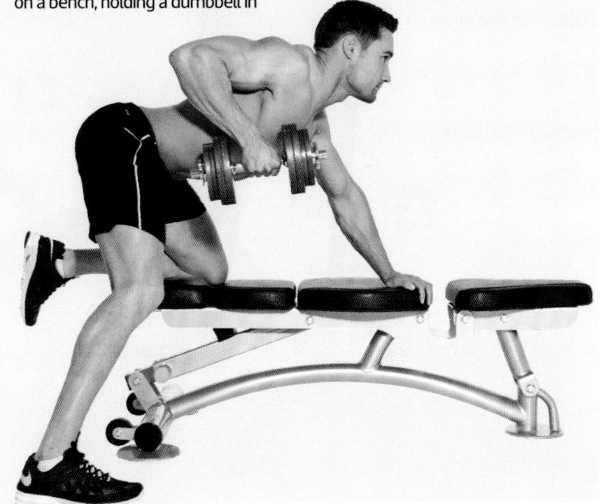

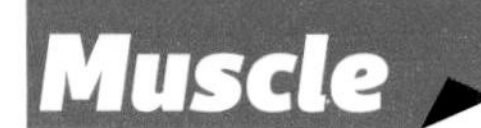

Abs

Do these five moves to build a rock-solid six-pack

Key move Medicine ball knee raise

It's vital to work your lower abs but all too easy to overlook them. The additional weight of the medicine ball forces them to work hard to raise your knees to your chest, while your core works to stabilise your upper body.

How to do it

- Hang from a pull-up bar with a medicine ball held securely between your knees.
- Bend your knees and use your lower abs to draw them up towards your chest.
- Once you have raised your knees as high as possible, pause, then slowly return to the start.

A

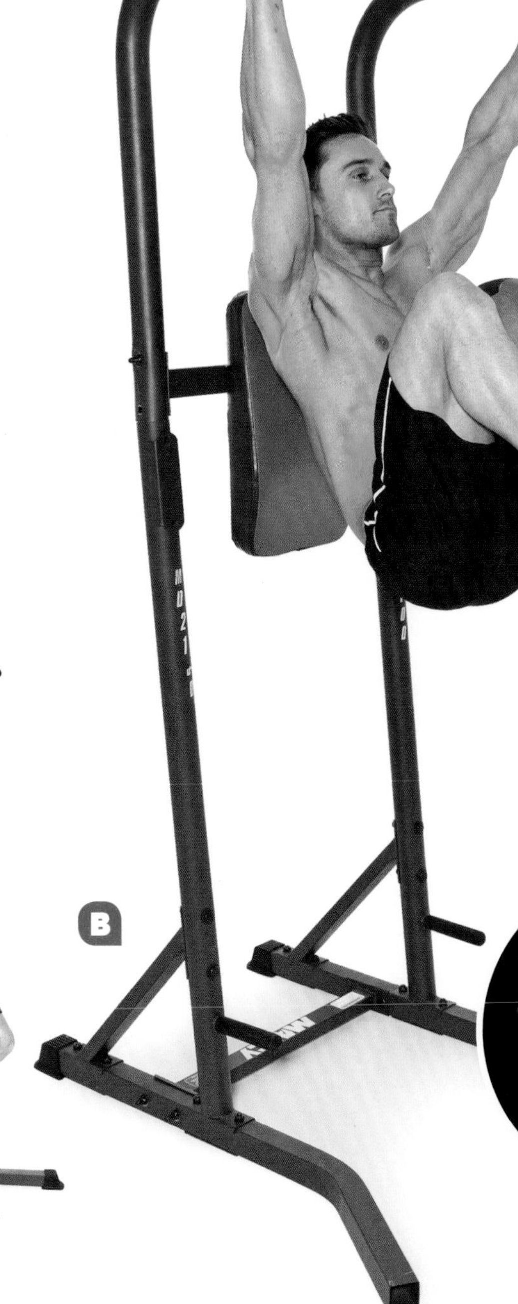

ABS TIP
Do a standalone abs workout or perform abs exercises after your heavy lifts. Doing them before can tire them out so you'll struggle when squatting, deadlifting or even benching.

'unch

his is the classic move for ırgeting your upper abs and still ne of the best, so it's an essential omponent of an abs workout.

łow to do it

Lie with your back flat on a mat with your knees bent at 90° and your feet flat on the floor. Place your fingers by your temples.
- Contract your abs to lift your shoulders up and curl your chest towards your knees, keeping your lower back on the mat.
- Pause at the top of the move and tense your abs, then lower slowly back to the start.

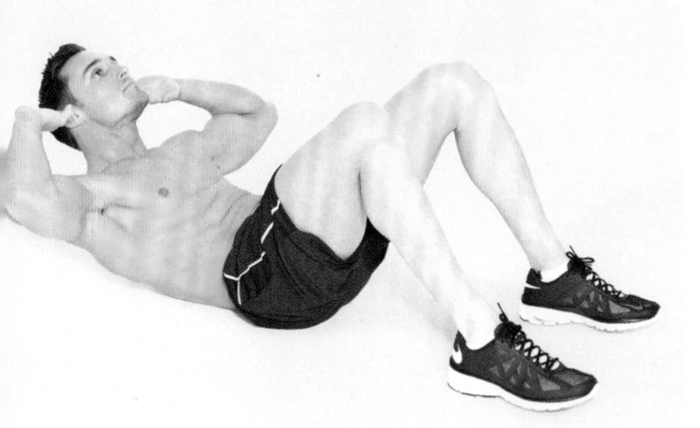

Reverse crunch

You place the emphasis on the lower part of your abs by hitting them from a different angle.

How to do it

- Start with your head and shoulders flat on the floor with your arms down by your sides, knees bent at 90° and feet flat on the floor.
- Contract your abs to lift your hips off the floor, then curl your knees towards your chest, keeping them bent at 90°.
- Pause at the top of the move, tense your abs, then lower your legs slowly back to the start.

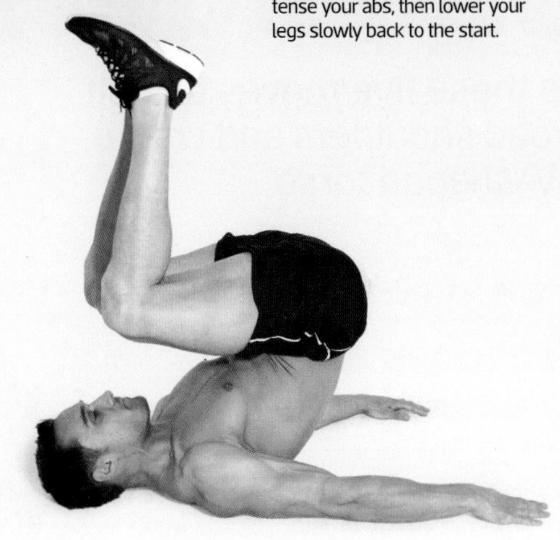

.ank

he plank is the classic stability nove, since every muscle must vork together to keep your torso table. It builds strength in deep-ying muscles, making many other noves easier, and strengthens he link between your upper nd lower body, which has huge ransferable value to every sport.

How to do it

- Hold your body in a straight line from head to heels with your elbows beneath your shoulders, your feet together, and your head looking down.
- Hold the position for as long as you can without letting your hips sag.

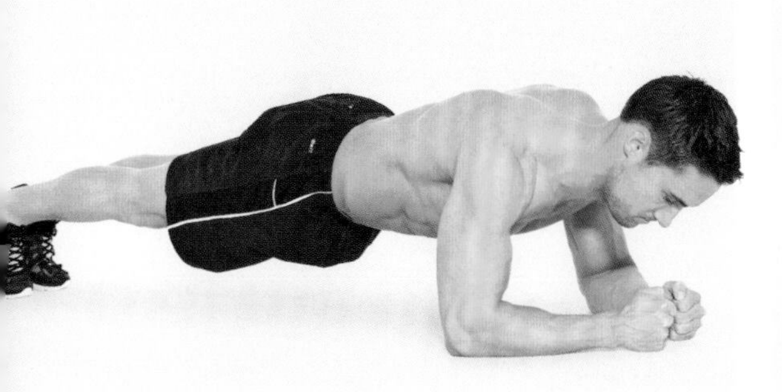

Jackknife

This advanced move, which requires flexibility as well as a strong core, hits both your upper and lower abs.

How to do it

- Lie flat on your back with your arms behind your head, off the floor, and your feet together, also off the floor.
- Contract your abs and bring your hands and feet up to meet above your stomach.
- Keep your legs as straight as you can and tense your abs at the top of the move, then slowly return to the start.

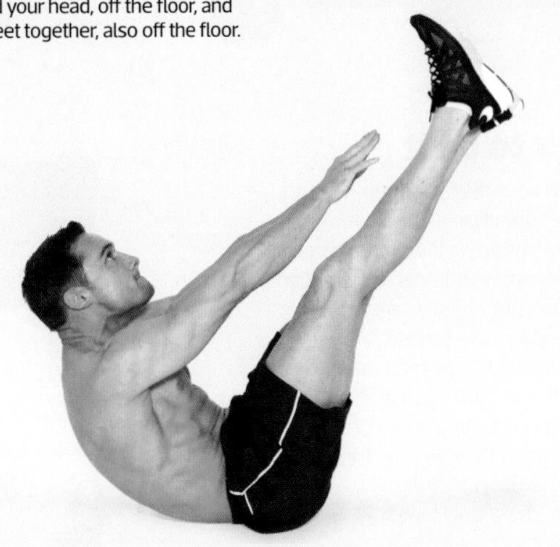

Shoulders

Do these five moves to built broad shoulders and create a V-shaped torso

Key move Barbell shoulder press

The shoulder press is a key upper-body lift if you want to add size and strength. It mainly works the front and middle deltoids, two of the three major muscles that make up your shoulders. Your triceps become involved as you straighten your arms, while your core must work hard throughout to stabilise your torso. It's a key move for creating impressively wide shoulders and will help improve your bench press.

SHOULDER PRESS TIP
The first rep will be the toughest because there's no bounce effect from the elasticity of the muscles. Use your legs to help initiate that tricky first rep and the rest will be a little easier.

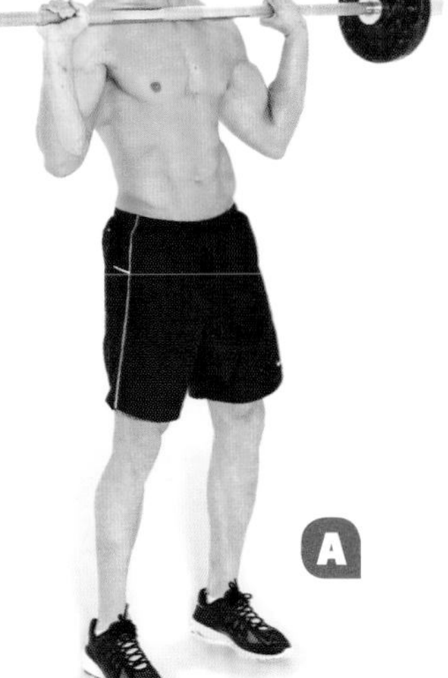
A

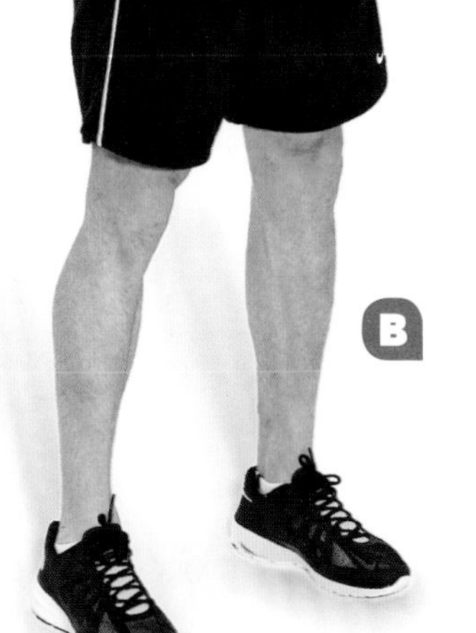
B

How to do it

- With your feet shoulder-width apart, position a bar on your upper chest, gripping it with hands just wider than shoulder-width apart.
- Keep your chest upright and your core braced.
- Press the bar directly upwards until your arms are extended overhead.
- As you lift, keep your core braced and don't tilt your hips forward.
- Lower the bar back to your chest and repeat.

Push press

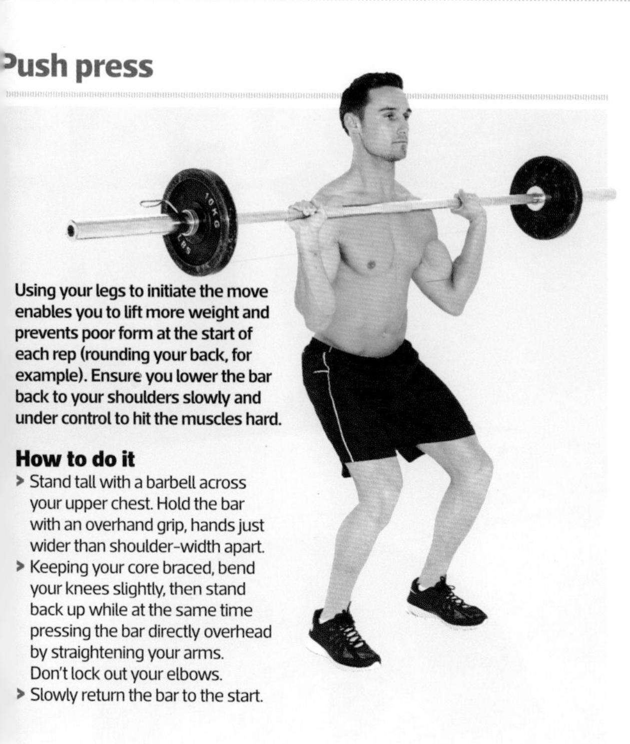

Using your legs to initiate the move enables you to lift more weight and prevents poor form at the start of each rep (rounding your back, for example). Ensure you lower the bar back to your shoulders slowly and under control to hit the muscles hard.

How to do it

- Stand tall with a barbell across your upper chest. Hold the bar with an overhand grip, hands just wider than shoulder-width apart.
- Keeping your core braced, bend your knees slightly, then stand back up while at the same time pressing the bar directly overhead by straightening your arms. Don't lock out your elbows.
- Slowly return the bar to the start.

Arnold press

This variation combines a pressing action with a rotational one to hit your deltoids from several angles.

How to do it

- Sit on an upright bench holding a dumbbell in each hand with your palms facing you.
- Keep your feet flat, your core braced, your back against the bench and your head looking forward.
- Press the weights up, rotating your palms so that you end the move with arms directly overhead with your palms facing away from you.
- Reverse back to the start.

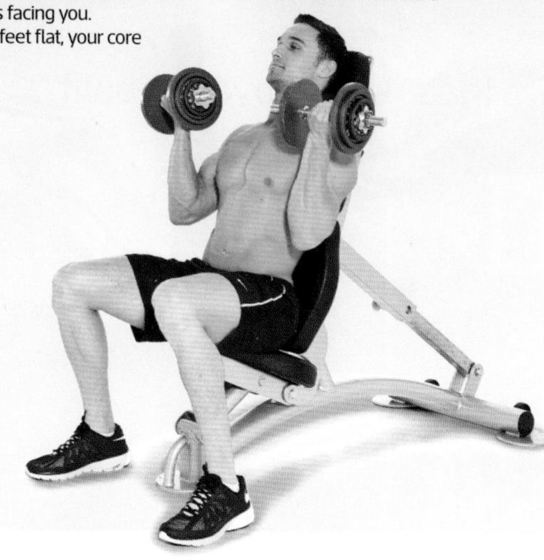

Cable lateral raise

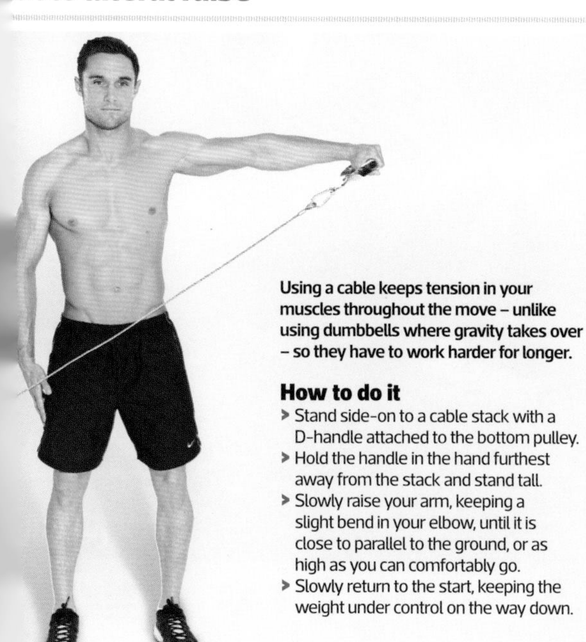

Using a cable keeps tension in your muscles throughout the move – unlike using dumbbells where gravity takes over – so they have to work harder for longer.

How to do it

- Stand side-on to a cable stack with a D-handle attached to the bottom pulley.
- Hold the handle in the hand furthest away from the stack and stand tall.
- Slowly raise your arm, keeping a slight bend in your elbow, until it is close to parallel to the ground, or as high as you can comfortably go.
- Slowly return to the start, keeping the weight under control on the way down.

Reverse dumbbell flye

This is a great move for targeting the muscles that make up the rear part of your shoulders. It's often neglected in favour of working the other muscles, but you need balanced growth to ensure that you get wide shoulders.

How to do it

- Lie flat on a bench, holding a dumbbell in each hand.
- Keeping a slight bend in your elbows, raise the weights out to the sides until they're at shoulder height, then return to the start.

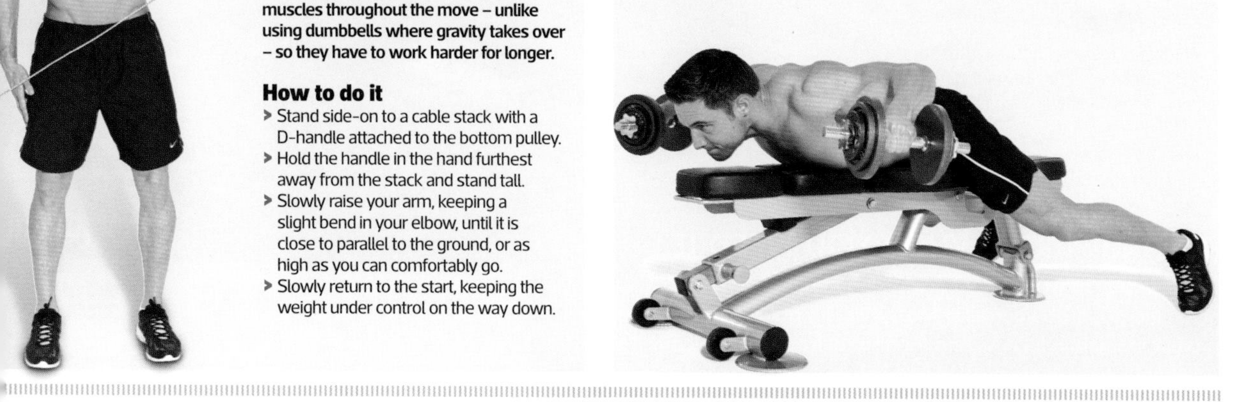

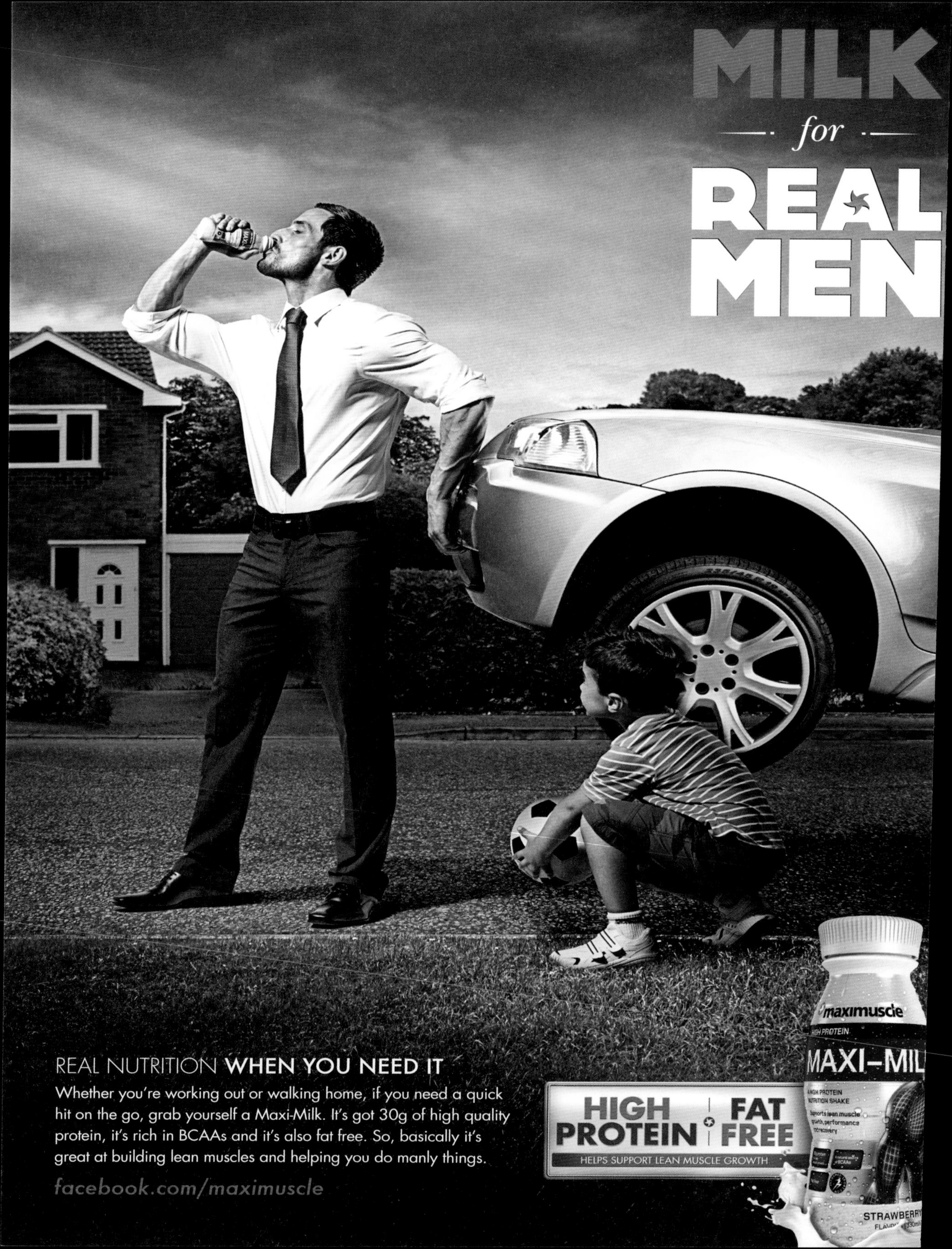

MILK
for
REAL
MEN
REAL NUTRITION WHEN YOU NEED IT
Whether you're working out or walking home, if you need a quick hit on the go, grab yourself a Maxi-Milk. It's got 30g of high quality protein, it's rich in BCAAs and it's also fat free. So, basically it's great at building lean muscles and helping you do manly things.
facebook.com/maximuscle
HIGH PROTEIN
FAT FREE
HELPS SUPPORT LEAN MUSCLE GROWTH
maximuscle
MAXI-MIL
STRAWBERRY

_ats

/ork the key muscles of your ack to add width to your torso

ey move Pull-up

ay be a bodyweight exercise, but the pull-up is
 seriously tough. The load on your muscles is
y high because you have to lift up and control
r entire weight against gravity. This has the huge
antage of building a strong, wide upper back,
ch helps create a desirable V-shaped torso.
venting your legs from swinging during the
rcise also gives your abs a good workout.

ow to do it

;rasp the bar with an overhand grip with your hands
vider than shoulder-width apart.
;tart from a dead hang with your arms fully extended.
'ull yourself up by squeezing your lats together.
)nce your chin is higher than your hands, pause briefly,
hen slowly lower yourself back to the start.

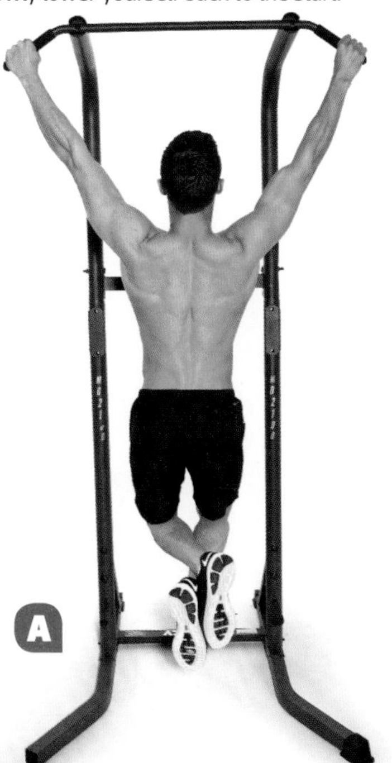

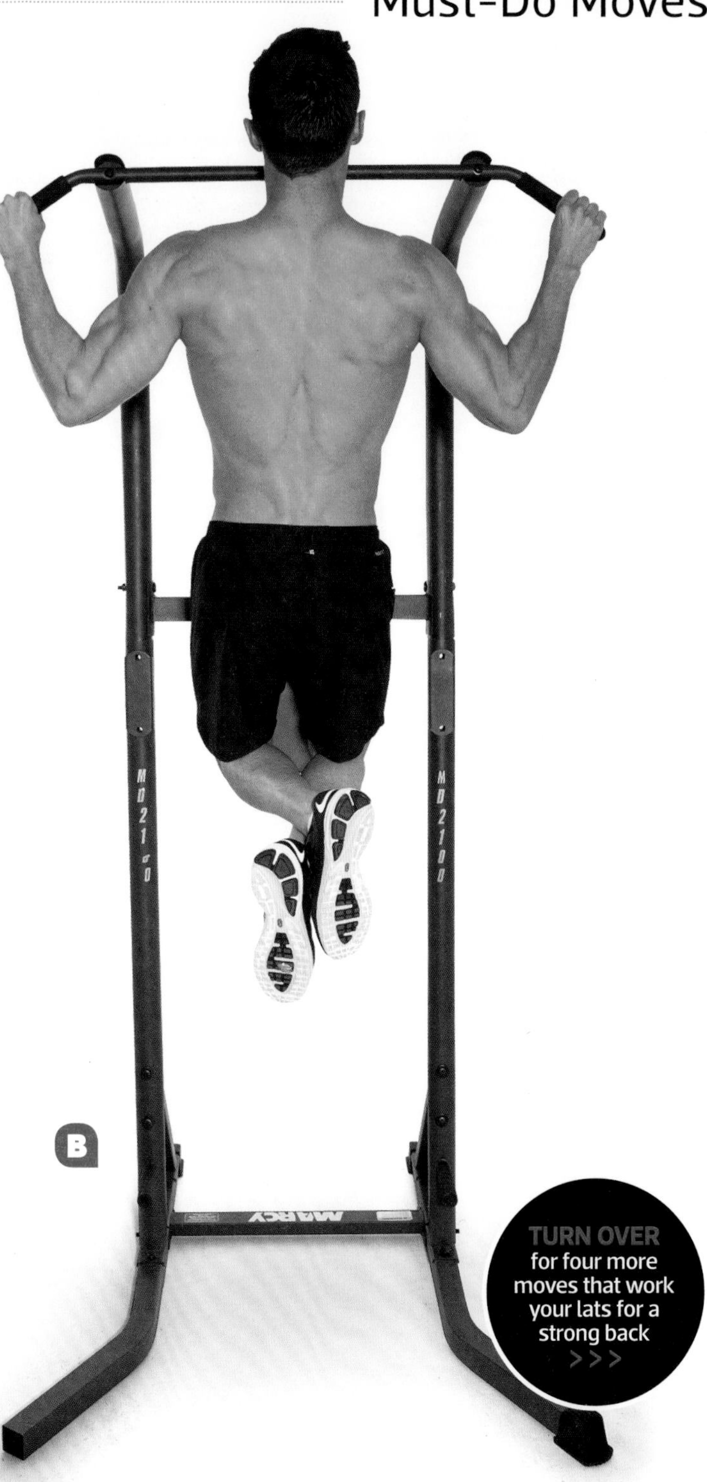

TURN OVER for four more moves that work your lats for a strong back >>>

Bent-over row

As well as the lats, this move works all the upper back's powerhouse muscles (traps, rhomboids and rear deltoids). The biceps assist the lift, while your abs work to keep your torso straight and stable.

How to do it

- Start with your core braced and your back straight.
- Bend your knees slightly and lean forward from the hips.
- Grip the bar with hands just wider than shoulder-width apart, letting it hang at knee level.
- Pull the bar up to your lower sternum, retracting your shoulder blades to allow the bar to come up to your chest, then lower the bar slowly to the start.

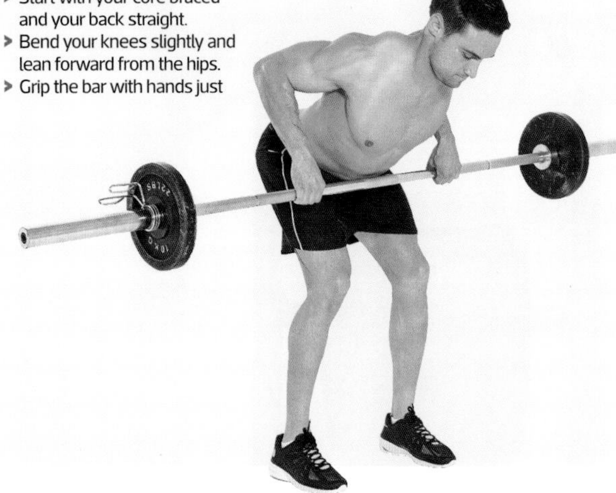

Straight-arm pull-down

Standing up and keeping your arms straight fully engages the lats and prevents your biceps – or any other back muscles – and momentum getting in on the act.

How to do it

- Stand tall in front of a cable machine with a straight bar attached to the top pulley.
- Holding the bar with an overhand grip, pull it down in an arc until it reaches the top of your thighs, keeping your arms straight throughout.
- Slowly return to the start.

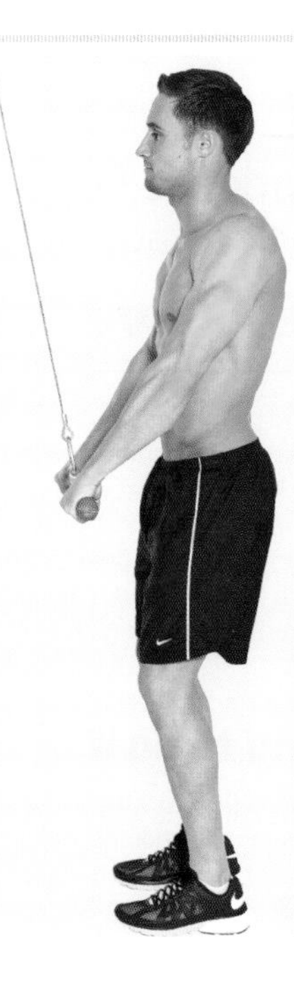

Dumbbell pull-over

Although it's a single-joint move, this exercise works a number of muscles, specifically the lats, lower chest and triceps.

How to do it

- Lie flat on a bench with your head and shoulders supported and your feet flat on the floor.
- Hold a single dumbbell over your chest with both hands and engage your core.
- Slowly lower the weight behind your head, keeping a slight bend in your elbows.
- Don't arch your back.
- Use your pecs to pull your arms back over your head to return to the start position.

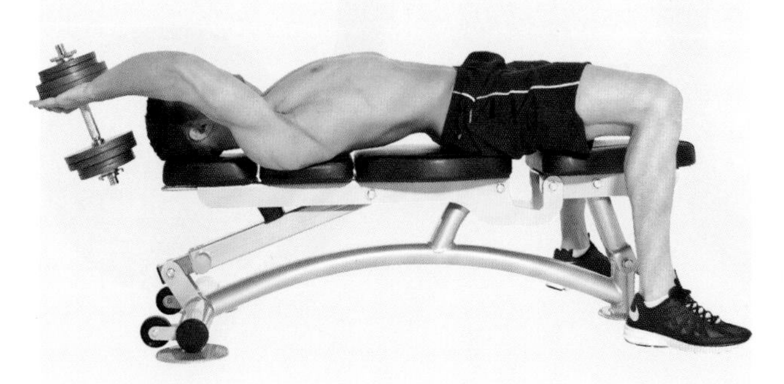

Lat pull-down

This works the same muscles as the pull-up but the machine allows you to adjust the resistance easily, so you can reduce or increase the weight and measure your progress in the exercise.

How to do it

- Sit on the seat and take an overhand wide grip on the bar.
- Look forward, retract your shoulder blades and keep your torso upright.
- Pull the bar down in front of you until it reaches your upper chest. Don't lean back to aid the movement.
- Squeeze your lats at the bottom of the move and return the bar slowly to the top.

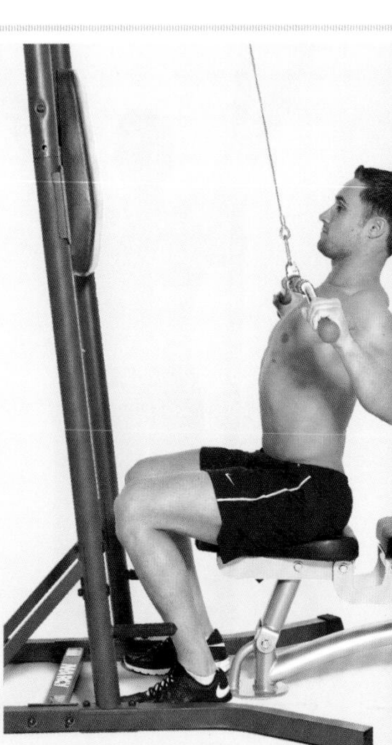

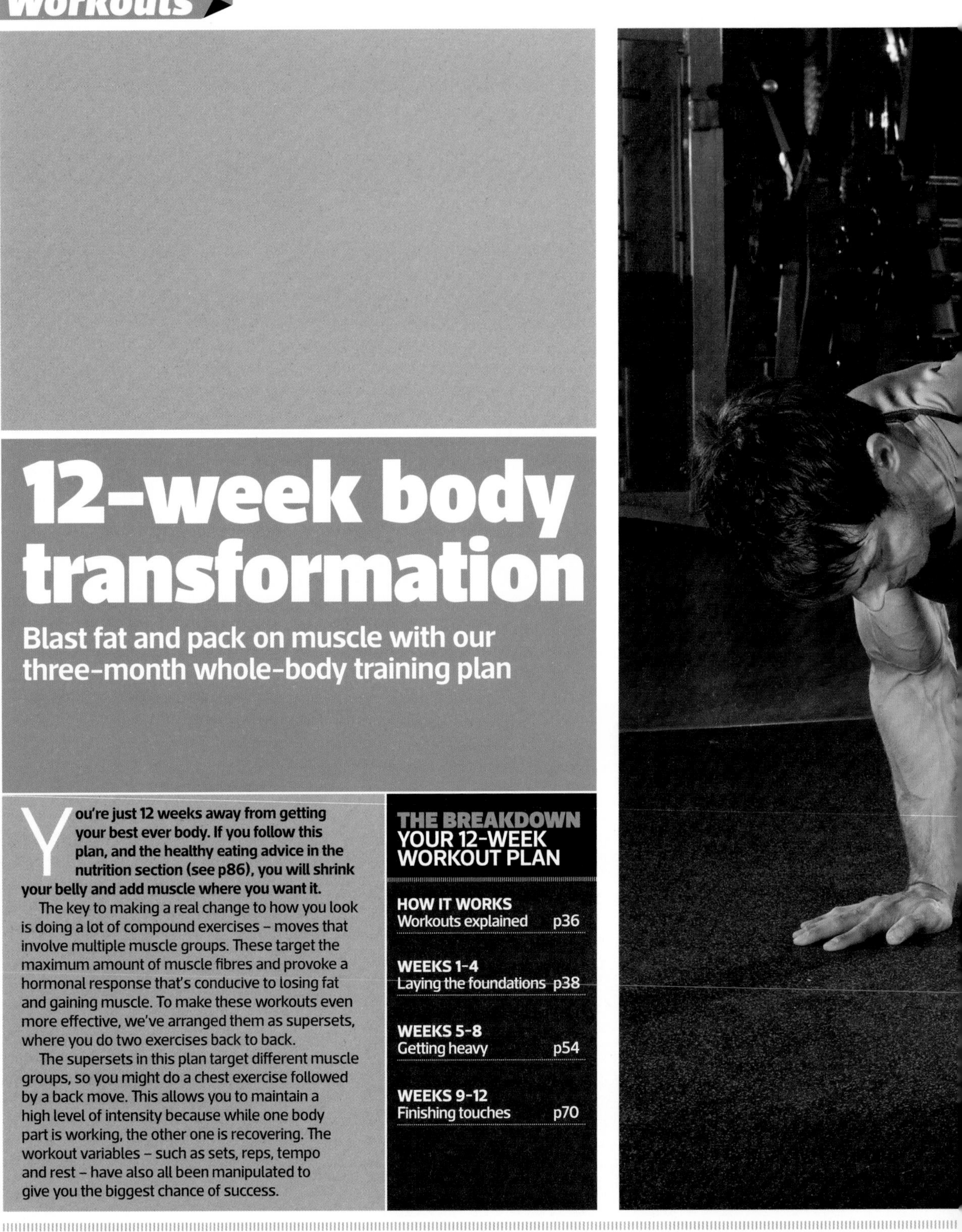

12-week body transformation

Blast fat and pack on muscle with our three-month whole-body training plan

You're just 12 weeks away from getting your best ever body. If you follow this plan, and the healthy eating advice in the nutrition section (see p86), you will shrink your belly and add muscle where you want it.

The key to making a real change to how you look is doing a lot of compound exercises – moves that involve multiple muscle groups. These target the maximum amount of muscle fibres and provoke a hormonal response that's conducive to losing fat and gaining muscle. To make these workouts even more effective, we've arranged them as supersets, where you do two exercises back to back.

The supersets in this plan target different muscle groups, so you might do a chest exercise followed by a back move. This allows you to maintain a high level of intensity because while one body part is working, the other one is recovering. The workout variables – such as sets, reps, tempo and rest – have also all been manipulated to give you the biggest chance of success.

THE BREAKDOWN
YOUR 12-WEEK WORKOUT PLAN

HOW IT WORKS
Workouts explained p36

WEEKS 1-4
Laying the foundations p38

WEEKS 5-8
Getting heavy p54

WEEKS 9-12
Finishing touches p70

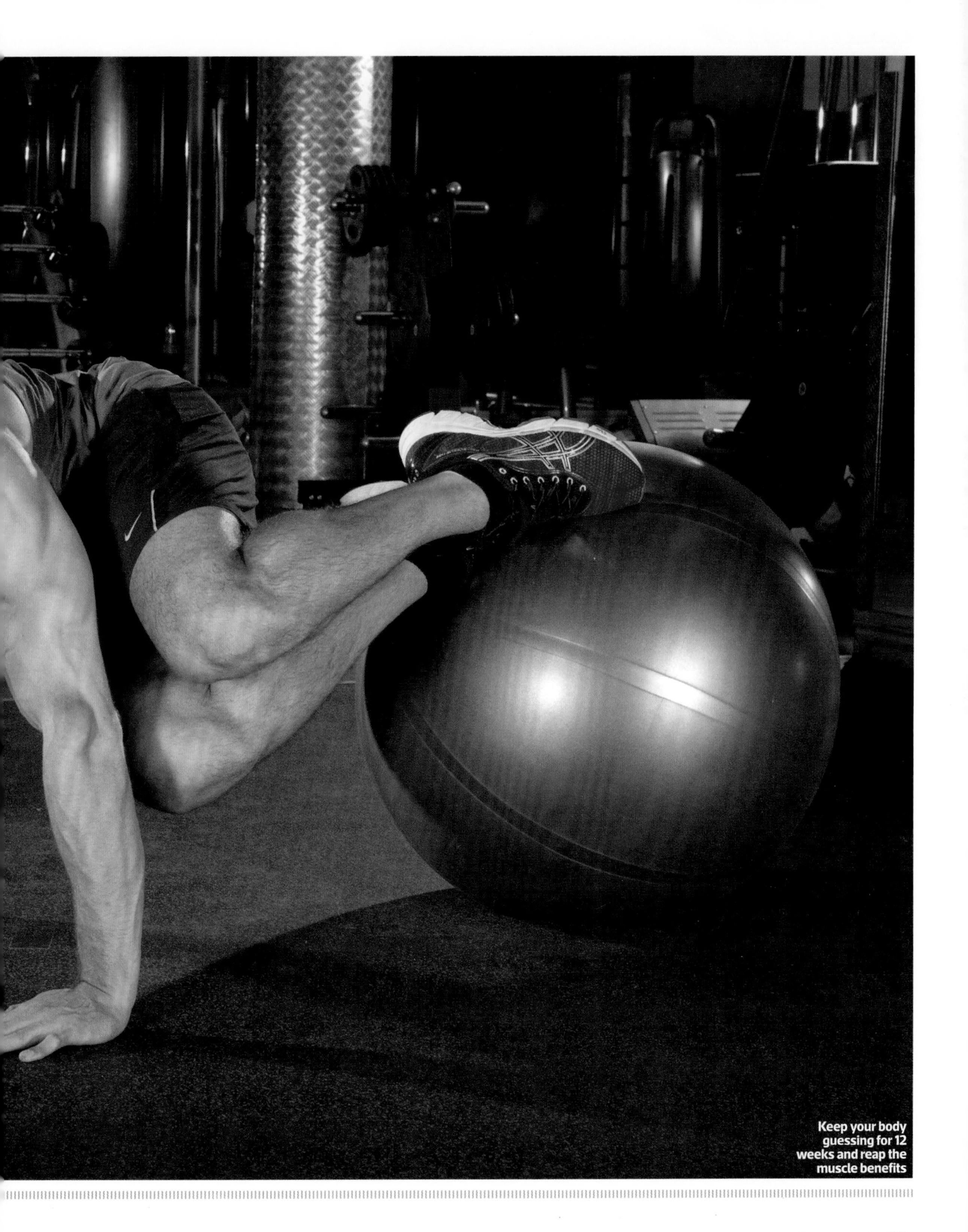
Keep your body guessing for 12 weeks and reap the muscle benefits

How to do the workouts

Here's everything you need to know to navigate your way through the plan

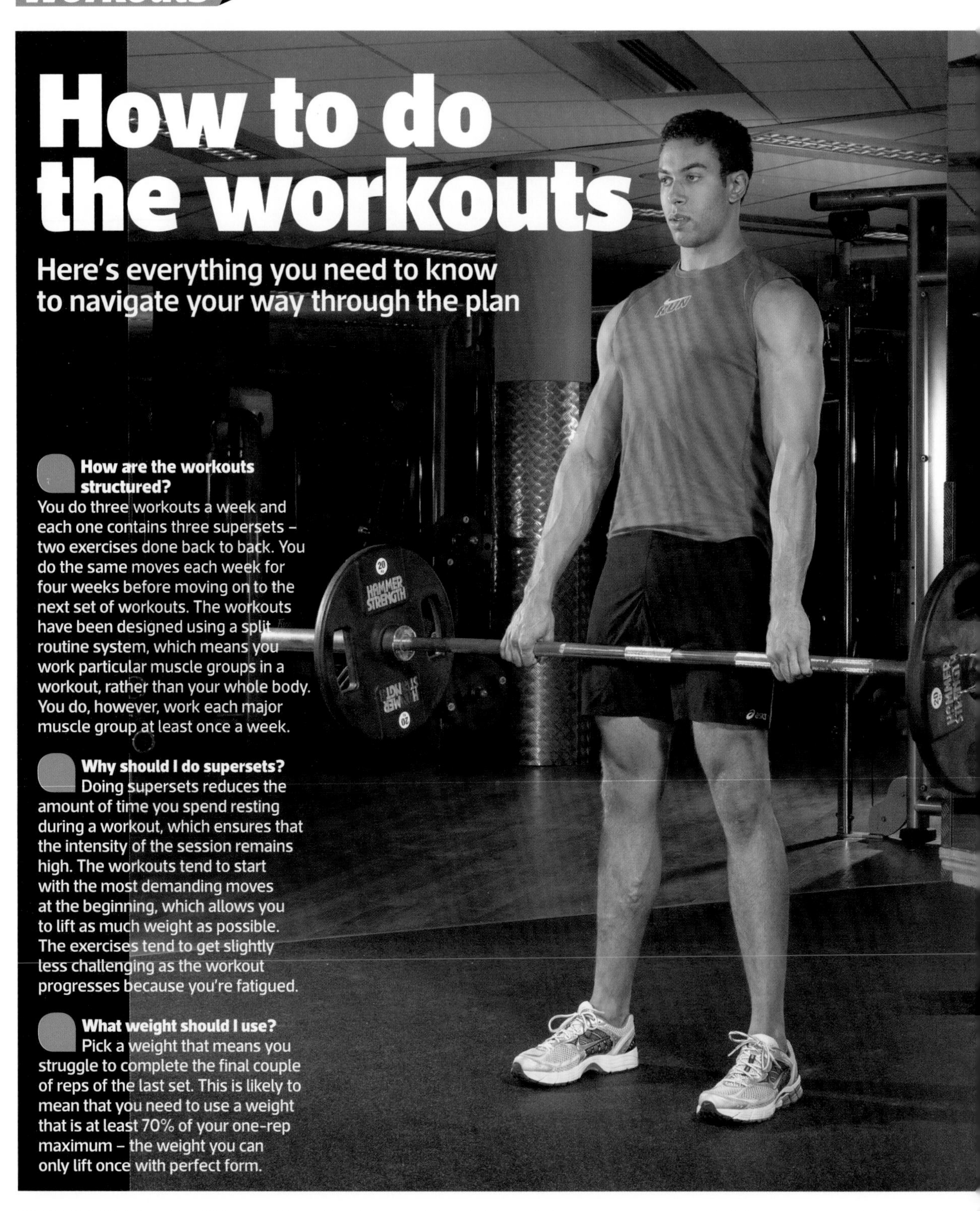

How are the workouts structured?
You do three workouts a week and each one contains three supersets – two exercises done back to back. You do the same moves each week for four weeks before moving on to the next set of workouts. The workouts have been designed using a split routine system, which means you work particular muscle groups in a workout, rather than your whole body. You do, however, work each major muscle group at least once a week.

Why should I do supersets?
Doing supersets reduces the amount of time you spend resting during a workout, which ensures that the intensity of the session remains high. The workouts tend to start with the most demanding moves at the beginning, which allows you to lift as much weight as possible. The exercises tend to get slightly less challenging as the workout progresses because you're fatigued.

What weight should I use?
Pick a weight that means you struggle to complete the final couple of reps of the last set. This is likely to mean that you need to use a weight that is at least 70% of your one-rep maximum – the weight you can only lift once with perfect form.

Using the workout tables

Here's the theory behind the routines you're going to be using for the next 12 weeks

Week
The reason you do the same workout each week is that three weeks isn't long enough for your body to get so comfortable with the exercises that it stops responding, particularly if you're adjusting other variables such as sets and rest times. By sticking with the same moves for three weeks you'll get better at the movement patterns involved in each exercise so you'll be able to lift heavier each week.

Reps
The number of times you perform an exercise in a set. All the rep counts are within a range that will result in hypertrophy (muscle growth). They vary because muscle groups respond in different ways. Those with more type II muscle fibres (responsible for fast, powerful movements) respond better to lower rep ranges than groups with more type I fibres (responsible for endurance efforts).

Sets
This is the number of groups of reps you perform. For each workout in the first week you perform two sets. This is because your body will have to get used to the movements and this is demanding. Once you're more familiar with the moves you increase the set count to three per exercise. If you're already familiar with the exercises in the plan, you can do three sets in the first week.

Tempo
This refers to the speed of the lift. It's important to stick to the right tempo for every part of the lift. The first number is the speed in seconds of the lowering part of a lift, such as lowering the bar to your chest in a bench press. The second is the pause at the bottom, the third is the lifting phase and the fourth is the pause between reps. 'X' means you should do that part as quickly as possible.

Rest
This is the rest you should take between supersets. Aim not to rest between the two exercises in a superset, then rest for the allotted time between supersets. Rest for two to three minutes between groups of supersets. The rest time decreases between week one and week two to make the workout more challenging and the rest times have been picked to maximise growth hormone release.

Heavy metal
Each workout includes a pair of heavy moves that work lots of muscles. This releases growth hormone, making the rest of the workout more effective at building muscle.

One-sided
Including unilateral - or one-sided - moves will balance out your body, ensuring that both sides are equally strong. Tackle your weakest side first for better results.

Use your body
Mastering bodyweight moves will give you great results – it'll help you to move your body as a single unit, and means that you'll be able to work out anywhere.

EXERCISE	WEEK	REPS	SETS	TEMPO	REST
SUPERSET 1					
1A Leg press	1 2 3 4	12 10 8 6	2 3 4 4	3010 3010 3010 3010	
1B Romanian deadlift	1 2 3 4	12 10 8 8	2 3 4 4	3010 3010 3010 3010	60 sec 60 sec 90 sec 90 sec
SUPERSET 2					
2A Side lunge	1 2 3 4	12 10 8 8	2 2 3 3	1010 1010 1010 1010	
2B One leg hamstring curl	1 2 3 4	8 10 8 10	2 2 3 3	2010 2010 2010 2010	60 sec 60 sec 90 sec 90 sec
SUPERSET 3					
3A Chin-up	1 2 3 4	3 4 4 5	4 4 5 5	4010 4010 4010 4010	
3B Dip	1 2 3 4	3 4 4 5	4 4 5 5	3010 3010 3010 3010	60 sec 60 sec 90 sec 90 sec

Lay the foundations

Use this month to nail your movement patters and set yourself up for real progress

Month one is where you lay the training foundations on which you can build solid muscle. It's vital that you do every move with good form because you're trying to establish perfect movement patterns. If you don't do things properly, your overall progress will be limited.

Workout 1

The first superset in this routine is a classic chest and back builder. With high reps in week one you won't lift a particularly heavy weight, but as the month progresses and the reps drop you should look to increase the load. The second superset works your chest and back again, but this time unilaterally (one side at a time), which is important for balanced muscle development. The final superset involves one bodyweight move – although it is a tricky one – and a machine exercise, so it's a sensible way to end your workout when you're tired.

Workout 2

In the first workout you targeted your chest and back so while those body parts are recovering it's time to hammer your legs and arms. The first superset uses front squats to work your quads and Romanian deadlifts to develop your hamstrings. Front squats are great because the position of the weight encourages you to use good form. The second superset also challenges the front and back of your thighs, this time with moves that are a test of stability and balance. You finish with a superset that focuses on your biceps and triceps.

Workout 3

The final workout focuses on the two muscle groups that you haven't yet worked: your shoulders and your abs. The shoulder joint is what's known as a freely moveable joint and that means it can be more injury-prone than other joints. For this reason, you start with a 'prehab' superset of internal and external cable rotations. They'll warm up the small muscles of the shoulder joint so that you can attack the shoulder press in the second set without risking injury. The abs superset at the end works your entire midsection, including your deep-lying core muscles and lower back.

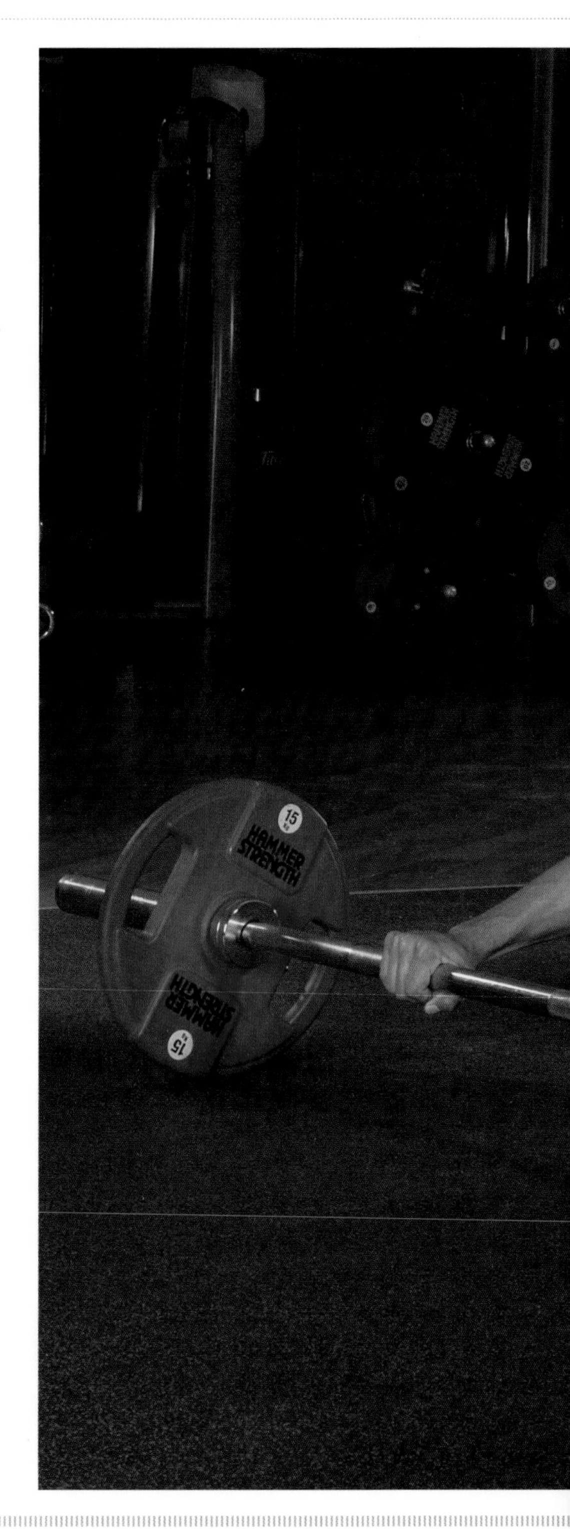

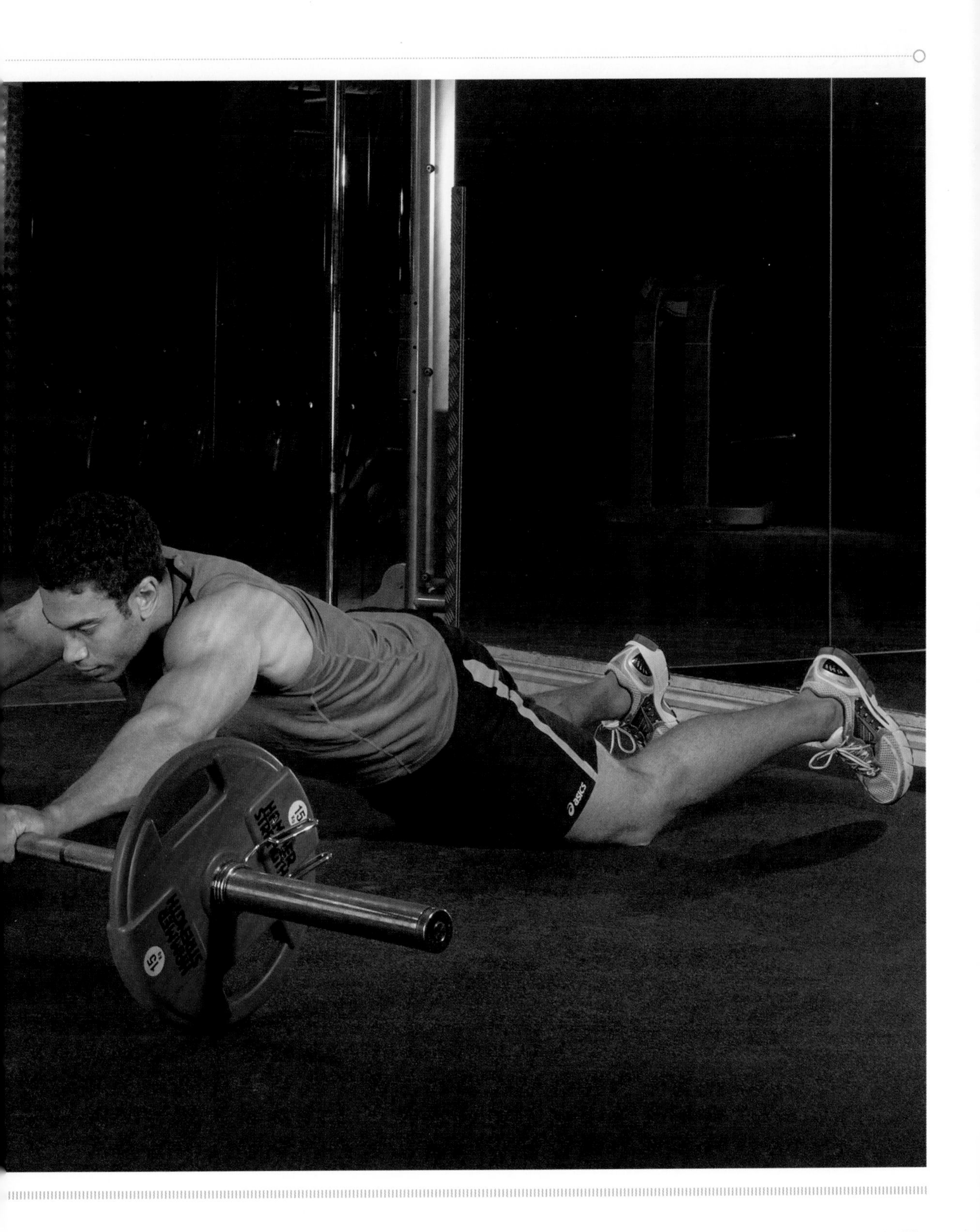

WORKOUT 1

Chest and back

EXERCISE	WEEK	REPS	SETS	TEMPO	REST
SUPERSET 1					
1A Incline bench press	1	12	2	3010	
	2	10	3	3010	
	3	8	4	3010	
	4	6	4	3010	
1B Bent-over row	1	12	2	3010	60sec
	2	10	3	3010	60sec
	3	8	4	3010	90sec
	4	8	4	3010	90sec
SUPERSET 2					
2A Alternating dumbbell press	1	12	2	2010	
	2	10	2	2010	
	3	8	3	2010	
	4	8	3	2010	
2B Renegade row	1	8	2	2010	60sec
	2	10	2	2010	60sec
	3	8	3	2010	90sec
	4	10	4	2010	90sec
SUPERSET 3					
3A Gym ball press-up	1	8	2	2010	
	2	10	2	2010	
	3	8	3	2010	
	4	10	3	2010	
3B One-arm lat pull-down	1	10 each side	2	3010	45sec
	2	10 each side	3	3010	60sec
	3	10 each side	3	3010	60sec
	4	8 each side	4	3010	90sec

Superset 1

1A Incline bench press

- Lie on a bench set at a 30-45° angle holding a barbell with an overhand grip, hands shoulder-width apart.
- Keep your feet flat on the floor and back against the bench.
- Slowly lower the bar down to your chest then press it directly back up.

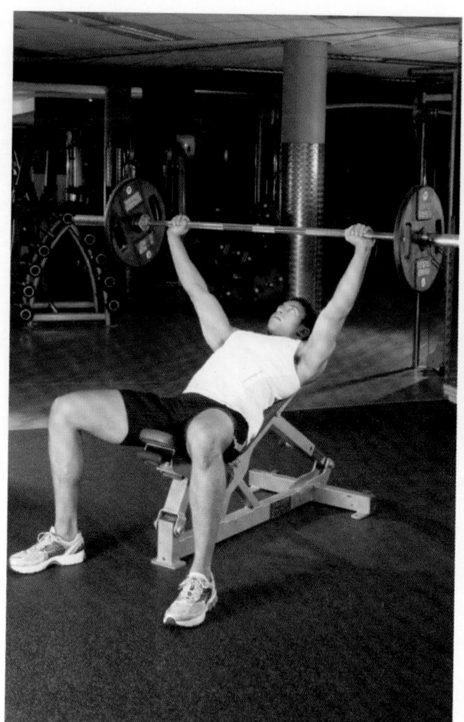

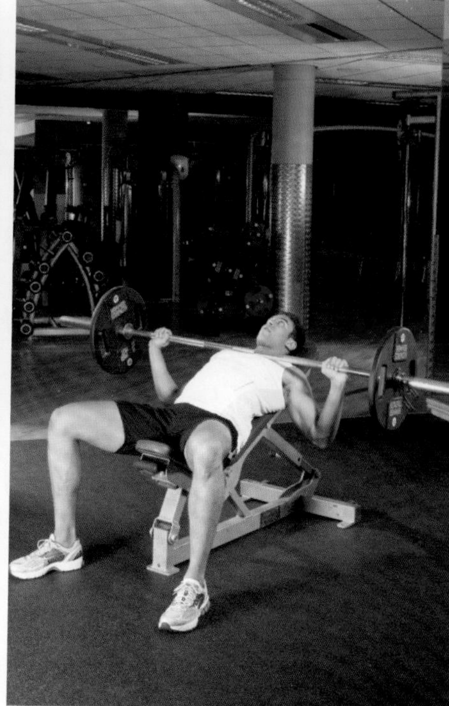

1B Bent-over row

- Start with your core braced, your back straight and your shoulder blades retracted.
- Grip the bar with your hands just wider than shoulder-width apart, letting them hang at knee level.
- Bend your knees slightly and lean forward from the hips.
- Pull the bar up to your lower sternum, retracting your shoulder blades to allow the bar to come up to your chest, then lower the bar slowly to the start.

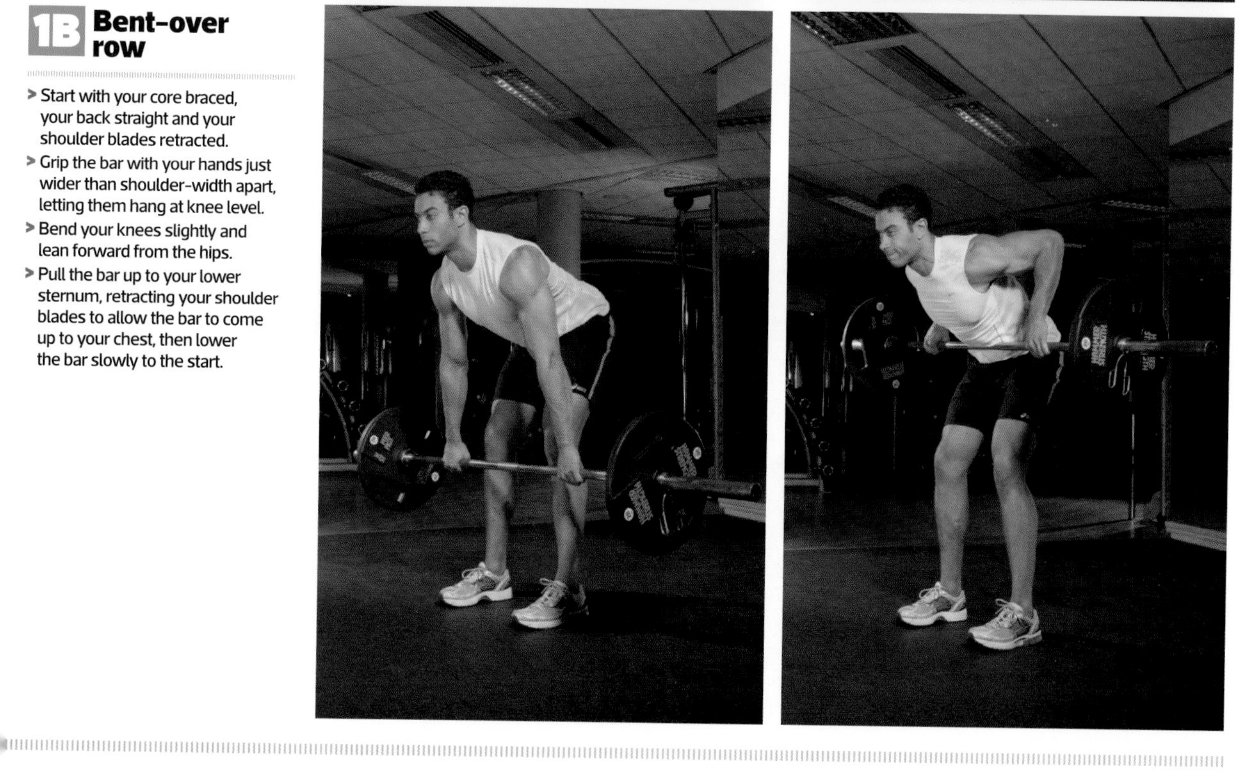

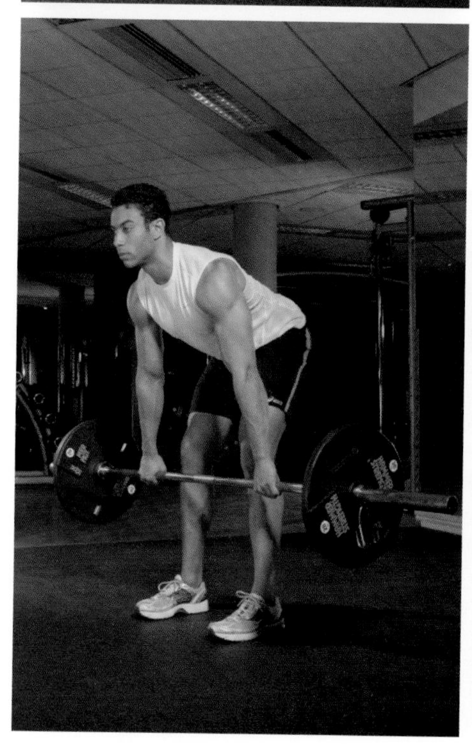

Superset 2

2A Alternating dumbbell press

- Lie on a flat bench with a dumbbell in each hand just wider than shoulder width.
- Keep your feet planted on the floor, and your glutes, upper back and head planted on the bench.
- Keeping one hand where it is, press the other weight up until your arm is almost fully extended.
- Slowly lower the weight back to the start position, then press up with the other arm. When you have returned to the start, that completes one rep.

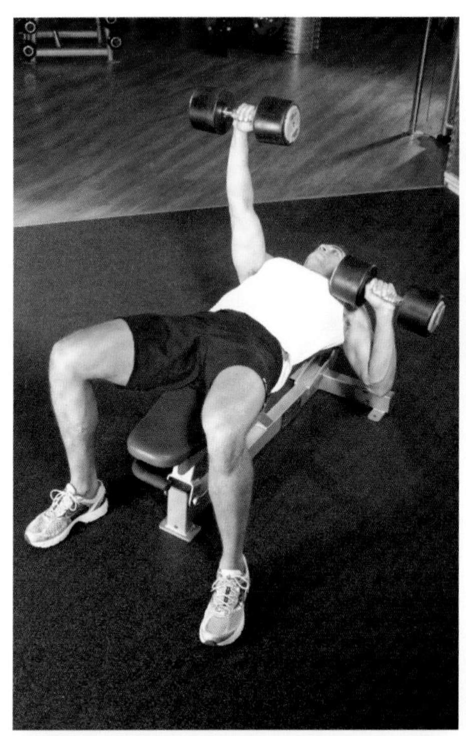

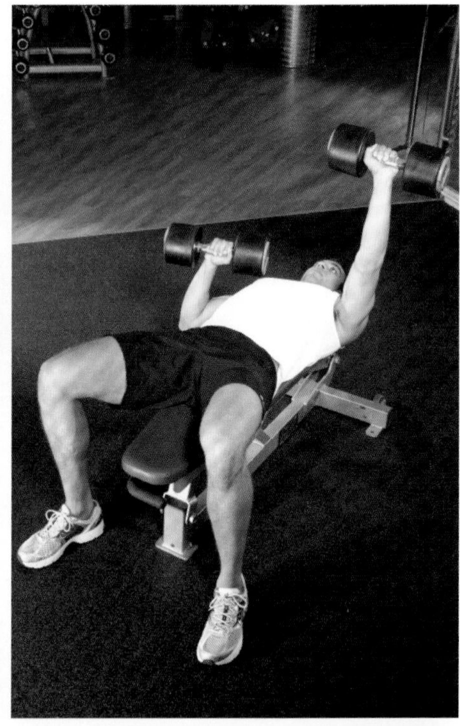

2B Renegade row

- Grab a dumbbell in each hand and assume a press-up position, making sure your feet are slightly wider than shoulder-width apart.
- Press up and lift one dumbbell up to your side, leading with your elbow, then lower back to the floor.
- Repeat with your other arm. When you have rowed both weights and returned to the start, that completes one rep.

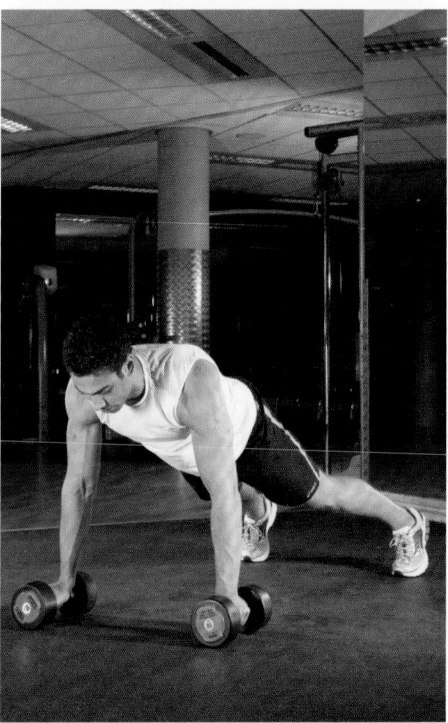

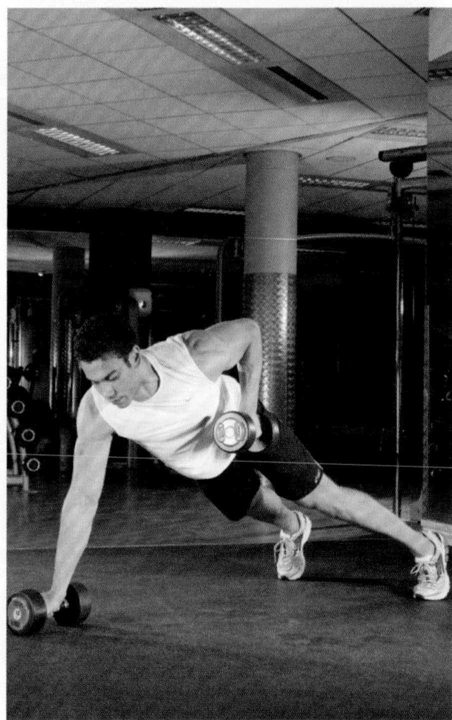

Superset 3

3A Gym ball press-up

- Assume a press-up position with your hands on a gym ball and your body in a straight line from head to heels.
- Slowly lower your chest down to the ball, then press back up.

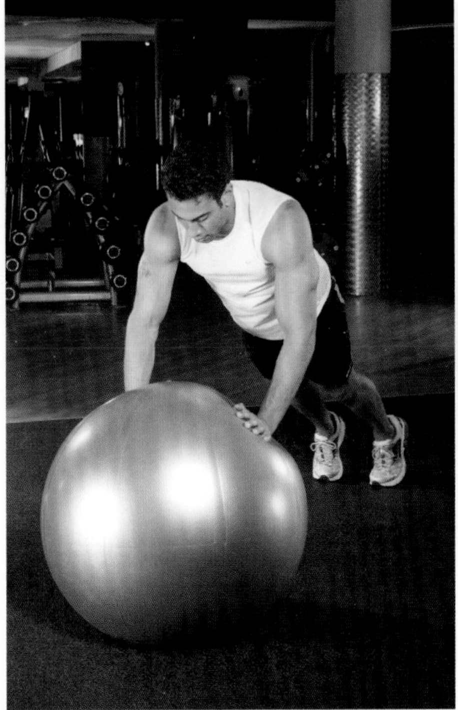

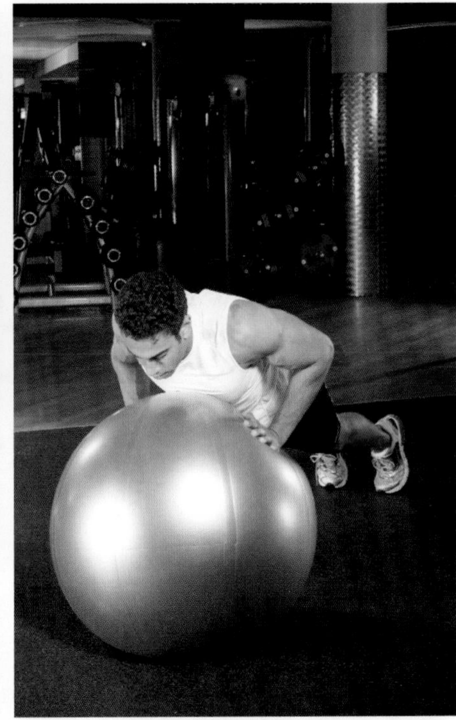

3B One-arm lat pull-down

- Sit on the seat and hold a D-handle in one hand.
- Look forward, retract your shoulder blades and keep your torso upright.
- Pull the handle down in front of you until it reaches your upper chest. Don't lean back to aid the movement.
- Squeeze your lats at the bottom of the move and return the bar slowly to the top.
- Complete all reps with one arm, then repeat with the other.

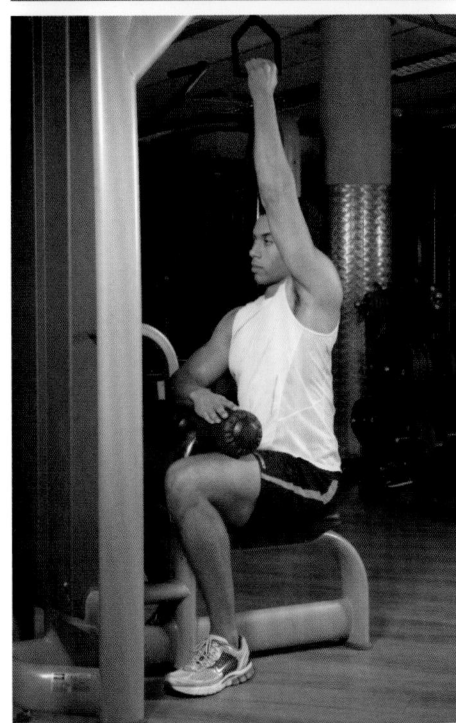

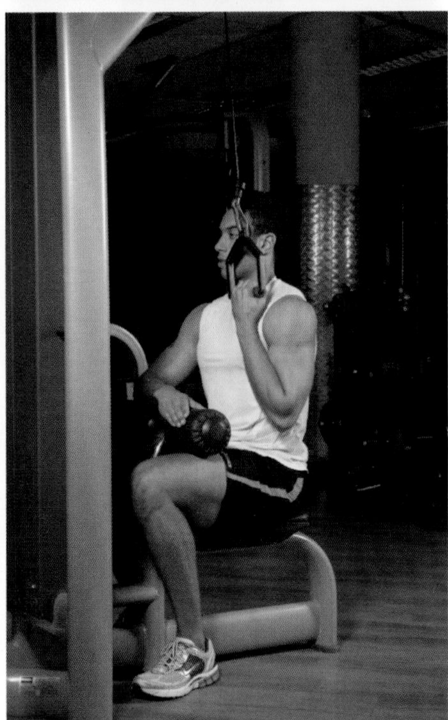

WORKOUT 2

Legs and arms

EXERCISE	WEEK	REPS	SETS	TEMPO	REST
SUPERSET 1					
1A Front squat	1 2 3 4	12 10 8 6	2 3 4 4	2010 2010 2010 2010	
1B Romanian deadlift	1 2 3 4	12 10 8 8	2 3 4 4	3010 3010 3010 3010	60sec 60sec 90sec 90sec
SUPERSET 2					
2A Bulgarian split squat	1 2 3 4	10 each side 12 each side 8 each side 8 each side	2 2 3 3	2010 2010 2010 2010	
2B Gym ball hamstring curl	1 2 3 4	8 10 8 10	2 2 3 3	2010 2010 2010 2010	60sec 60sec 90sec 90sec
SUPERSET 3					
3A Incline biceps curl	1 2 3 4	8 10 8 10	2 2 3 3	4010 4010 4010 4010	
3B Overhead triceps extension	1 2 3 4	10 each side 10 each side 10 each side 8 each side	2 3 3 4	3010 3010 3010 3010	45sec 45sec 60sec 60sec

Superset 1

1A Front squat

- Rest the bar on the front of your shoulders, gripping it with your elbows pointing forward and feet shoulder-width apart.
- Maintain a natural arch in your back and core braced throughout the move.
- Squat down until your thighs are at least parallel to the floor.
- Push back up through your heels.

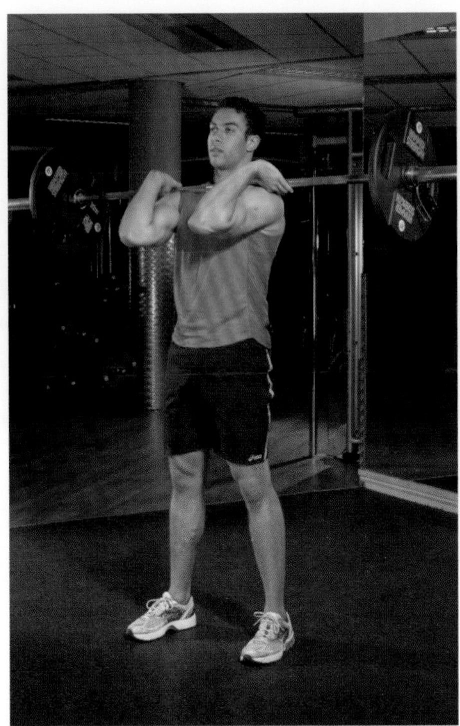

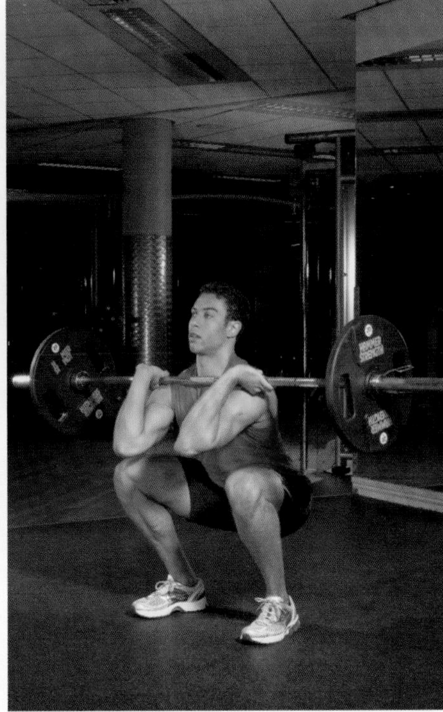

1B Romanian deadlift

- Stand tall holding a barbell with an overhand grip just outside your hips, feet shoulder-width apart. Stand with your shoulder blades retracted, torso upright, core braced and a natural arch in your back.
- Initiate the move by slowly leaning forward from the hips, not the waist, and lower the bar slowly down the front of your shins until you feel a strong stretch in your hamstrings.
- Reverse the move back to the start.

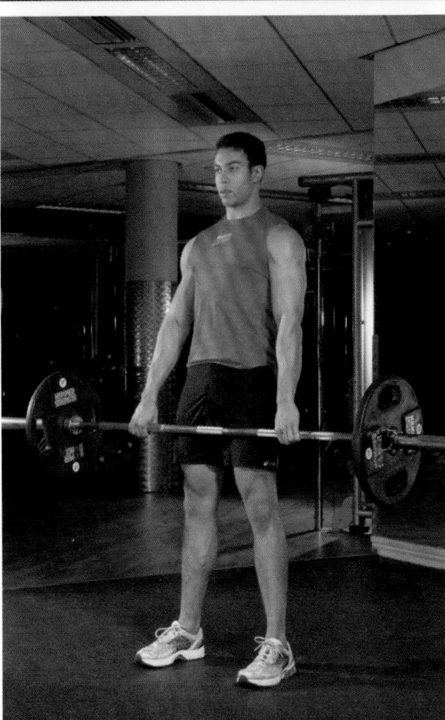

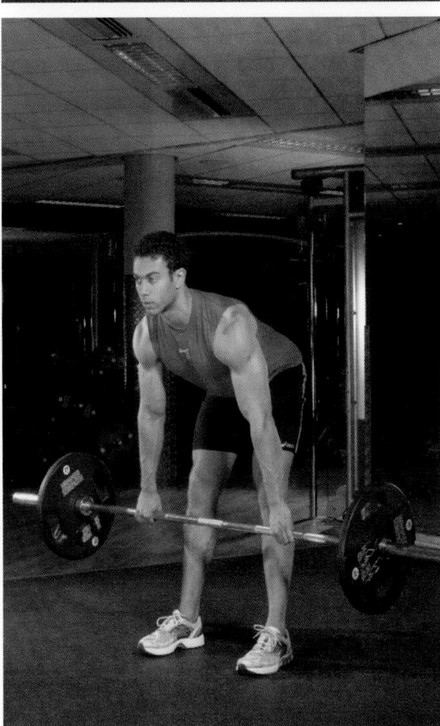

Superset 2

2A Bulgarian split squat

- Hold a barbell across the back of your shoulders and rest your back foot on a bench. Your front leg should be about a metre in front of the bench with toes pointing ahead.
- Keeping your torso upright and head facing forward, bend your front leg until your thigh is parallel to the floor.
- Keep your knee in line with your toes and don't let it travel beyond your toes.

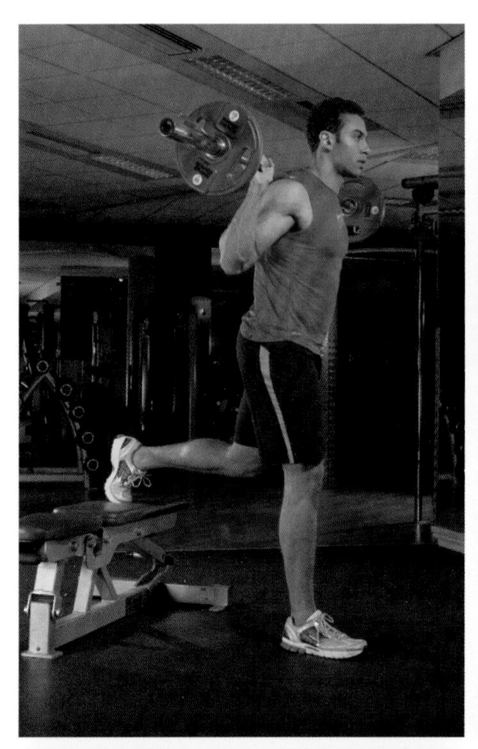

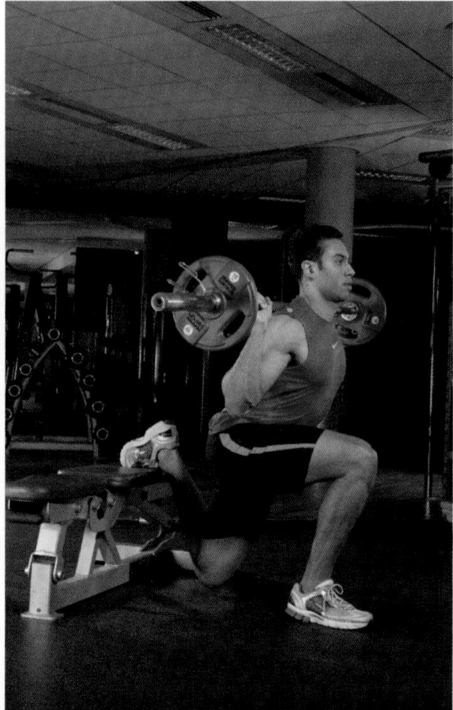

2B Gym ball hamstring curl

- Lie with your head, shoulders and upper back on a gym mat and your feet together on top of a gym ball. Your body should form a straight line from head to heels.
- Keeping your back straight, raise your hips and drag the ball in towards your backside with your heels.
- Pause briefly at the top of the move, then slowly return to the start.

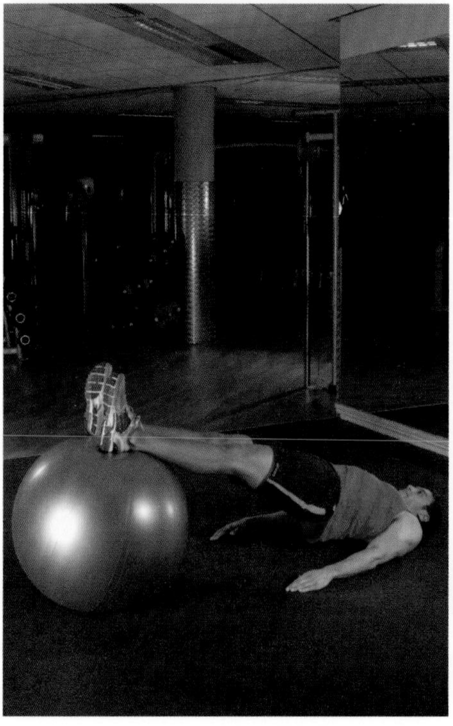

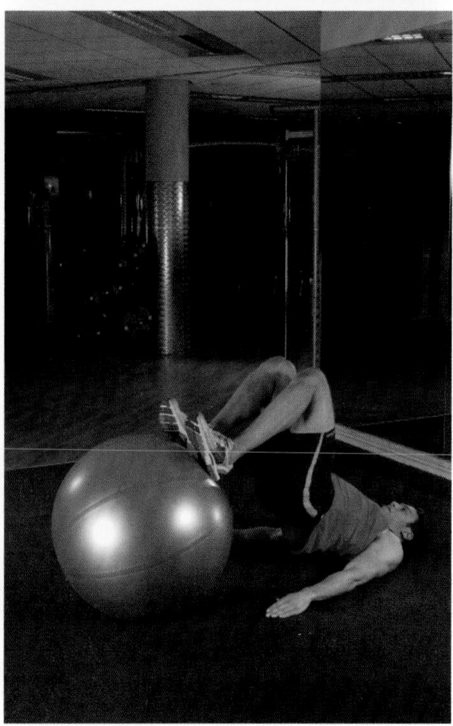

Superset 3

3A Incline biceps curl

- Sit on an incline bench holding a dumbbell in each hand.
- Slowly curl the weights up, keeping your elbows close to your sides.
- Lower back to the start.

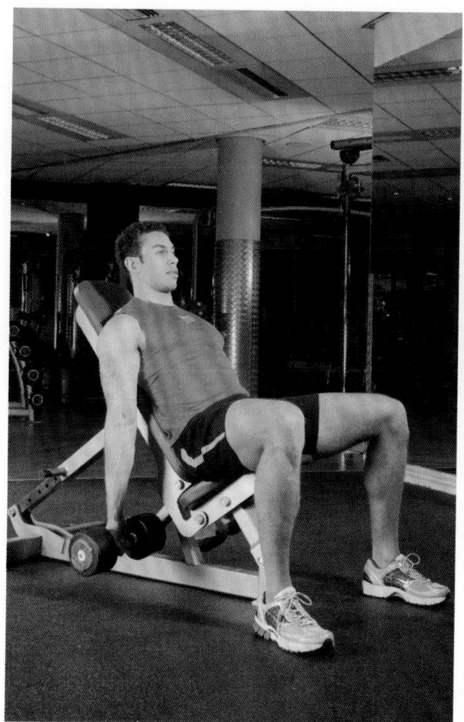

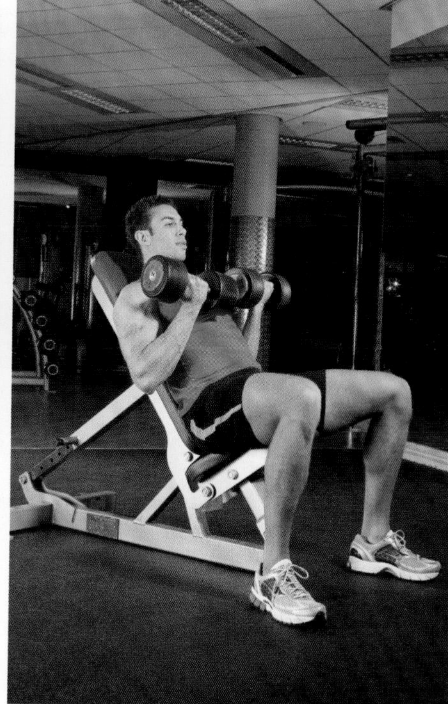

3B Overhead triceps extension

- Sit on a bench with on arm behind you and hold a dumbbell above your head in the other hand.
- Keeping your elbow pointing up, lower the weight behind your head.
- Return to the start.
- When you have completed all the reps with one arm, switch to the other.

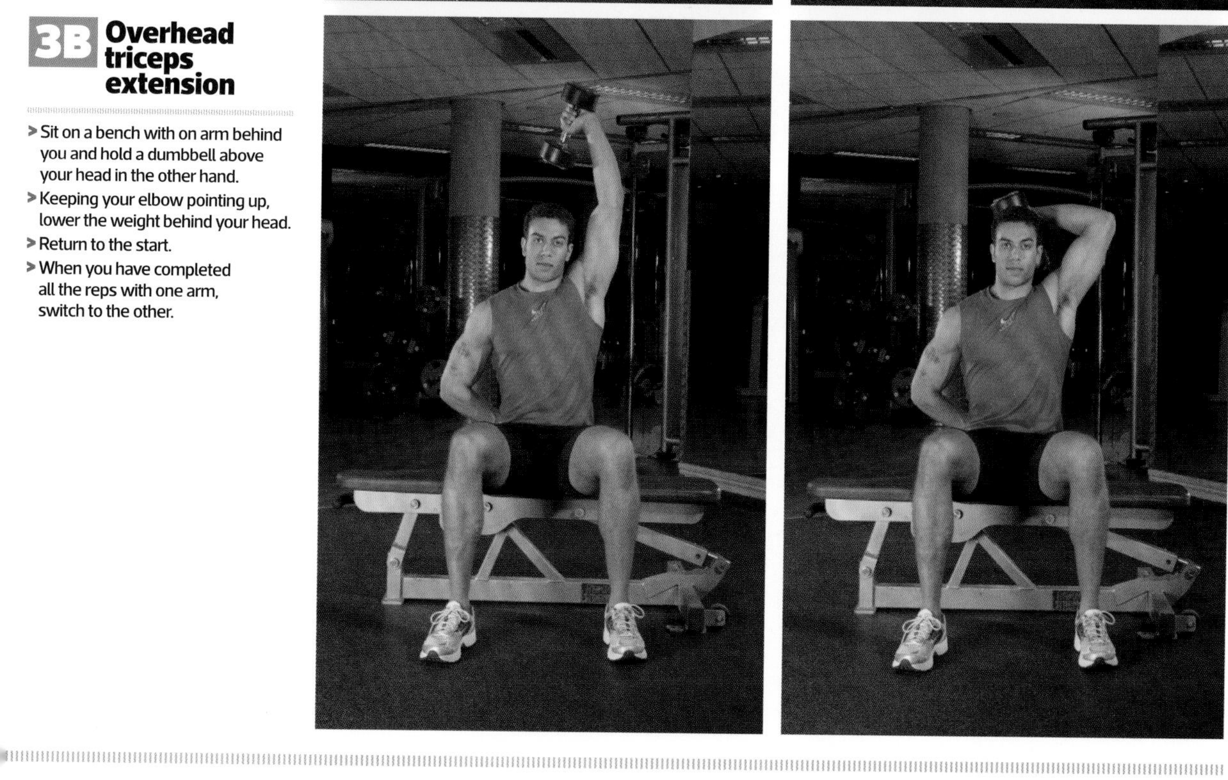

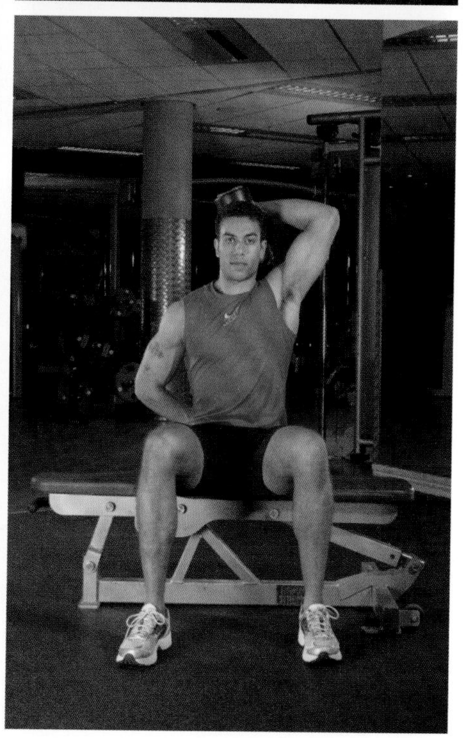

WORKOUT 3

Shoulders and abs

EXERCISE	WEEK	REPS	SETS	TEMPO	REST
SUPERSET 1					
1A Internal cable rotation	1 2 3 4	12 each side 12 each side 12 each side 12 each side	2 2 2 2	3010 3010 3010 3010	
1B External cable rotation	1 2 3 4	12 each side 12 each side 12 each side 12 each side	2 2 2 2	3010 3010 3010 3010	60sec 60sec 60sec 60sec
SUPERSET 2					
2A Push press	1 2 3 4	10 12 10 12	2 2 3 4	2010 2010 2010 2010	
2B Halo	1 2 3 4	8 10 8 10	2 2 3 3	2010 2010 2010 2010	60sec 60sec 90sec 90sec
SUPERSET 3					
3A Barbell rollout	1 2 3 4	8 10 8 10	2 2 3 3	4010 4010 4010 4010	
3B Gym ball Russian twist	1 2 3 4	10 10 10 8	2 3 3 4	3010 3010 3010 3010	45sec 45sec 60sec 60sec

Superset 1

1A Internal cable rotation

- Set the handle on a cable machine so it's in line with your lower chest and grasp it with your palm facing out and elbow bent at 90°.
- Pull the handle towards your chest, keeping the 90° bend in your elbow.
- Slowly return to the start and repeat.
- When you have completed all the reps with one arm, switch to the other.

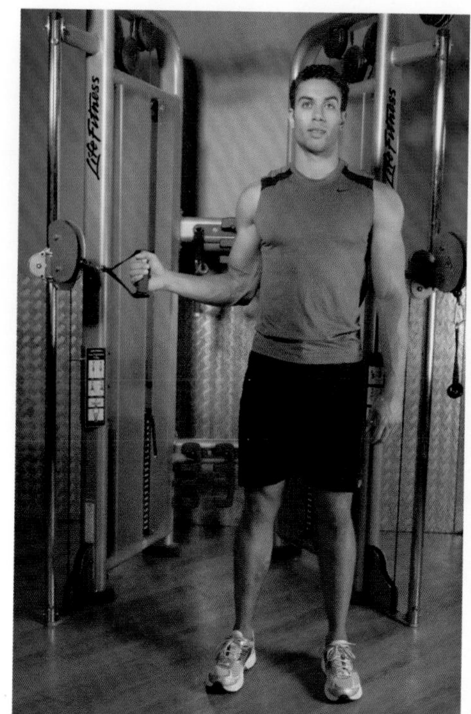

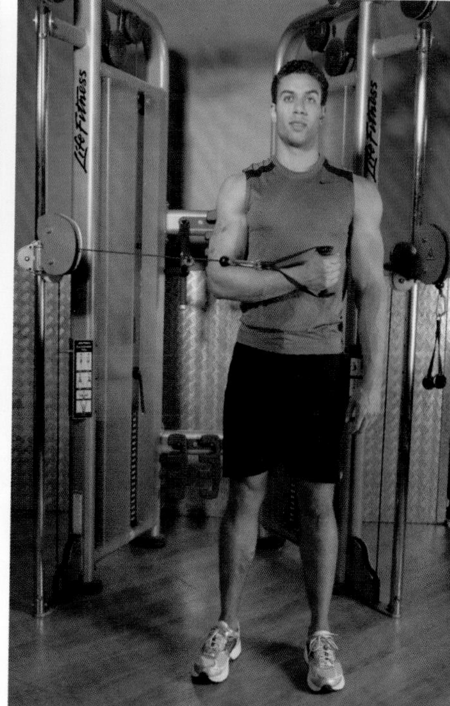

1B External cable rotation

- Set the handle on a cable machine so it's in line with your lower chest and grasp it with your opposite hand, meaning your arm comes across your chest, palm facing you and elbow bent at 90°.
- Pull the handle away from your chest, keeping the 90° bend in your elbow.
- Slowly return to the start and repeat.
- When you have completed all the reps with one arm, switch to the other.

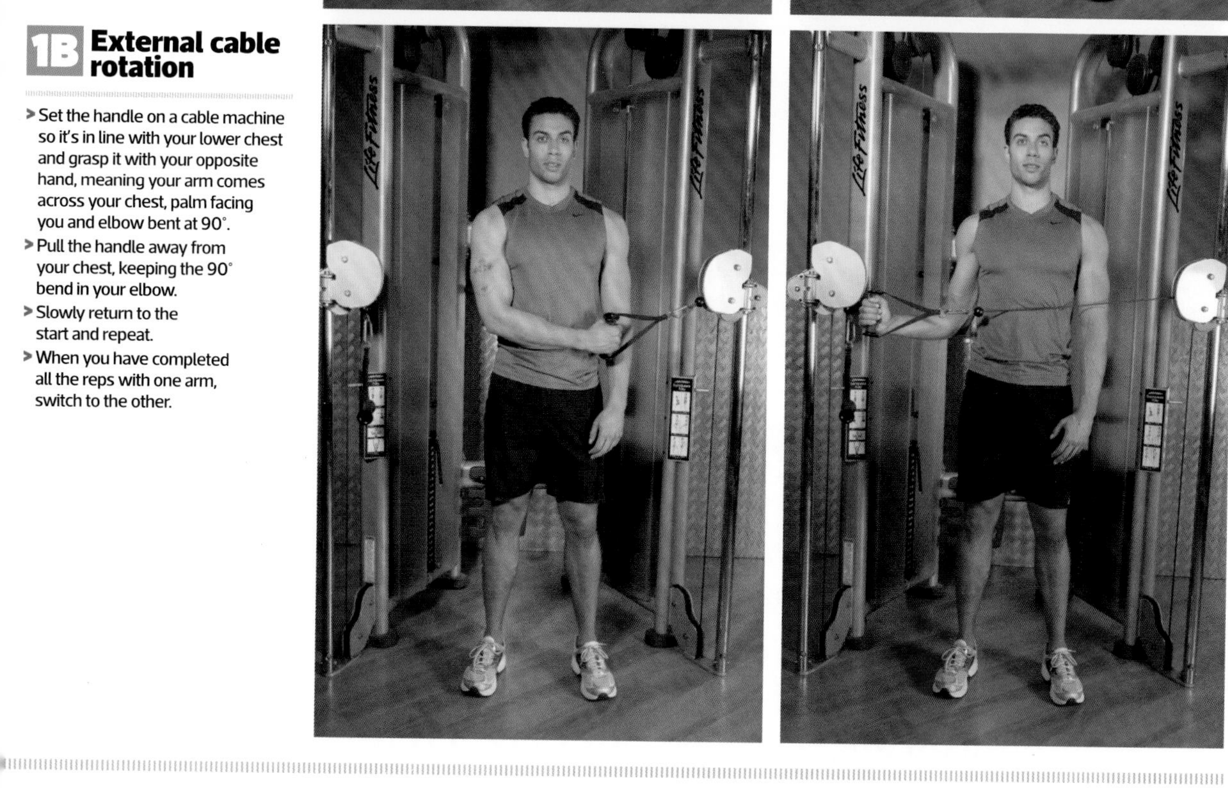

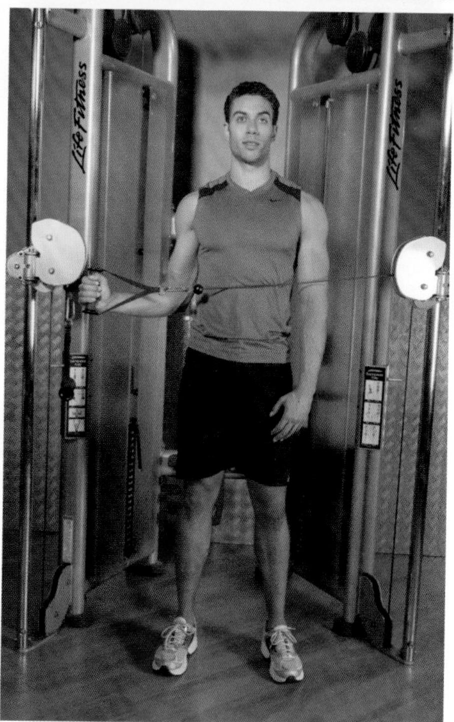

Superset 2

2A Push press

- Stand tall with a barbell across your upper chest. Hold the bar with an overhand grip just wider than shoulder-width apart.
- Keeping your core braced, bend your knees slightly, then stand up straight again while at the same time pressing the bar directly overhead by straightening your arms. Don't lock out your elbows.
- Slowly return the bar back to the start.

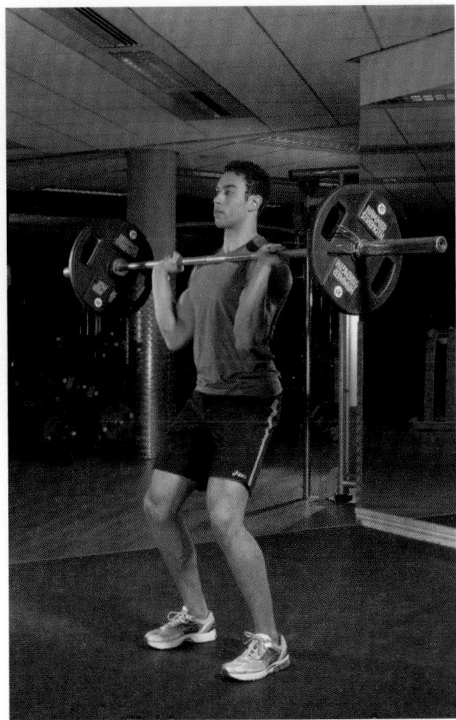

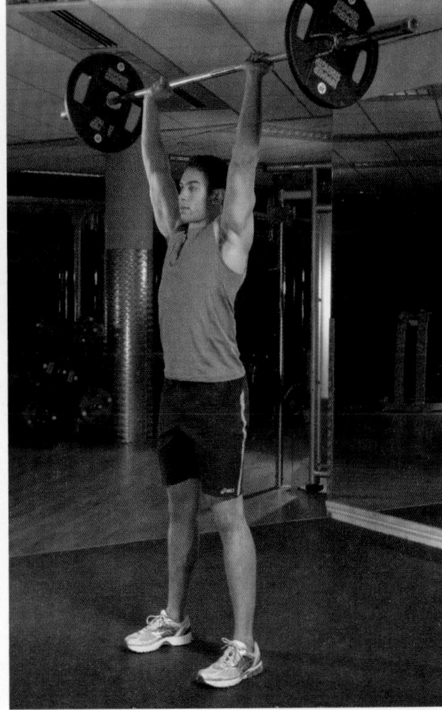

2B Halo

- Hold a weight plate directly above your head.
- Rotate it around your head, keeping your core braced throughout.

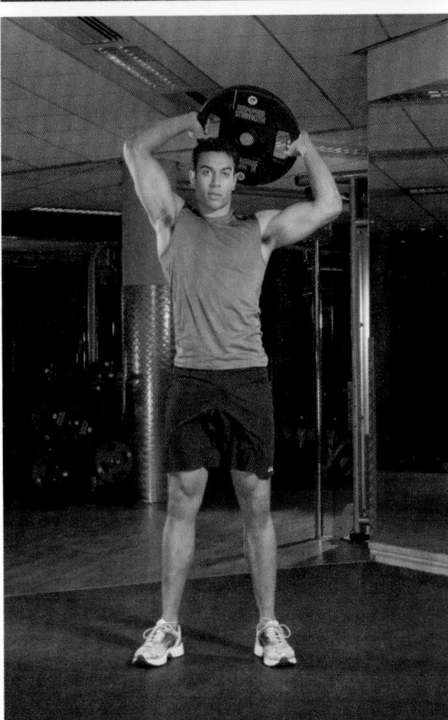

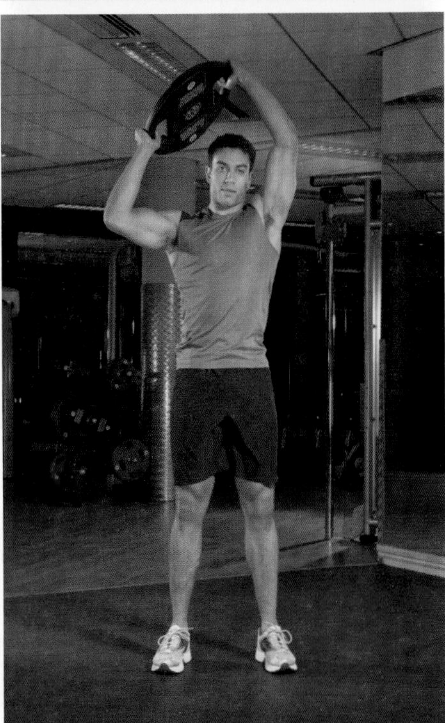

Superset 3

3A Barbell rollout

- Kneel in front of a barbell and grip the bar with hands shoulder-width apart.
- Roll the bar forwards as far as you can to lower your chest towards the floor, then contract your abs to return to the start.

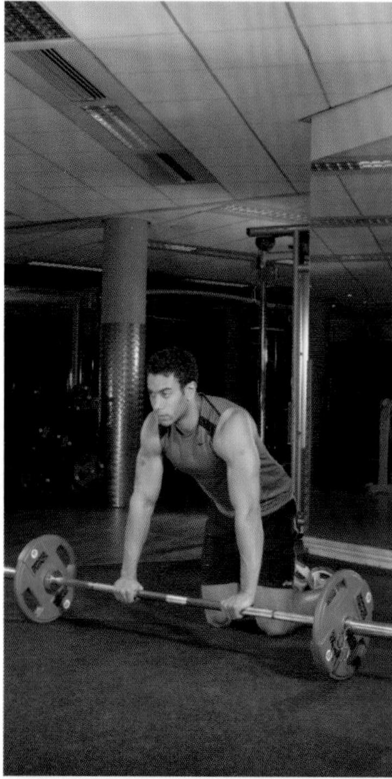

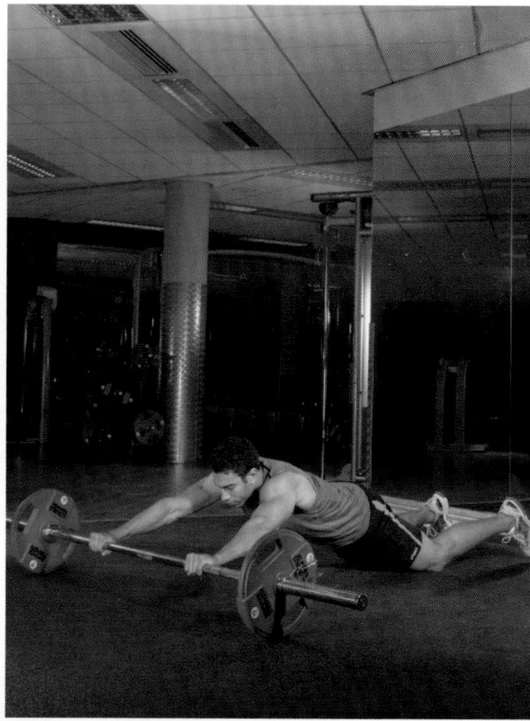

3B Gym ball Russian twist

- Lie back on a gym ball with knees bent, holding a dumbbell with both hands.
- Twist your torso from side to side, controlling the weight throughout.
- Alternate sides. When you return to the middle after twisting to each side, that completes one rep.

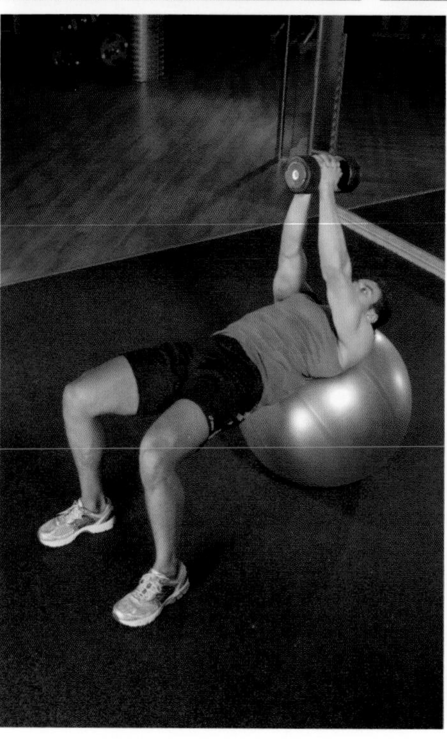

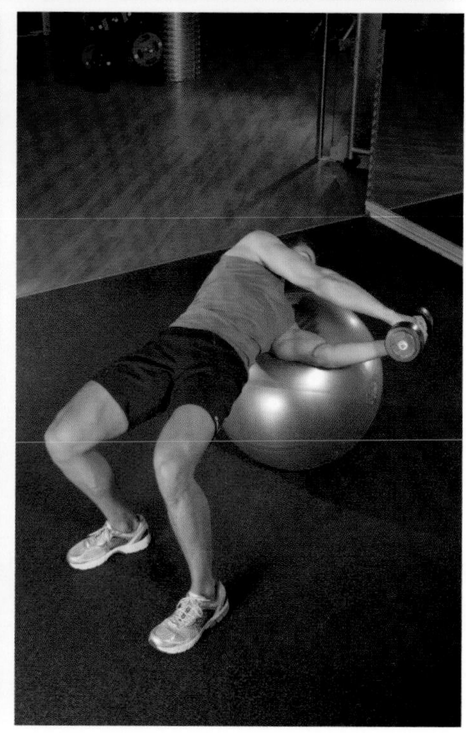

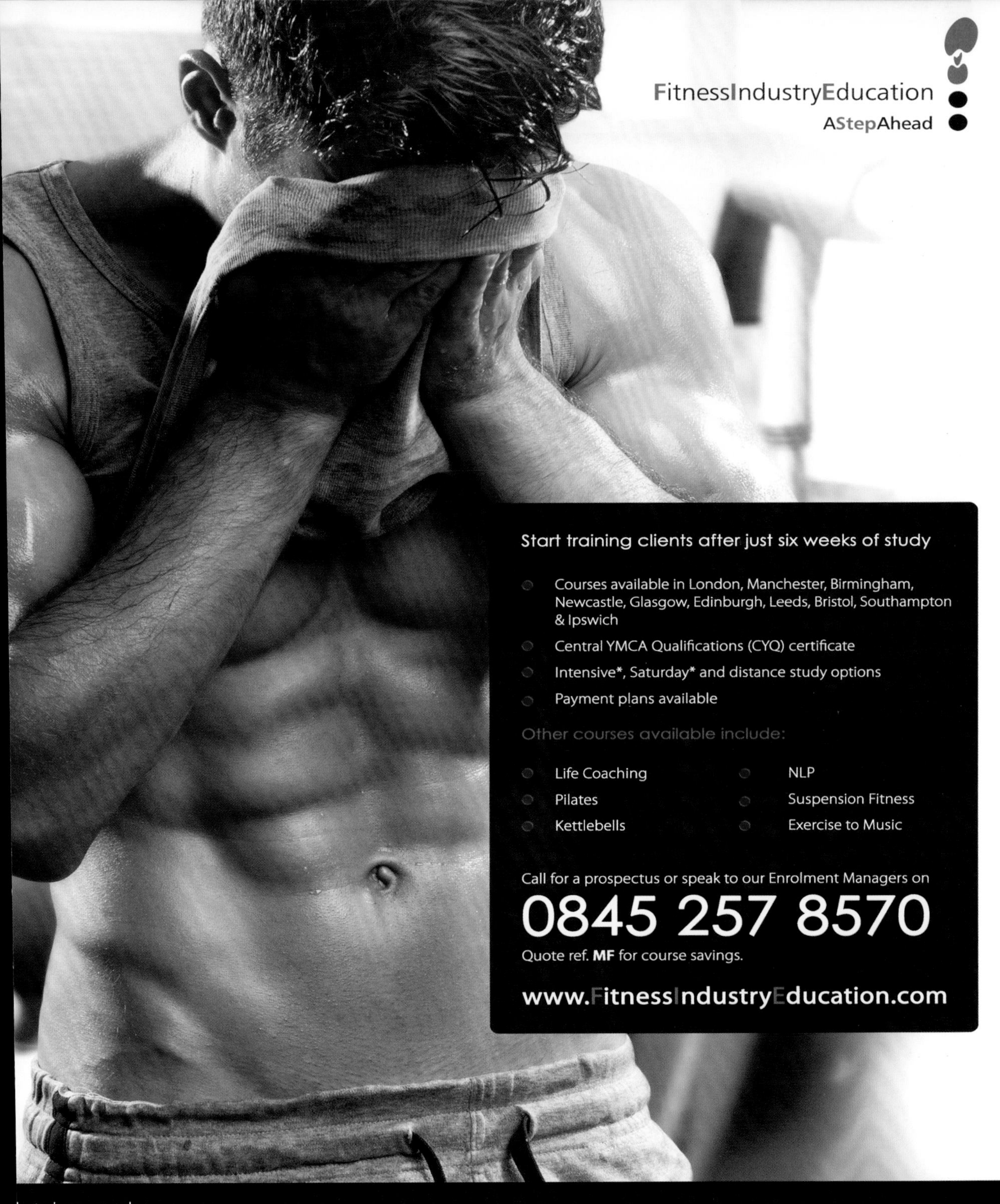

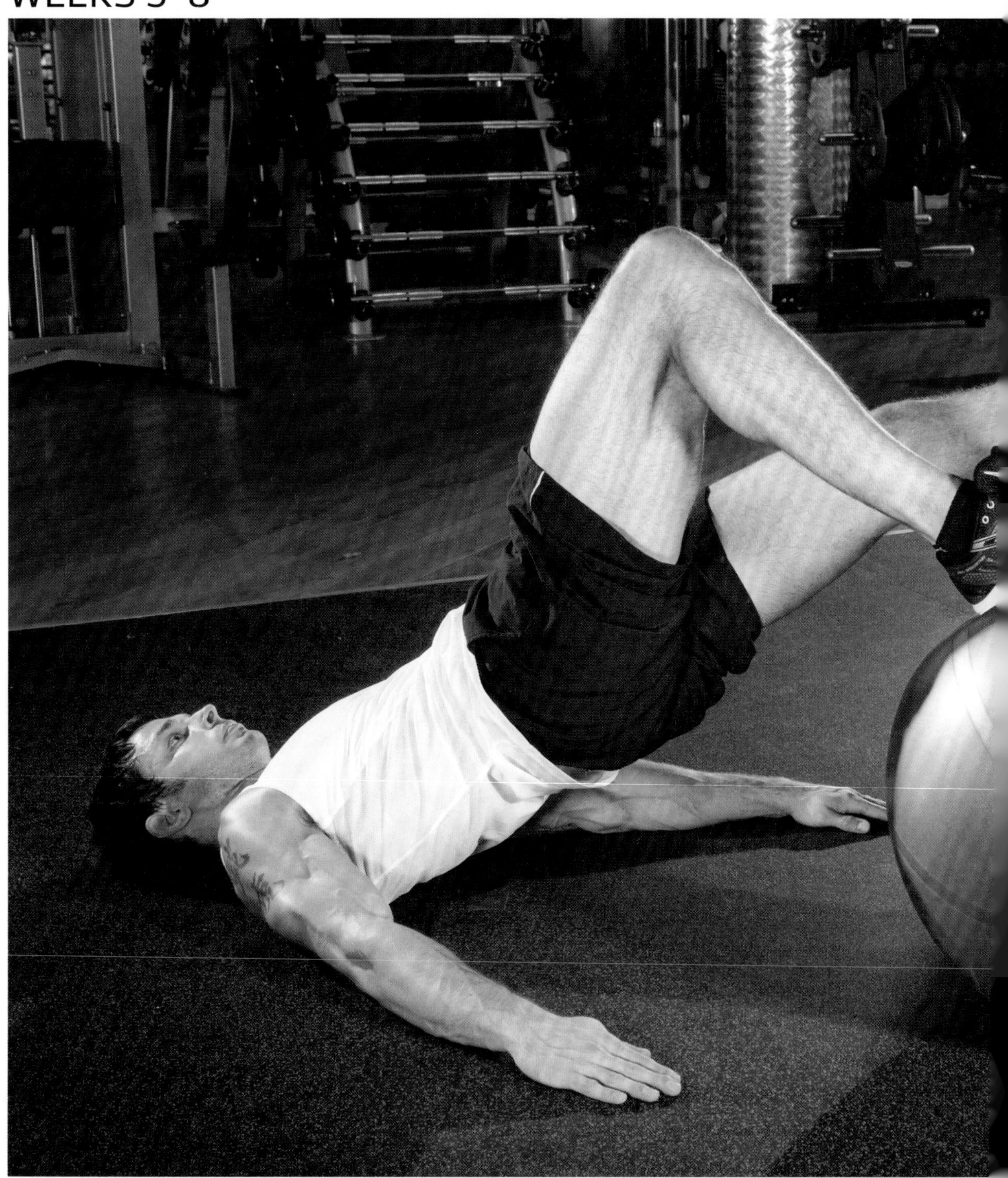

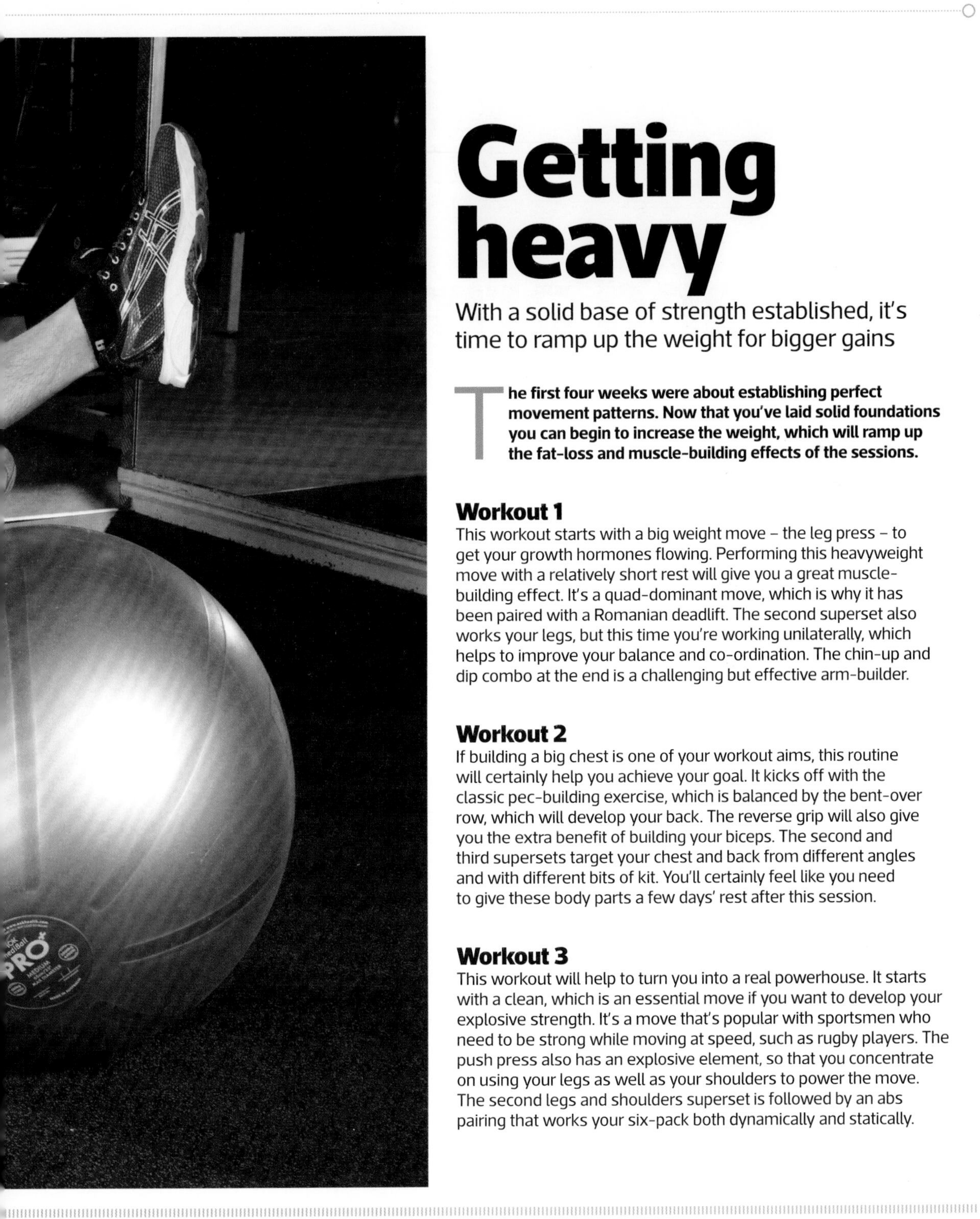

Getting heavy

With a solid base of strength established, it's time to ramp up the weight for bigger gains

The first four weeks were about establishing perfect movement patterns. Now that you've laid solid foundations you can begin to increase the weight, which will ramp up the fat-loss and muscle-building effects of the sessions.

Workout 1

This workout starts with a big weight move – the leg press – to get your growth hormones flowing. Performing this heavyweight move with a relatively short rest will give you a great muscle-building effect. It's a quad-dominant move, which is why it has been paired with a Romanian deadlift. The second superset also works your legs, but this time you're working unilaterally, which helps to improve your balance and co-ordination. The chin-up and dip combo at the end is a challenging but effective arm-builder.

Workout 2

If building a big chest is one of your workout aims, this routine will certainly help you achieve your goal. It kicks off with the classic pec-building exercise, which is balanced by the bent-over row, which will develop your back. The reverse grip will also give you the extra benefit of building your biceps. The second and third supersets target your chest and back from different angles and with different bits of kit. You'll certainly feel like you need to give these body parts a few days' rest after this session.

Workout 3

This workout will help to turn you into a real powerhouse. It starts with a clean, which is an essential move if you want to develop your explosive strength. It's a move that's popular with sportsmen who need to be strong while moving at speed, such as rugby players. The push press also has an explosive element, so that you concentrate on using your legs as well as your shoulders to power the move. The second legs and shoulders superset is followed by an abs pairing that works your six-pack both dynamically and statically.

WORKOUT 1

Legs and arms

EXERCISE	WEEK	REPS	SETS	TEMPO	REST
SUPERSET 1					
1A Leg press	1	12	2	3010	
	2	10	3	3010	
	3	8	4	3010	
	4	6	4	3010	
1B Romanian deadlift	1	12	2	3010	60sec
	2	10	3	3010	60sec
	3	8	4	3010	90sec
	4	8	4	3010	90sec
SUPERSET 2					
2A Side lunge	1	12	2	1010	
	2	10	2	1010	
	3	8	3	1010	
	4	8	3	1010	
2B One-leg hamstring curl	1	8	2	2010	60sec
	2	10	2	2010	60sec
	3	8	3	2010	90sec
	4	10	3	2010	90sec
SUPERSET 3					
3A Chin-up	1	3	4	4010	
	2	4	4	4010	
	3	4	5	4010	
	4	5	5	4010	
3B Dip	1	3	4	3010	60sec
	2	4	4	3010	60sec
	3	4	5	3010	90sec
	4	5	5	3010	90sec

Superset 1

1A Leg press

- Lie on the leg press machine following the instructions to position yourself safely and correctly with legs straight.
- With your feet hip-width apart, lower the weights towards you until your legs are bent.
- Return to the start.

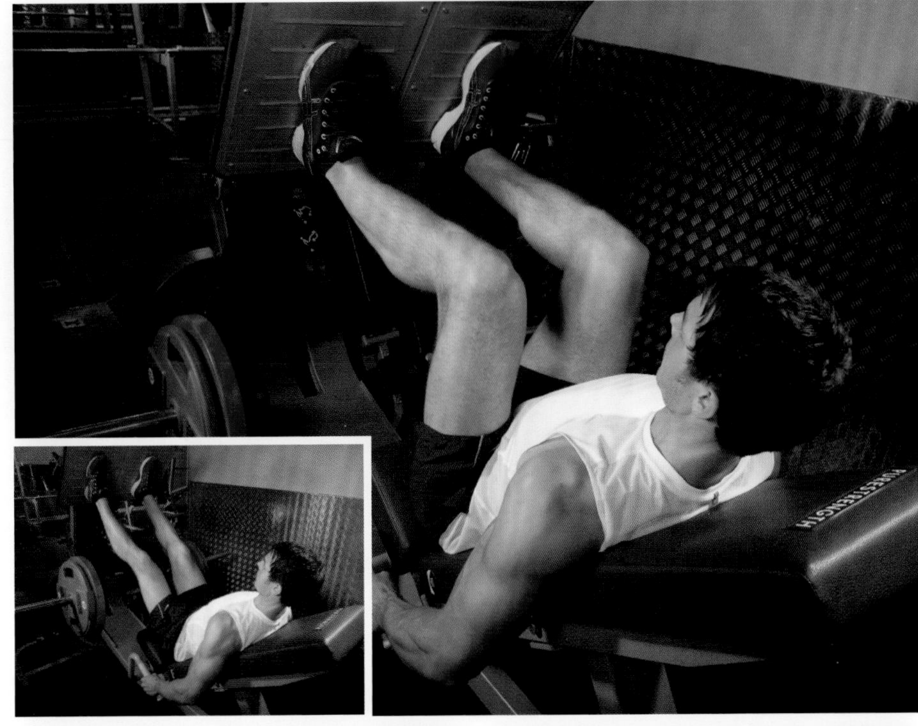

1B Romanian deadlift

- Stand tall holding a barbell with an overhand grip just outside your hips, feet shoulder-width apart. Stand with your shoulder blades retracted, torso upright, core braced and a natural arch in your back.
- Initiate the move by slowly leaning forward from the hips, not the waist, and lower the bar slowly down the front of your shins until you feel a strong stretch in your hamstrings.
- Reverse the move back to the start and push your hips forward to reset the start position.

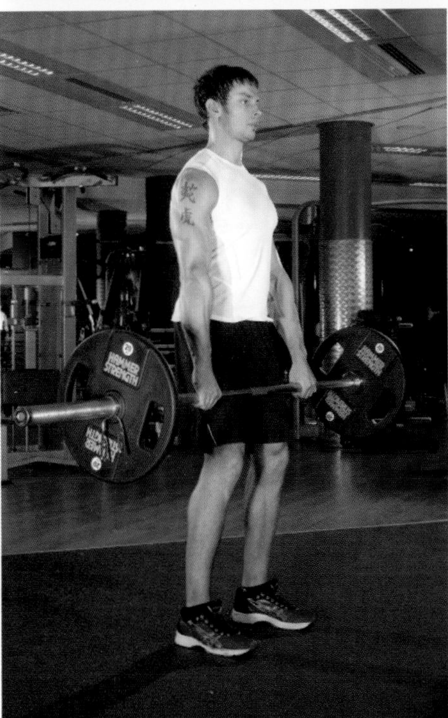

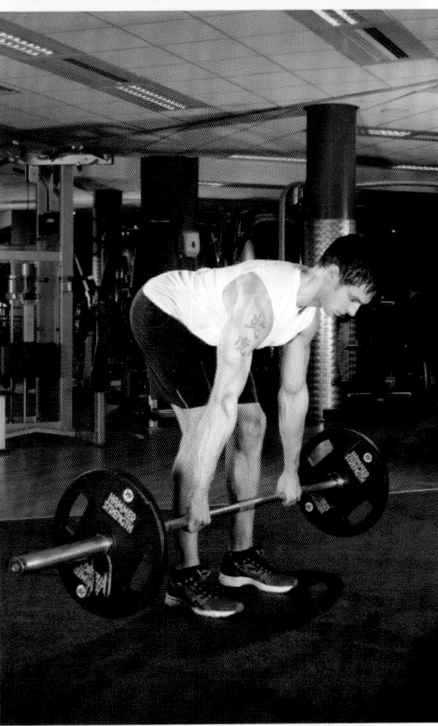

Superset 2

2A Side lunge

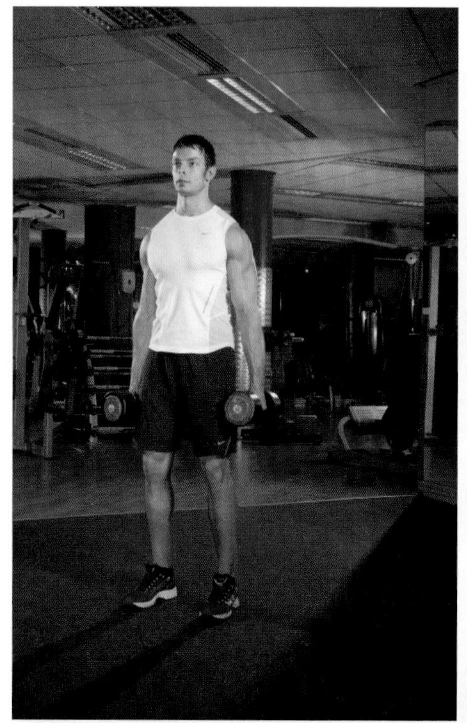

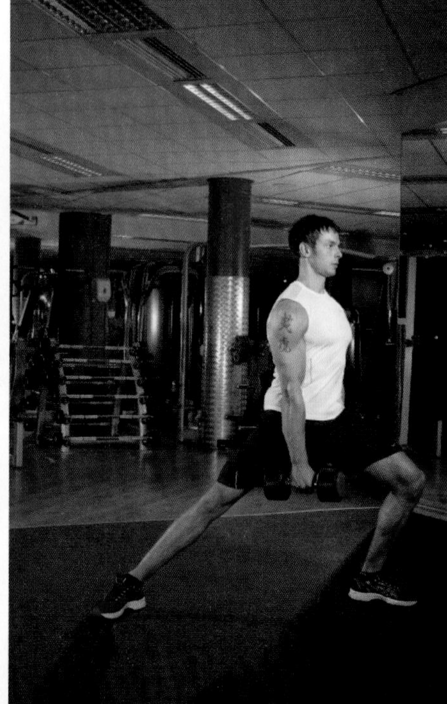

- Stand tall with feet close together, holding a dumbbell in each hand.
- Keeping your core braced and head facing forward, take a big step to one side and lower your body down towards the leading leg, with your knee in line with your toes.
- Push back off the leading leg and repeat on the other side. When you return to the start position after lunging to both side, that completes one rep.

2B One-leg gym ball hamstring curl

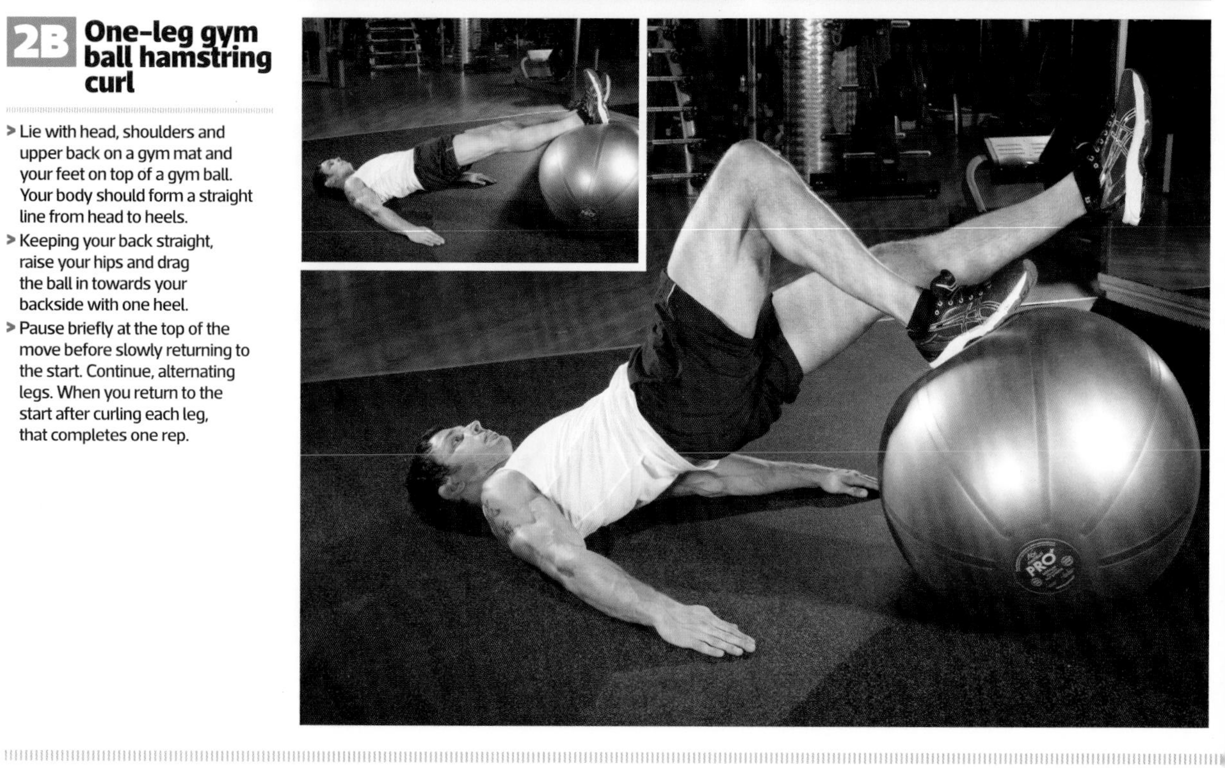

- Lie with head, shoulders and upper back on a gym mat and your feet on top of a gym ball. Your body should form a straight line from head to heels.
- Keeping your back straight, raise your hips and drag the ball in towards your backside with one heel.
- Pause briefly at the top of the move before slowly returning to the start. Continue, alternating legs. When you return to the start after curling each leg, that completes one rep.

Superset 3

3A Chin-up

- Grab the bar with an underhand grip with your hands slightly wider than shoulder-width apart.
- Start from a dead hang with your arms fully extended.
- Pull yourself up by squeezing your lats together.
- Once your chin is higher than your hands pause briefly, before slowly lowering yourself back to the start.

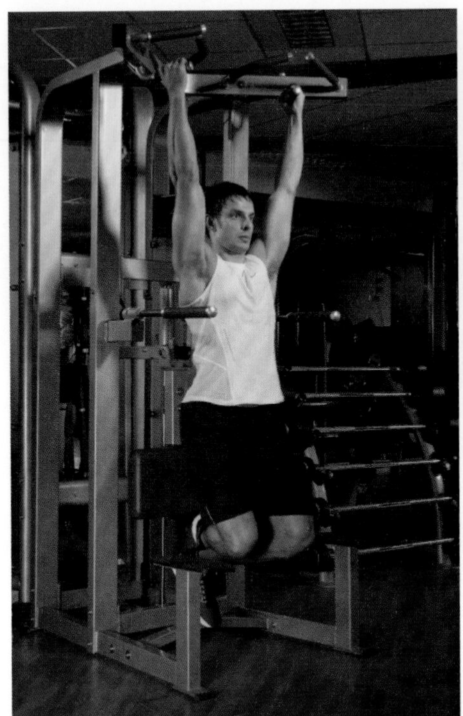

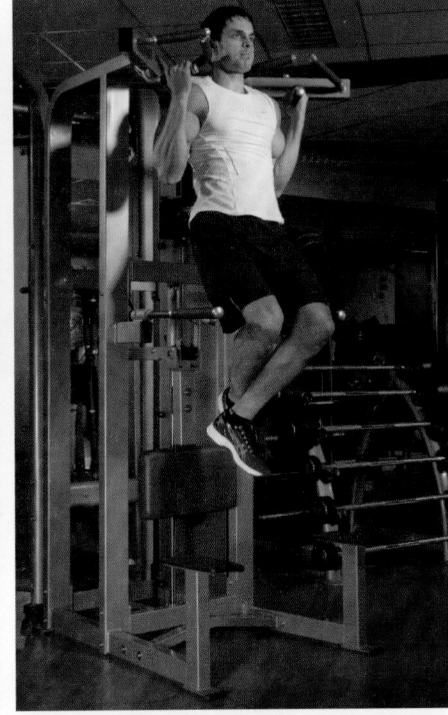

3B Dip

- Grip parallel bars, keeping your body upright.
- With your elbows pointing straight back, lower your body as far down as you can comfortably go without stressing your shoulders.
- Keep your core braced and don't swing your legs for momentum.

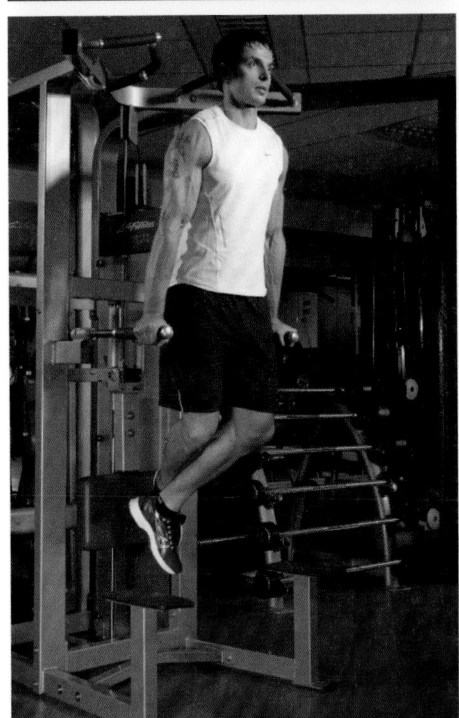

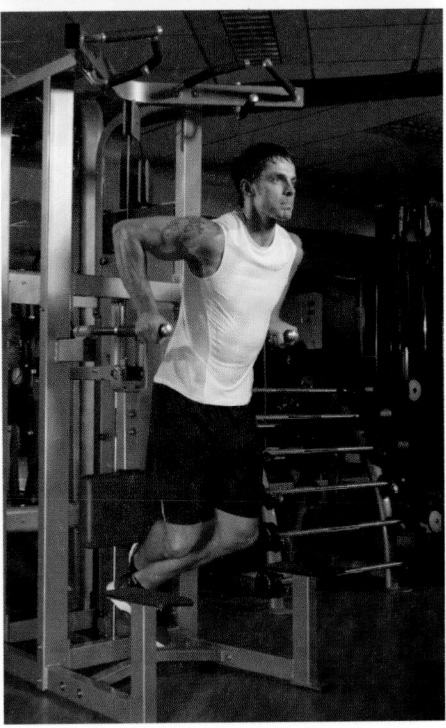

WORKOUT 2

Chest and back

EXERCISE	WEEK	REPS	SETS	TEMPO	REST
SUPERSET 1					
1A Bench press	1 2 3 4	12 10 8 6	2 3 4 4	3010 3010 3010 3010	
1B Reverse-grip bent-over row	1 2 3 4	12 10 8 8	2 3 4 4	3010 3010 3010 3010	60sec 60sec 90sec 90sec
SUPERSET 2					
2A Dumbbell flye	1 2 3 4	10 12 8 8	2 2 3 3	3010 3010 3010 3010	
2B Standing cable row	1 2 3 4	8 10 8 10	2 2 3 3	2010 2010 2010 2010	60sec 60sec 90sec 90sec
SUPERSET 3					
3A Cable crossover	1 2 3 4	8 10 8 10	2 2 3 3	4010 4010 4010 4010	
3B Inverted row	1 2 3 4	8 8 8 8	2 2 3 3	3010 3010 3010 3010	45sec 45sec 60sec 60sec

Superset 1

1A Bench press

- Lie on the bench with your feet on the floor, directly underneath your knees.
- Your head, upper back and glutes should be flat against the bench. Brace your core and maintain a natural arch in your back.
- Hold the bar with an overhand grip that is wider than shoulder-width apart.
- Slowly lower the bar to your chest, taking your elbows out to 90°, until the bar is almost touching the middle of chest or just over your nipples.
- Pause briefly, then drive your feet hard into the floor and push the bar back strongly to the start position.

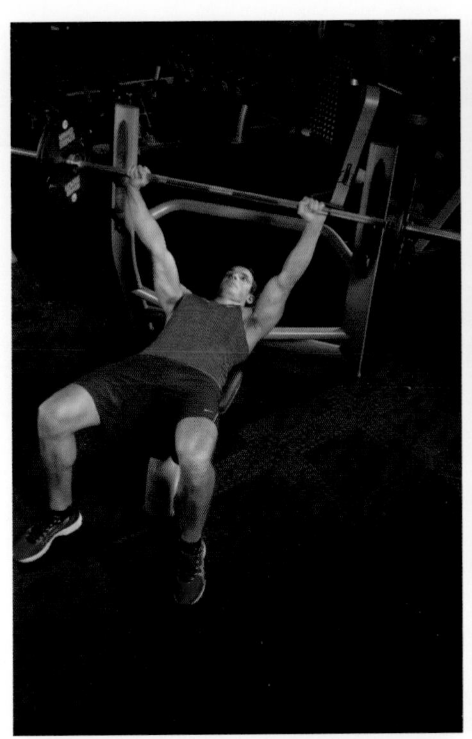

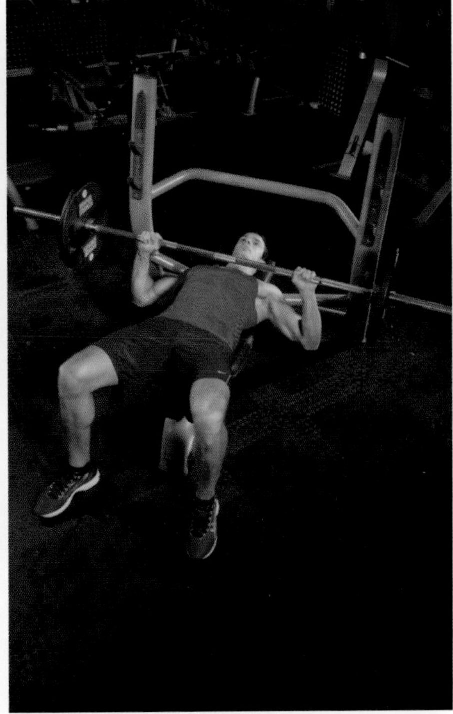

1B Reverse-grip bent-over row

- Start with your core braced, your back straight and your shoulder blades retracted.
- Bend your knees slightly and lean forward from the hips.
- Grip the bar with an underhand grip with hands just wider than shoulder-width apart letting them hang at knee level.
- Pull the bar up to your lower sternum, retracting your shoulder blades to allow the bar to come up to the chest, then lower the bar slowly to the start.

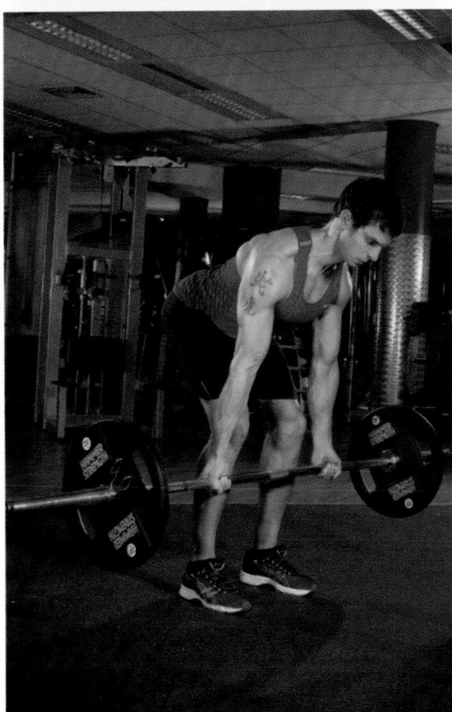

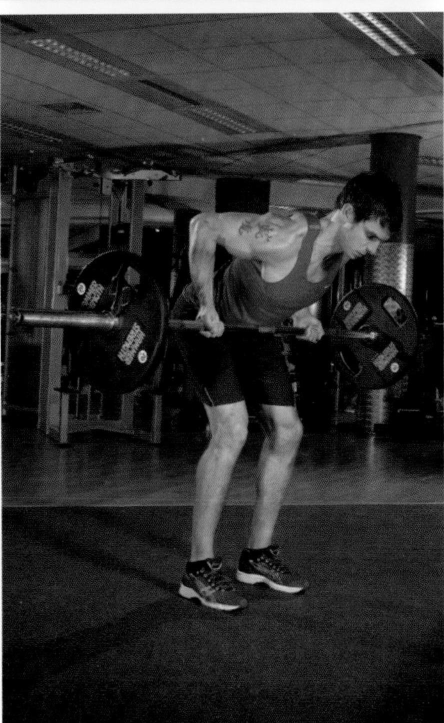

Superset 2

2A Gym ball dumbbell flye

- Lie on a gym ball holding a dumbbell in each hand directly above your chest. with palms facing.
- Make sure your head and shoulders are supported on the bench and that your feet are flat on the floor.
- Keeping a slight bend in your elbows, slowly lower the weights out to the side as far as is comfortable. Don't arch your back.
- Use your pecs to reverse the movement to raise the weights back to the top.

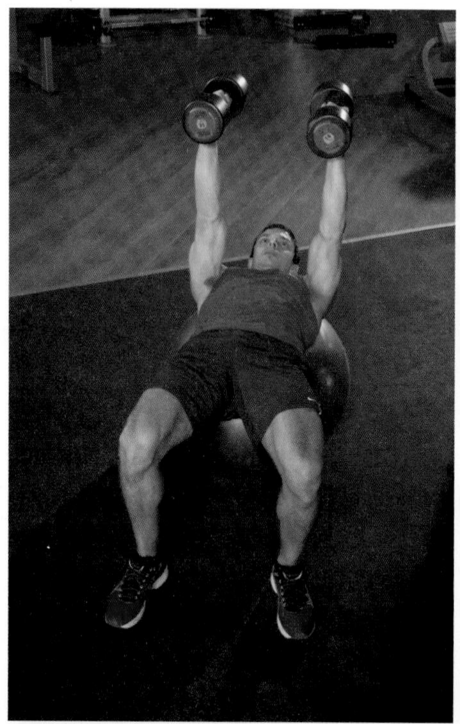

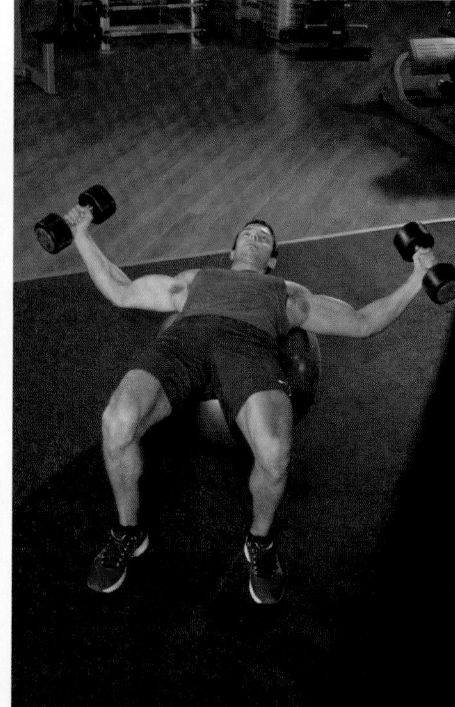

2B Standing cable row

- Stand at a cable machine with a straight bar attachment at chest height.
- With an overhand grip, pull the bar into your chest.
- Pause briefly then return to the start.

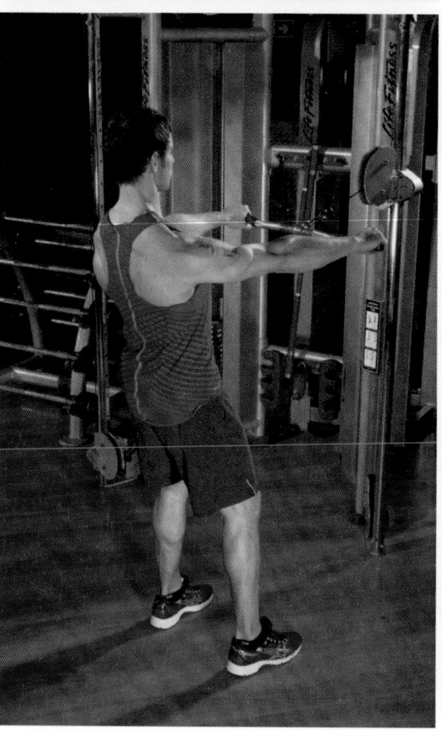

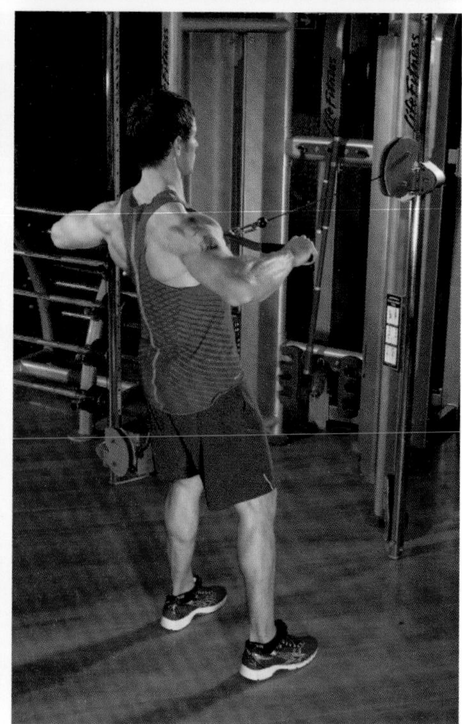

Superset 3

3A Cable crossover

- Stand in the middle of a cable machine with a split stance holding a D-handle attachment in each hand, with the cable set above shoulder height.
- Keeping a natural arch in your back, core braced and upper body still, bring your hands down in an arc to meet in front of you.
- Pause briefly and squeeze your chest muscles, then return slowly to the start with the weight under full control.

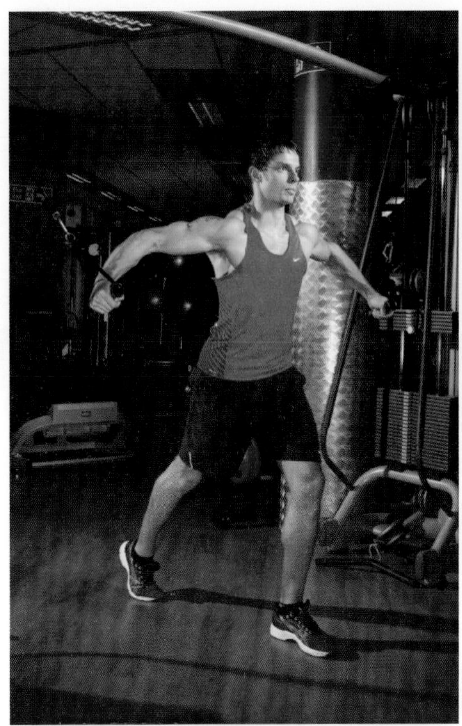

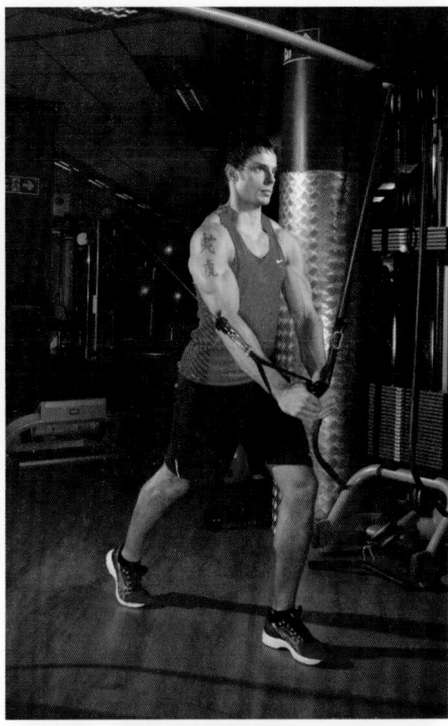

3B Inverted row

- Set a Smith machine bar at about chest height. Lie underneath the bar on the floor with your feet on a bench and hold it with an overhand grip, hands just wider than shoulder-width apart.
- Keeping your hips in line with your torso, pull your body up to the bar until you touch it with your chest.
- Lower yourself slowly back to the starting position.

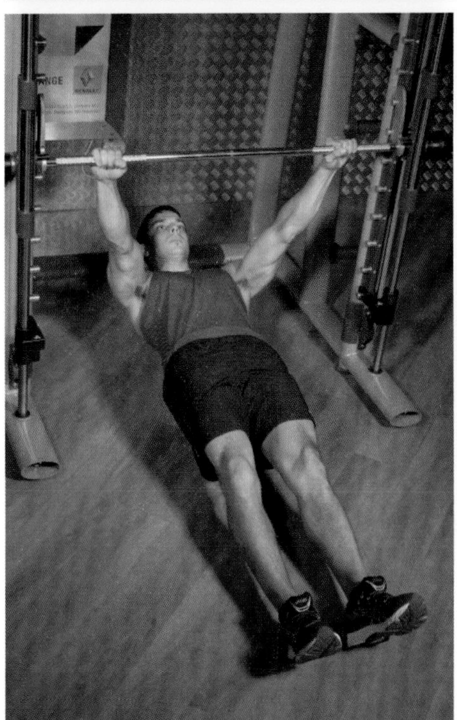

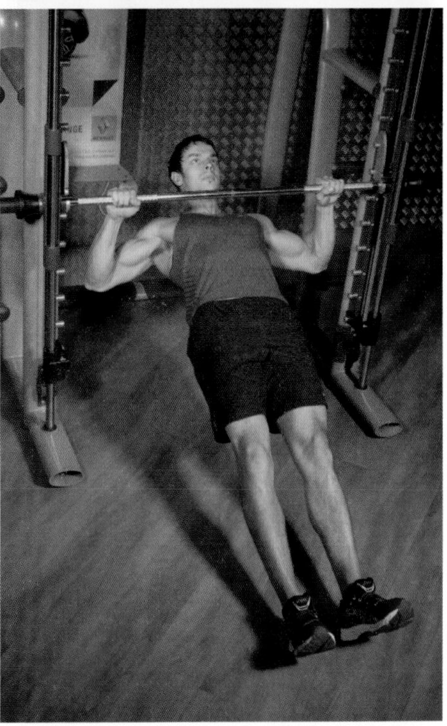

WORKOUT 3

Legs, shoulders and abs

EXERCISE	WEEK	REPS	SETS	TEMPO	REST
SUPERSET 1					
1A Clean	1 2 3 4	10 3 4 5	2 8 6 5	10X0 10X0 10X0 10X0	
1B Push press	1 2 3 4	10 8 6 5	2 3 4 5	2010 2010 2010 2010	60sec 60sec 90sec 90sec
SUPERSET 2					
2A Cable lunge press	1 2 3 4	10 each side 12 each side 10 each side 8 each side	2 2 3 4	2010 2010 2010 2010	
2B Alternating wide press	1 2 3 4	8 10 8 10	2 2 3 3	2010 2010 2010 2010	60sec 60sec 90sec 90sec
SUPERSET 3					
3A Gym ball jackknife twist	1 2 3 4	5 5 6 6	4 5 5 5	2010 2010 2010 2010	
3B Plank	1 2 3 4	30sec 30sec 45sec 45sec	2 2 3 3		45sec 45sec 60sec 60sec

Superset 1

1A Clean

- Stand with your shins touching the bar and feet hip-width apart.
- Squat down and hold the bar with an overhand grip.
- Keeping your core braced, your chest up and a natural arch in your back, lift the bar off the ground by driving up through your heels.
- Once the bar reaches your hips, rise up on tiptoes, shrug your shoulders powerfully and pull the bar up higher, leading with your elbows.
- As the bar travels towards shoulder height, squat back down under the bar and rotate your elbows forward so you catch it on your fingers and the front of your shoulders.
- From there, bend your knees slightly and then straighten them while pressing the bar directly above your head by straightening your arms. Reverse the move back to the start.

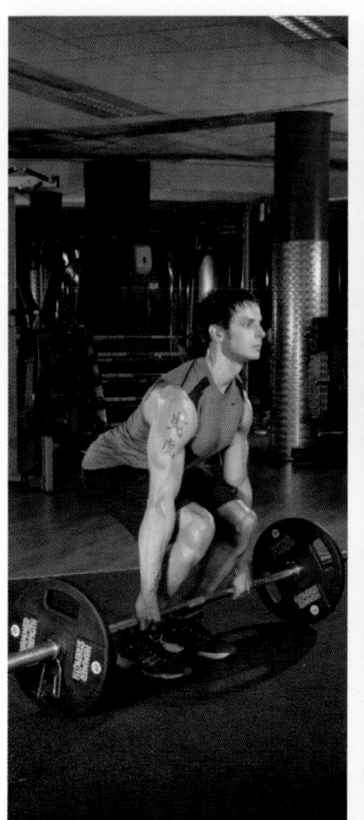

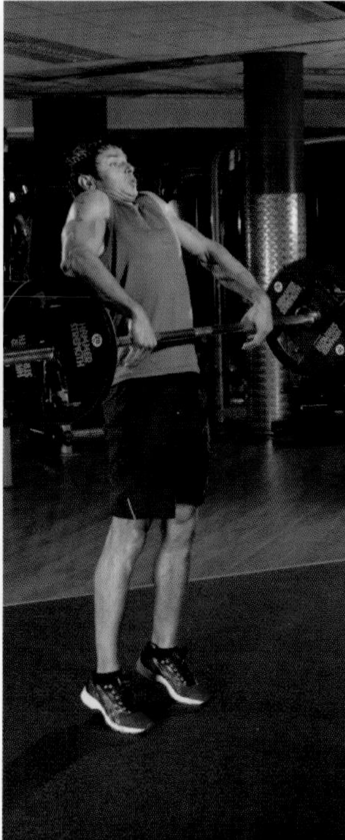

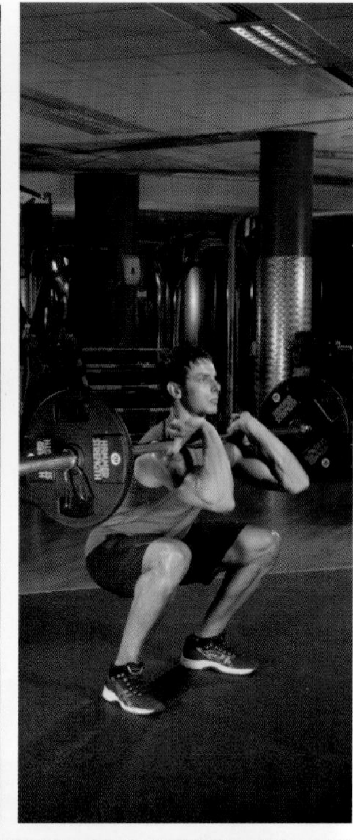

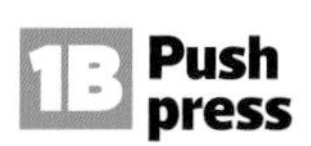

1B Push press

- Stand tall with a barbell across your upper chest. Hold the bar with an overhand grip, hands just wider than shoulder-width apart.
- Keeping your core braced, bend your knees slightly, then stand up straight again while at the same time pressing the bar directly overhead by straightening your arms. Don't lock out your elbows.
- Slowly return the bar back to the start.

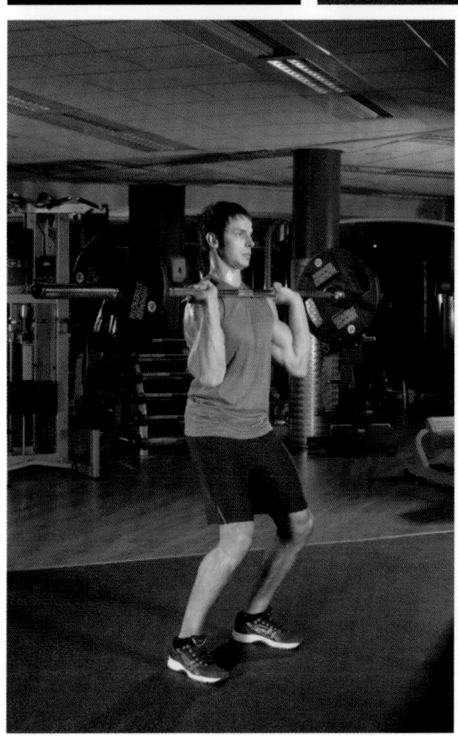

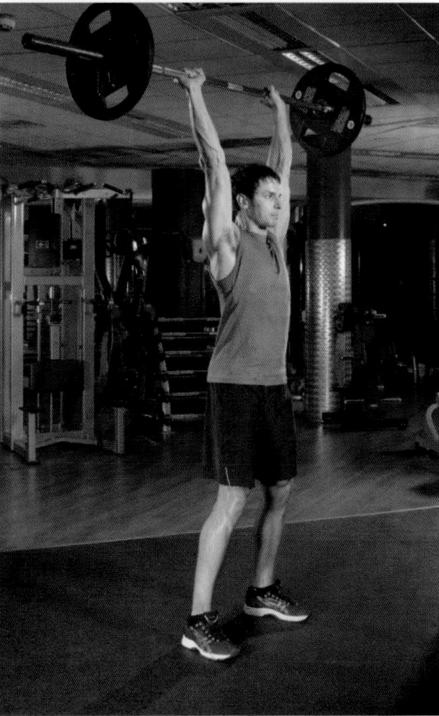

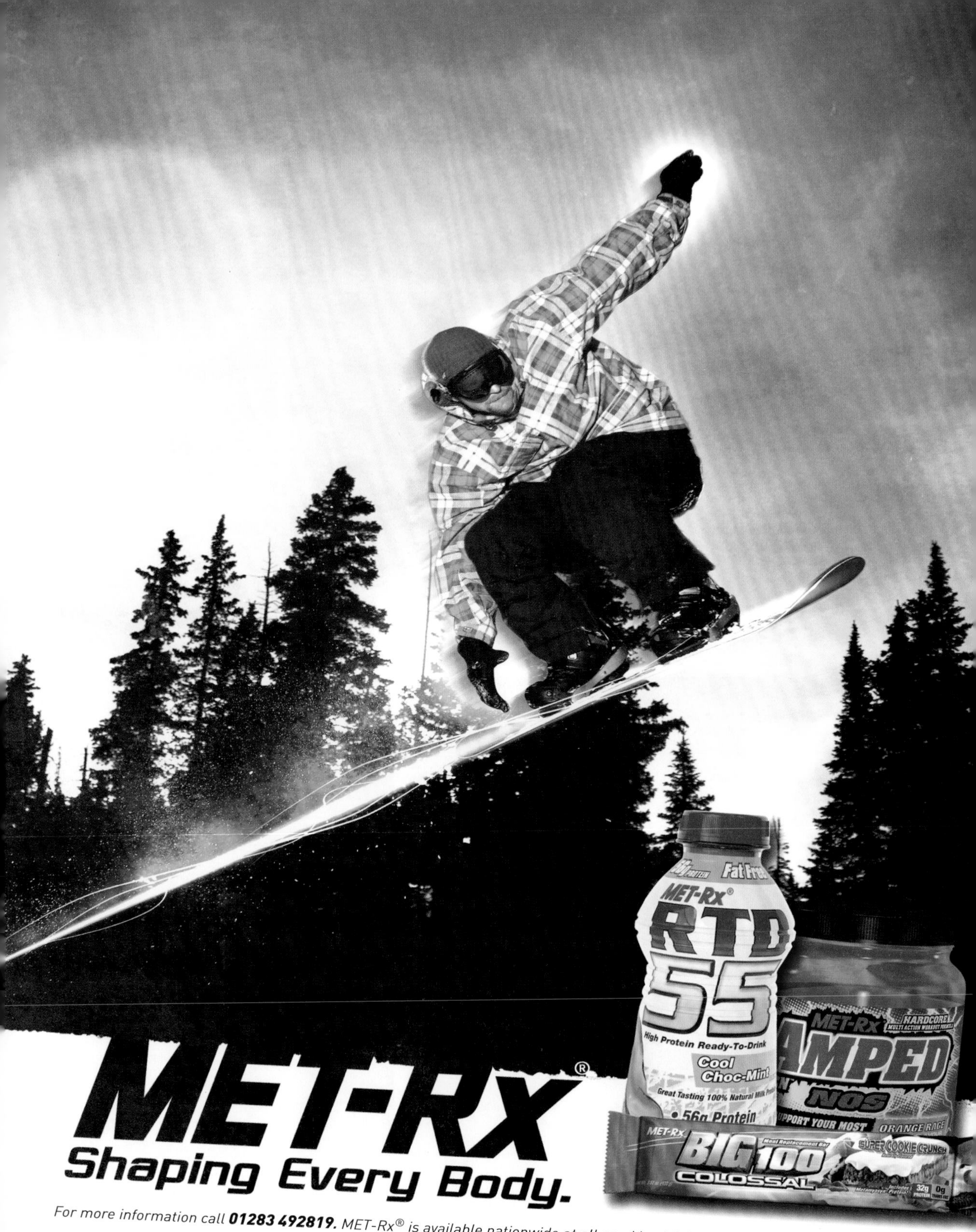
MET-Rx®
RTD 55
56g PROTEIN
Fat Free
High Protein Ready-To-Drink
Cool Choc-Mint
Great Tasting 100% Natural Milk Protein
• 56g Protein
MET-Rx
HARDCORE
AMPED
NOS
ORANGE RAGE
MET-Rx
BIG 100
COLOSSAL
SUPER COOKIE CRUNCH
MET-RX®
Shaping Every Body.

Superset 2

2A Cable lunge press

- Stand with your back to a cable machine, holding a D-handle attached to the low pulley in one hand.
- Lower into a lunge position, leading with the leg opposite the hand holding the handle and holding your empty hand out straight in front of you.
- Press the handle up and forward, rising out of the lunge and bringing your empty hand down as you do so.
- Lower back into the lunge and repeat. Complete all the reps on one side, then switch sides.

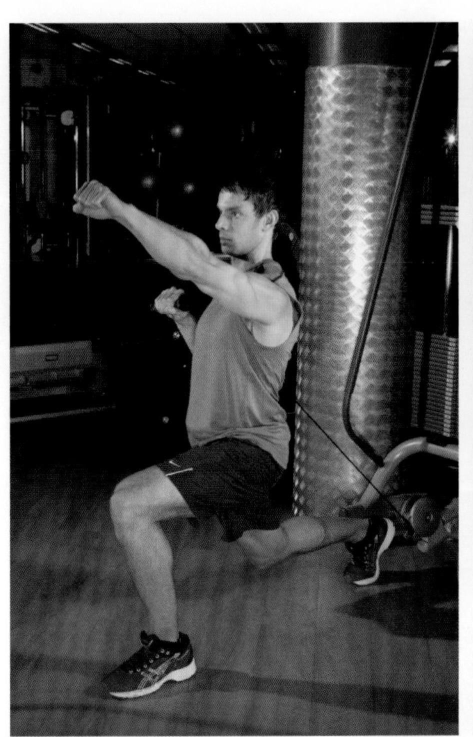

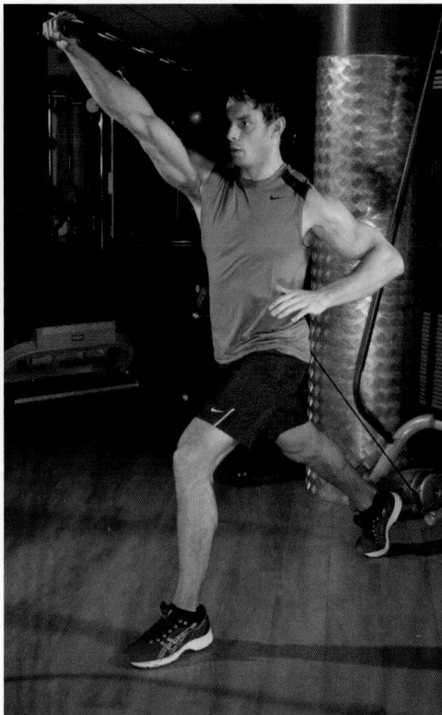

2B Alternating wide press

- Stand with feet shoulder-width apart with a dumbbell held in each hand at shoulder height.
- One hand at a time, press the dumbbell up and out to the side at a 45° angle.
- Slowly return to the start and repeat with the other arm. When you have returned to the start position after pressing with each arm, that completes one rep.

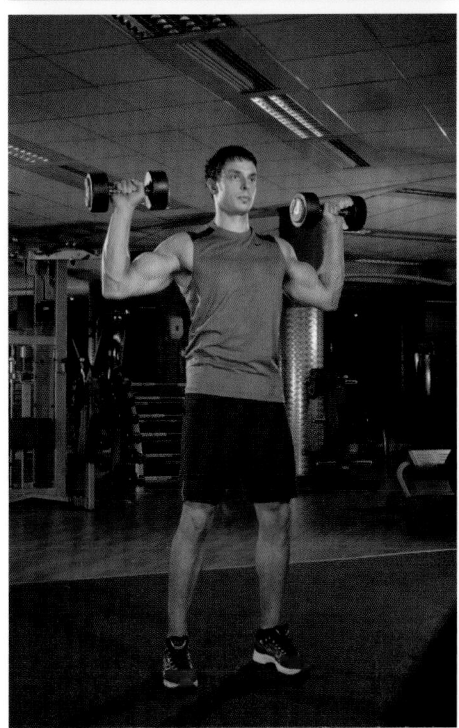

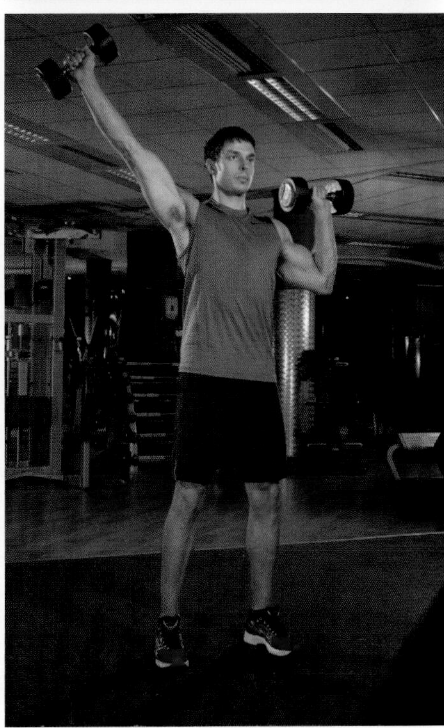

Superset 3

3A Gym ball jackknife twist

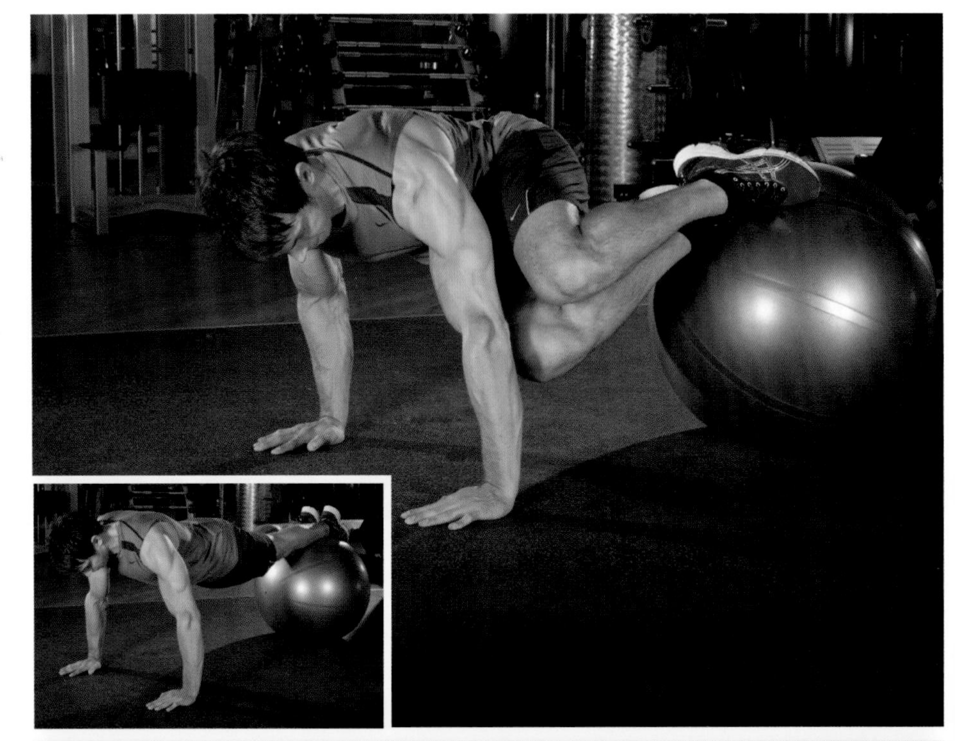

- Start in a press-up position with your shins resting on a gym ball and your body in a straight line from head to heels.
- Contract your abs to draw your knees in towards your chest, then twist out to the side. Reverse back to the start then repeat, twisting to the other side. When you return to the start position after twisting to each side, that completes one rep.

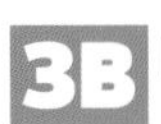

3B Plank

- Assume a press-up position but with your feet, elbows and forearms on the floor so your body forms a straight line from head to heels.
- Hold the position for as long as you can and don't let your hips sag.

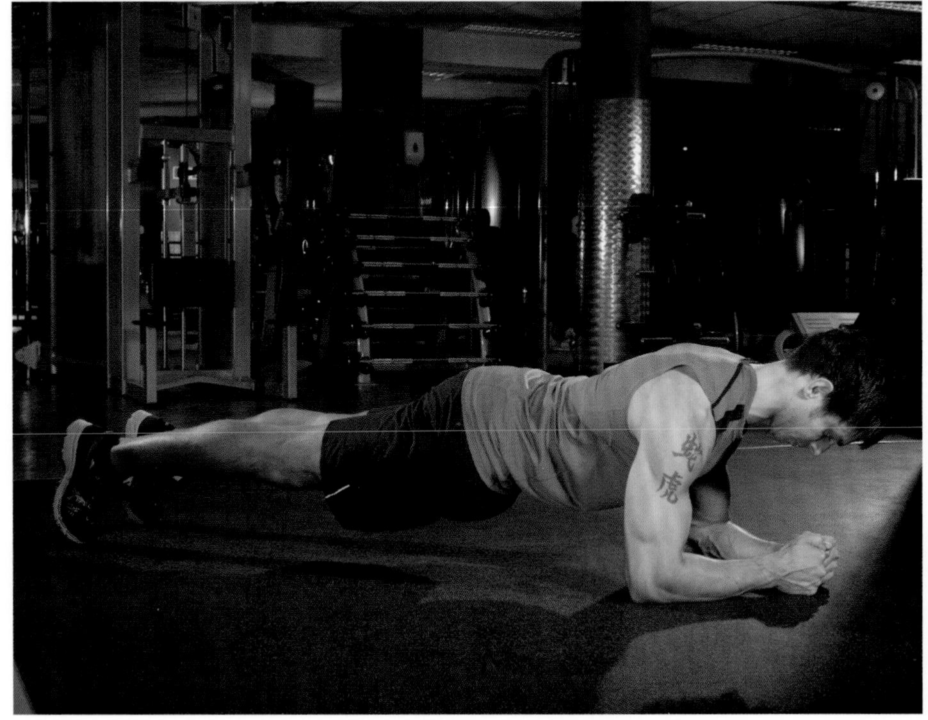

Finishing touches

Your body is strong, conditioned and used to training. It's time for the final push

By now you should have noticed increases in your strength, so take advantage of that by lifting as much weight as possible to maximise your muscle growth potential. As in the first two months, you'll do a split routine that focuses on a couple of major muscle groups in each session.

Workout 1

The deadlift is king of the barbell muscle-builders, because when your form is good it allows you to lift more weight than any other move. The high pull that follows is a tough exercise because it involves moving the bar through a big range of motion at speed, which will get your heart rate racing. The second superset pairs a unilateral leg exercise with a shoulder move that also involves alternating sides, so you get balanced muscle growth. The final set of moves involves the taxing push press with the calf raise, which is less punishing but allows you to target your calves.

Workout 2

The previous workout will have taken a lot out of you because it involves a lot of difficult moves. This session focuses on the glory muscles of the arms and abs, but it's no easier. The first superset will target your back and biceps as well as your chest, core and triceps. The second set is a bit easier because it involves fewer muscles, but it will really zone in on your arms. The final superset works your often overlooked lower abs before finishing with a classic static hold.

Workout 3

The final session in this programme involves your chest and back. The incline variation of the bench press will develop your upper pecs and the front of your shoulders. The cable pull-over in the second set will simultaneously work both your chest and your back, while the fold dip will fatigue your chest, triceps and abs. The gym ball flye is a great way of isolating your chest muscles and taking them to fatigue so don't be surprised if you can only manage fairly light weights. The final move is a safe way of finishing off your back muscles.

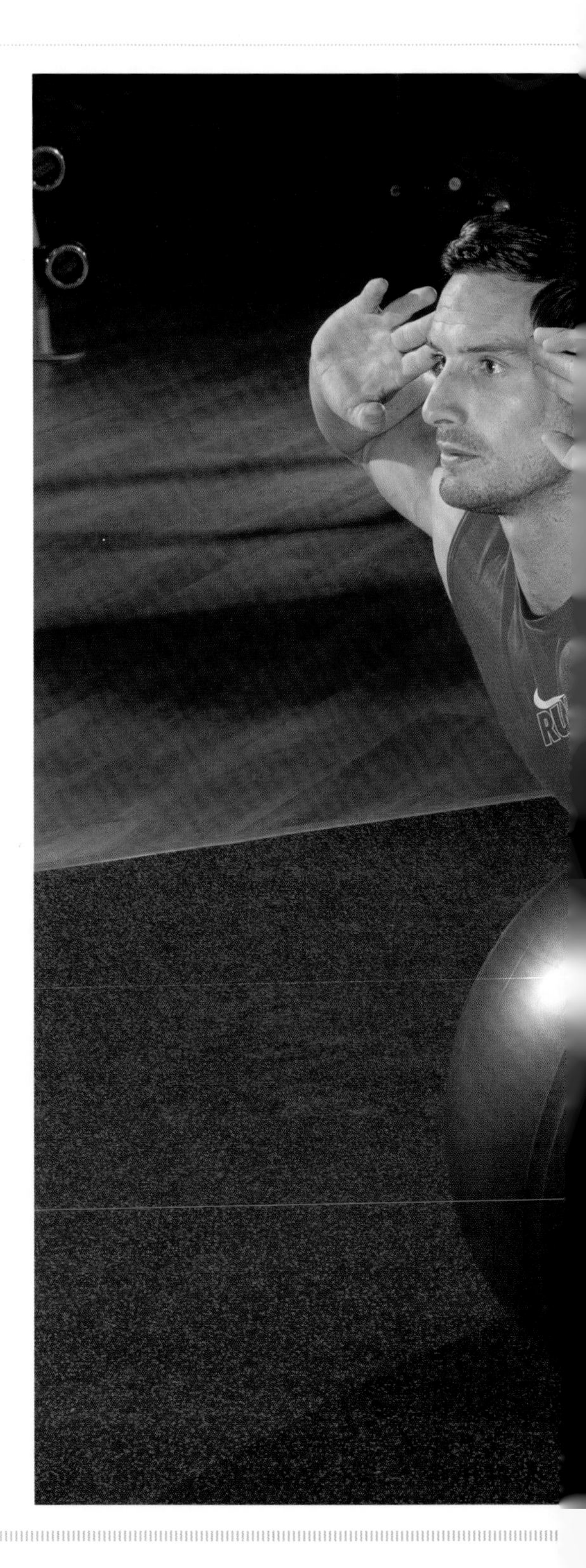

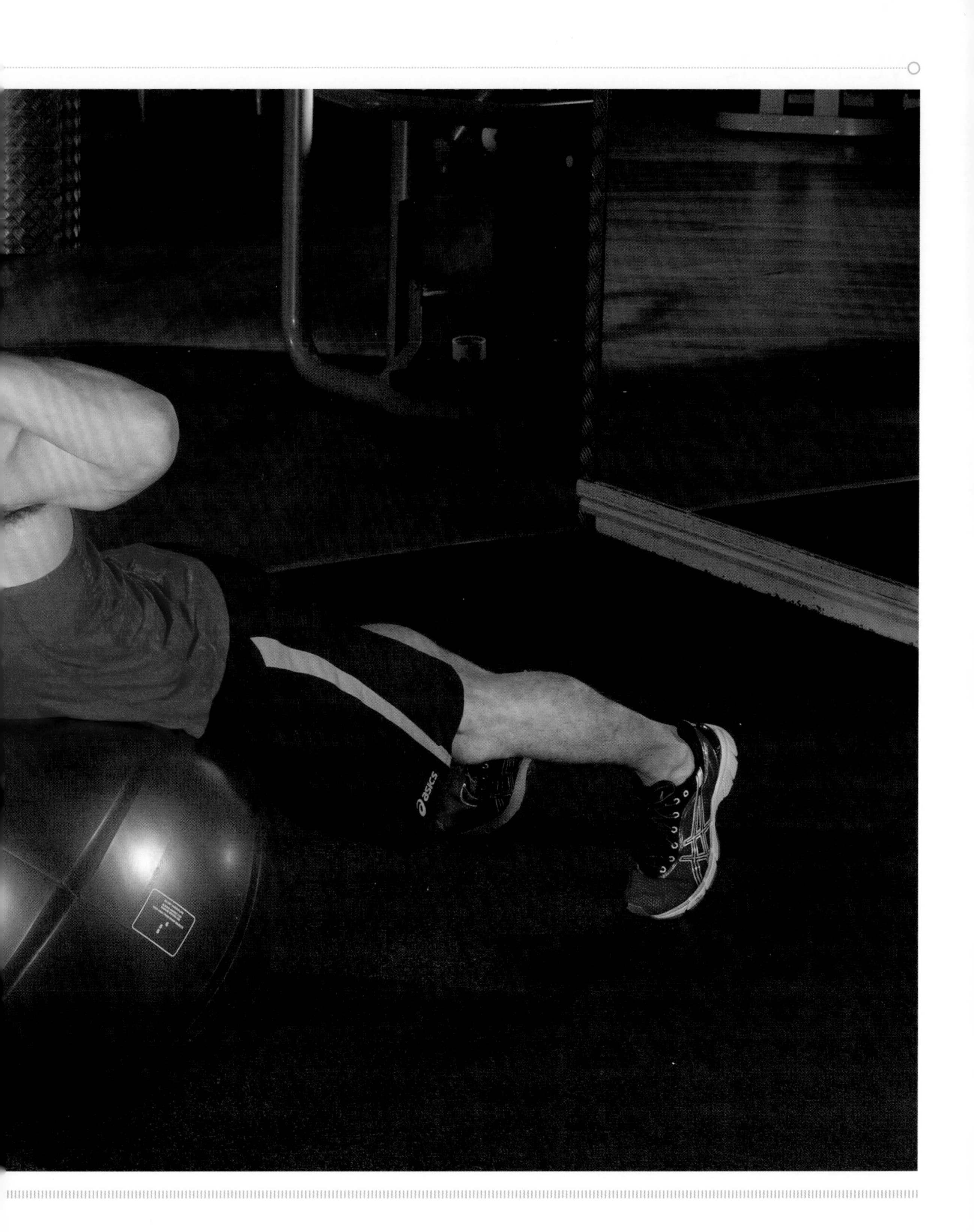
asics

WORKOUT 1

Legs and shoulders

EXERCISE	WEEK	REPS	SETS	TEMPO	REST
SUPERSET 1					
1A Deadlift	1 2 3 4	10 10 8 6	2 3 4 4	2010 2010 2010 2010	
1B High pull	1 2 3 4	12 10 8 8	2 3 4 4	2010 2010 2010 2010	60sec 60sec 90sec 90sec
SUPERSET 2					
2A Side step-up	1 2 3 4	12 each side 10 each side 8 each side 8 each side	2 2 3 3	1010 1010 1010 1010	
2B Front/lateral raise	1 2 3 4	8 10 8 10	2 2 3 3	3010 3010 3010 3010	60sec 60sec 90sec 90sec
SUPERSET 3					
3A Push press	1 2 3 4	8 8 6 6	2 3 4 4	1010 1010 1010 1010	
3B Calf raise	1 2 3 4	10 each side 10 each side 10 each side 10 each side	2 2 3 3	3010 3010 3010 3010	60sec 60sec 90sec 90sec

Superset 1

1A Deadlift

- Grip the bar just outside your knees with your core braced, your shoulders retracted and over the bar and your back flat.
- Use your glutes to power the initial lift, pushing down through your heels.
- Keep the bar close to your body and, as it passes your knees, push your hips forward. Keep your shoulders back throughout the move.

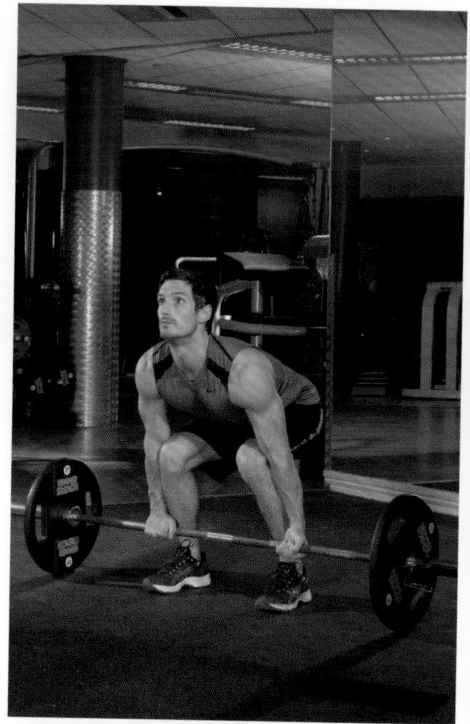

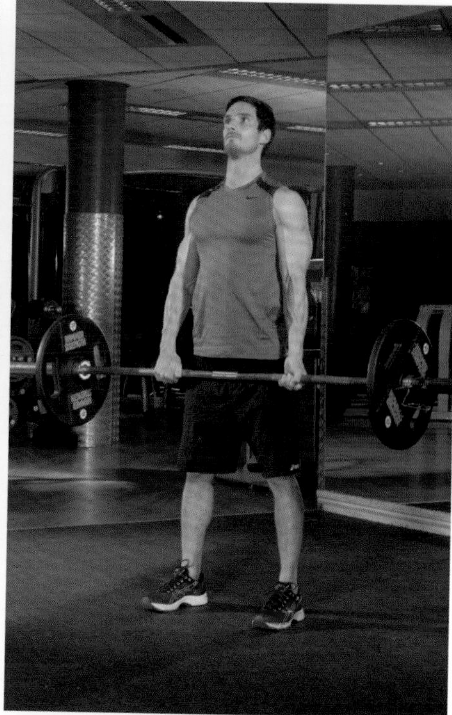

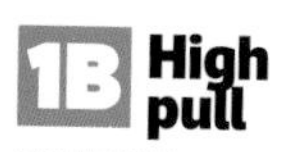

1B High pull

- Hold a barbell at knee height, gripping the bar with hands shoulder-width apart and keeping your back straight and core braced.
- Lift the weight, leading with your elbows, to your upper chest and extend your body until you are up on your toes.
- Slowly lower the weight back to the start.

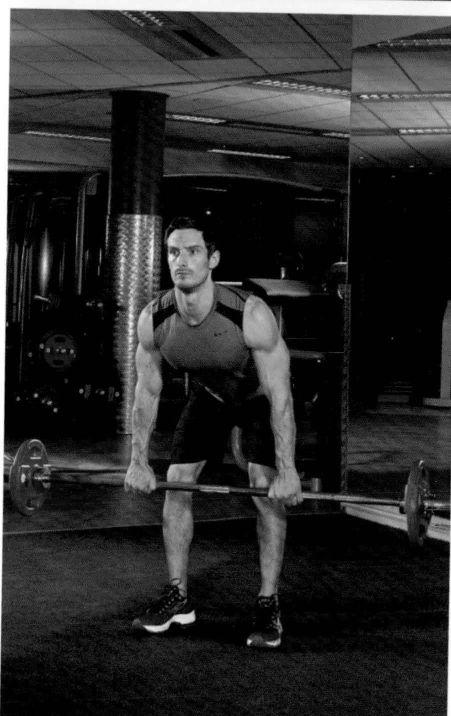

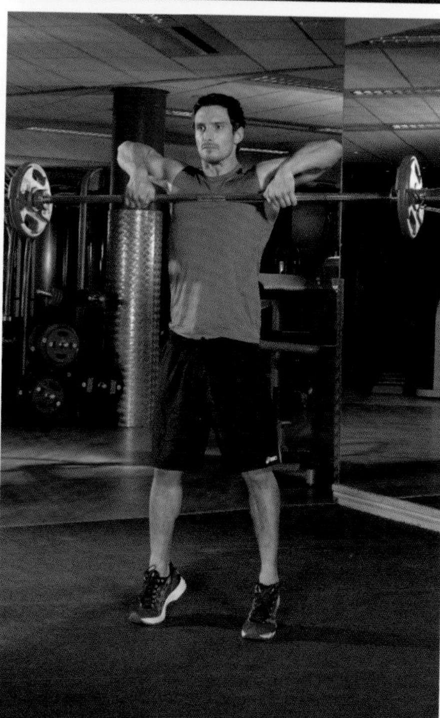

WEEKS 9-12

Superset 2

2A Side step-up

- Stand side-on to a box that is about knee height.
- Step up on the box with one foot. Drive your body up but don't place your free foot on the box.
- Return to the start. Complete a set on one side, then switch sides.

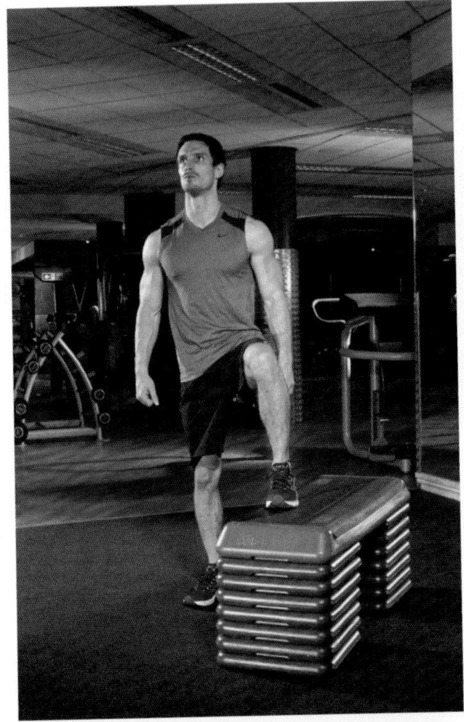

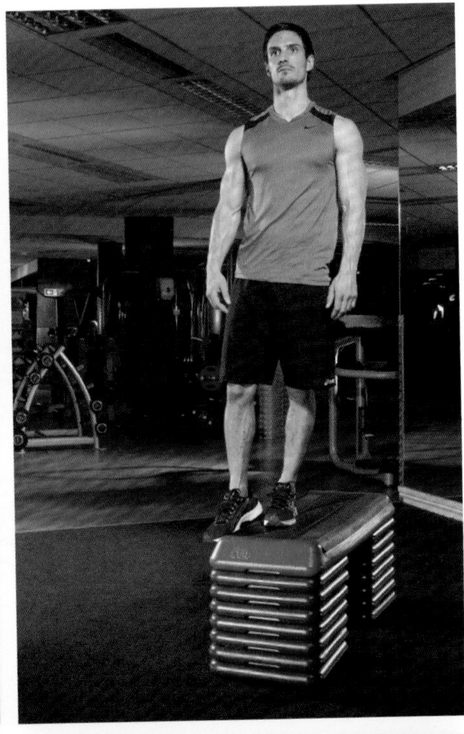

2B Front/lateral raise

- Stand tall with core braced and feet apart, holding a light dumbbell in each hand by your sides with palms facing each other.
- Keeping your arms straight, raise one dumbbell in front of you and the other to one side, using your muscles and not momentum.
- Stop at shoulder height, then lower slowly.
- Raise the dumbbell you raised in front to the side and vice vera. When you return to the start position, that completes one rep.

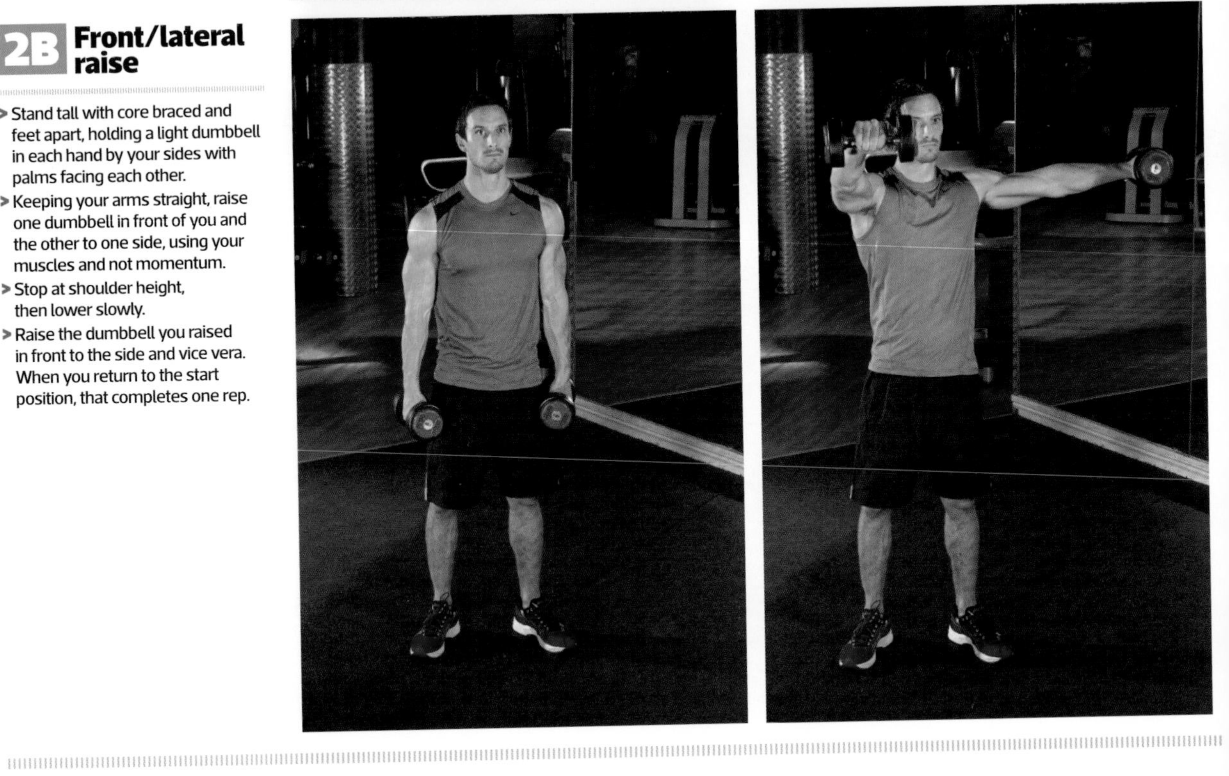

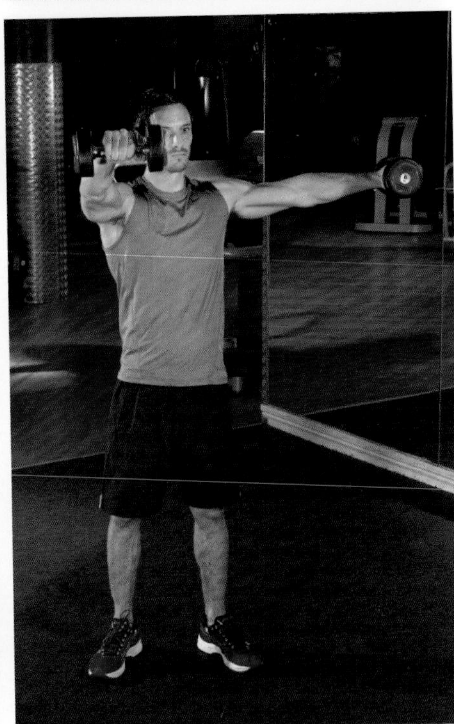

Superset 3

3A Push press

- Hold the bar on your upper chest, gripping the bar with hands just wider than shoulder-width apart.
- Keeping your core braced, bend your knees and lower into a quarter-squat then push up with your knees and arms at the same time to raise the bar directly overhead.
- Lower the weight back to the start and go directly into the next rep.

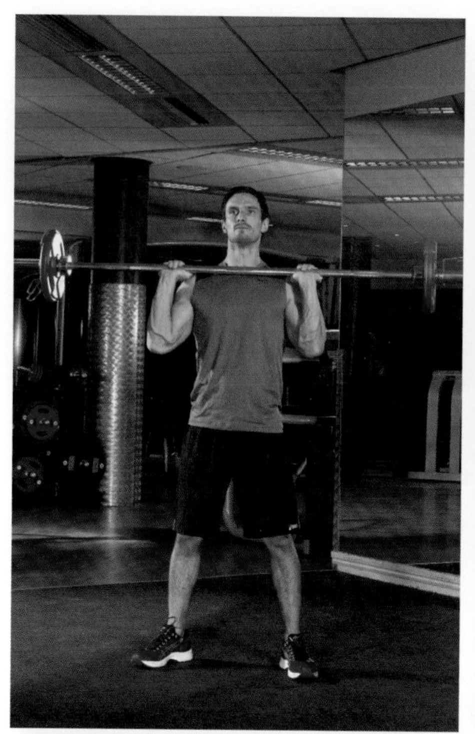

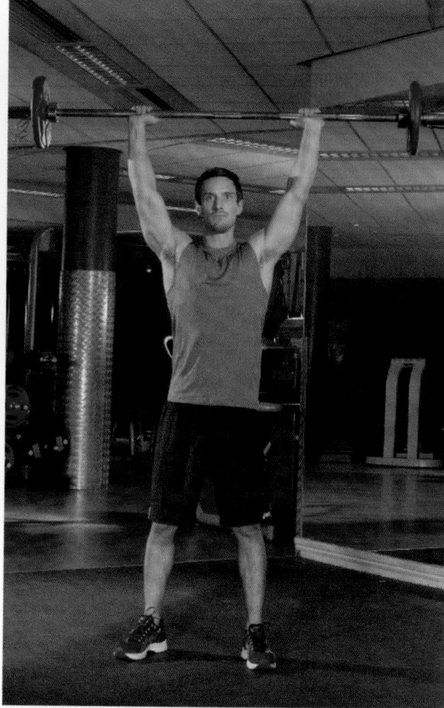

3B Calf raise

- Place the ball of your foot on the edge of a step and let your non-working foot hang free. Hold a dumbbell by your side and, if necessary, hold a wall for balance.
- Push up until your heel is as high as it can go, holding the tension at the top of the move.
- Lower slowly to the start. Complete a set on one side, then switch sides.

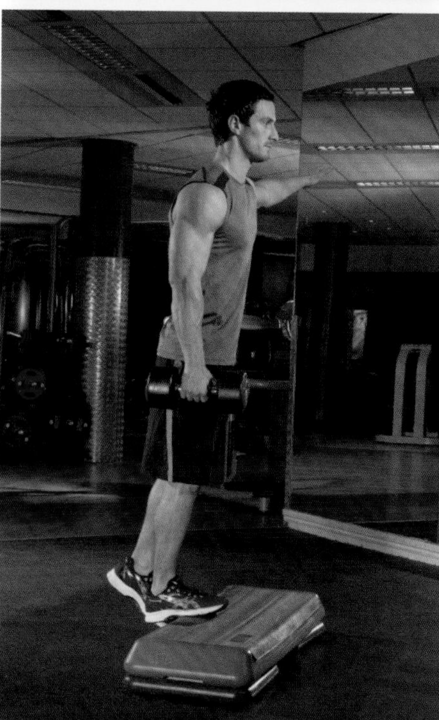

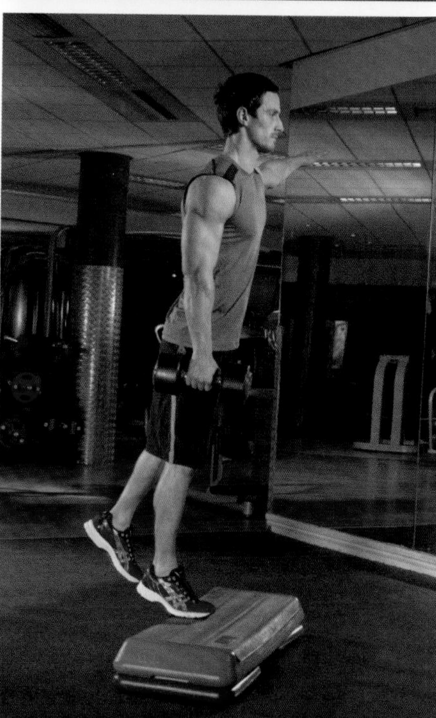

WORKOUT 2

Arms and abs

EXERCISE	WEEK	REPS	SETS	TEMPO	REST
SUPERSET 1					
1A Chin-up	1 2 3 4	4 4 5 5	4 4 5 5	3010 3010 3010 3010	
1B Medicine ball press-up	1 2 3 4	8 10 8 10	2 2 3 3	3010 3010 3010 3010	60sec 60sec 90sec 90sec
SUPERSET 2					
2A Preacher curl	1 2 3 4	10 12 8 8	2 2 3 3	3010 3010 3010 3010	
2B Gym ball triceps extension	1 2 3 4	8 10 8 10	2 2 3 3	3010 3010 3010 3010	60sec 60sec 90sec 90sec
SUPERSET 3					
3A Hanging leg raise	1 2 3 4	8 10 8 10	2 2 3 3	3010 3010 3010 3010	
3B Gym ball back extension	1 2 3 4	10 12 10 12	2 2 3 3	2010 2010 2010 2010	45sec 45sec 60sec 60sec

Superset 1

1A Chin-up

- Hang from a bar with your hands 30cm apart or from chin-up handles, using an underhand grip.
- Maintain a natural arch in your back – don't hunch forwards – and don't let your legs swing.
- Curl yourself up the bar, leading with your chest and focusing on pulling with your biceps.
- Once your chin is above your hands slowly lower yourself back to the start.

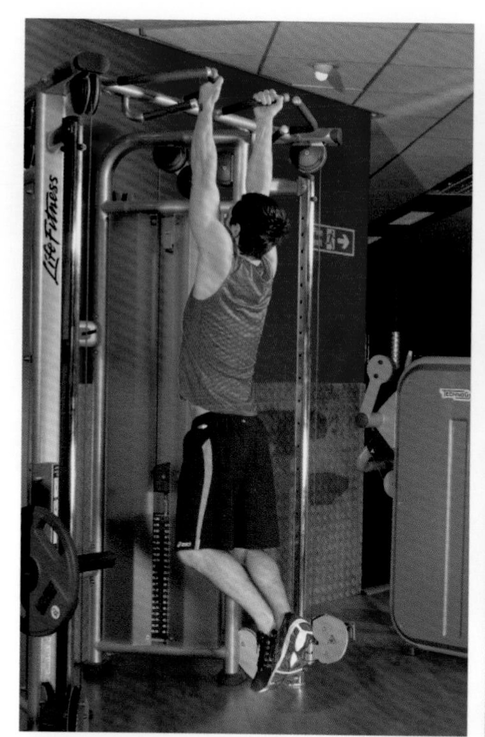

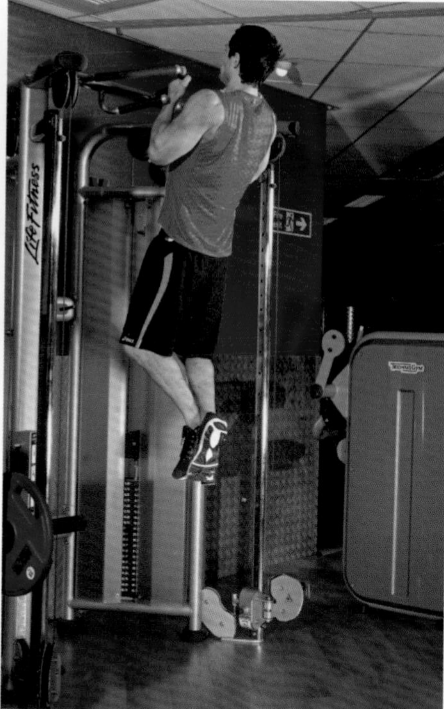

1B Medicine ball press-up

- Start in a press-up position but with your hands either side of a medicine ball, rather than flat on the floor.
- Keeping your body in a straight line from head to heels, lower your chest until it touches the ball before powering back up strongly.

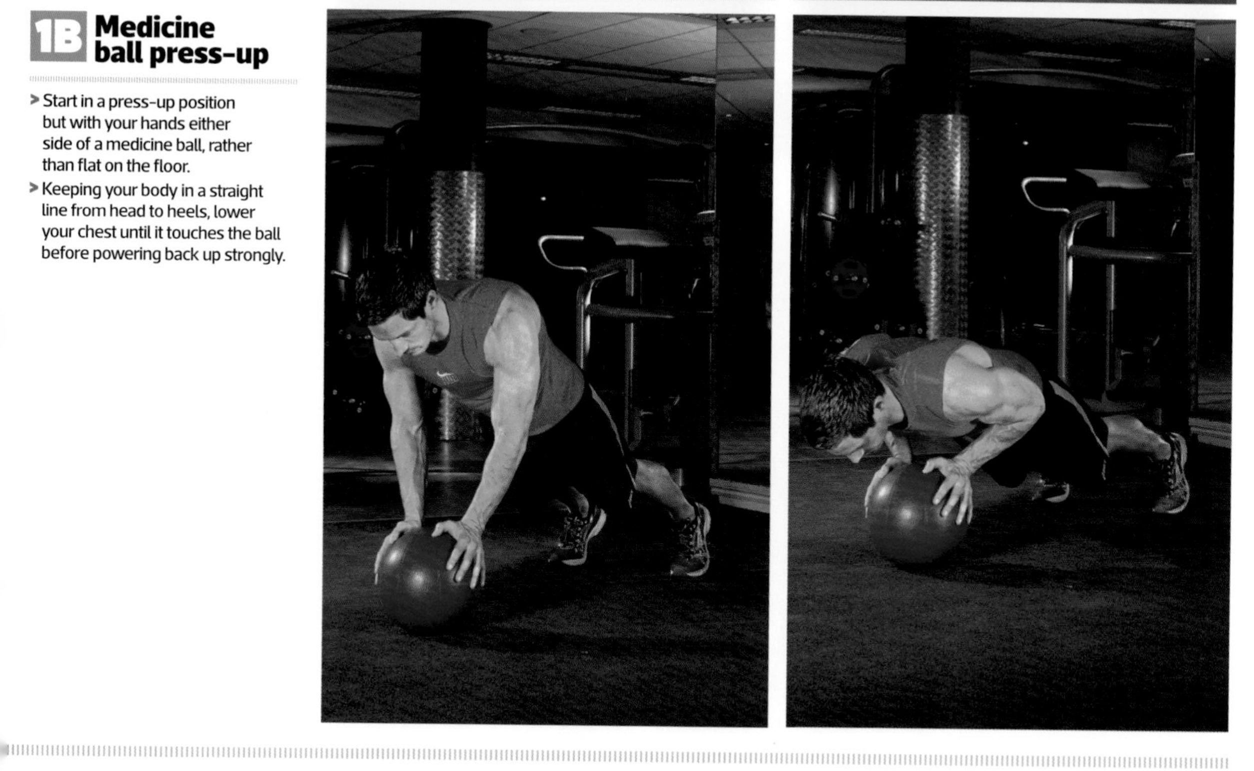

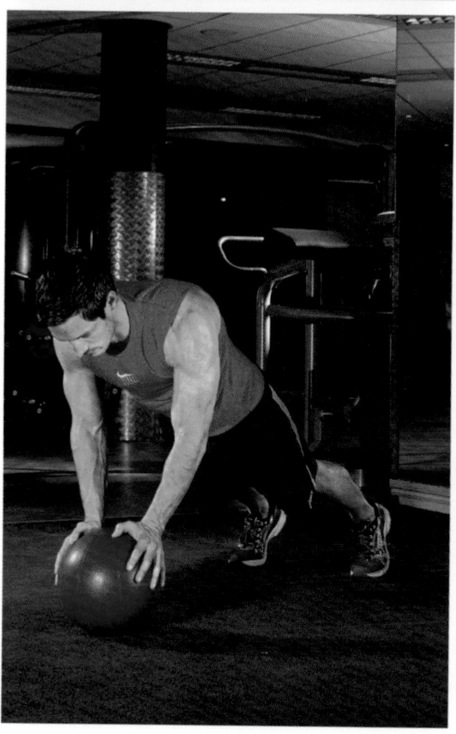

Superset 2

2A EZ-bar preacher curl

> Sit at a preacher bench and hold an EZ-bar with an underhand grip.
> Keeping your torso against the bench, slowly curl the bar up towards your face.
> At the top, squeeze your biceps muscles before slowly returning the bar back down.

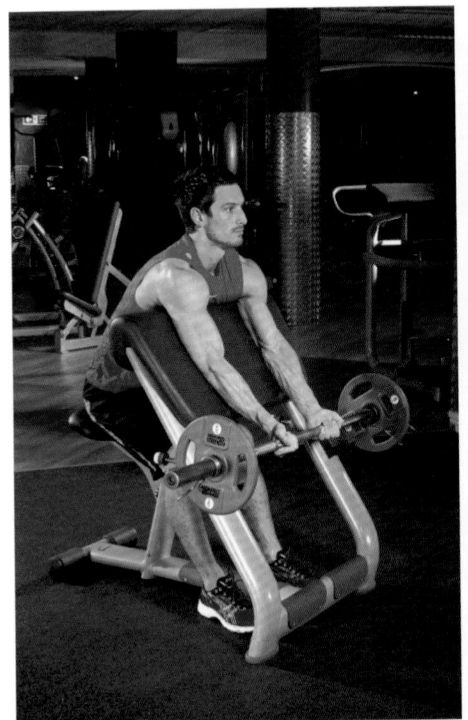

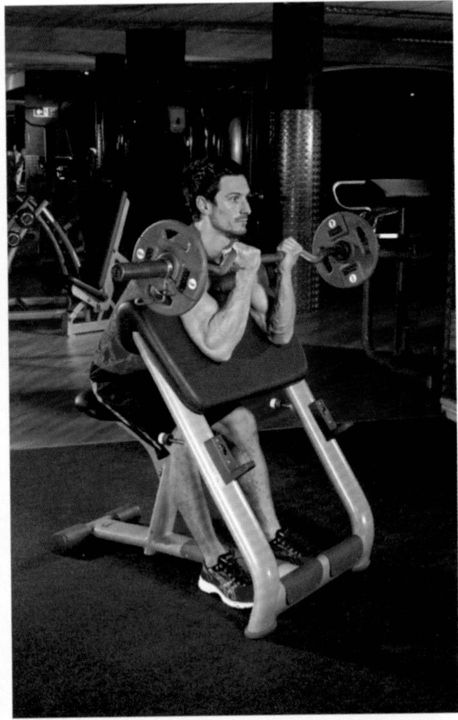

2B Gym ball triceps extension

> Lie with your upper back on a gym ball, holding a dumbbell in each hand directly above your chest.
> Keeping your elbows pointing to the ceiling, slowly lower the weights down to the side of your head.
> Slowly return to the start.

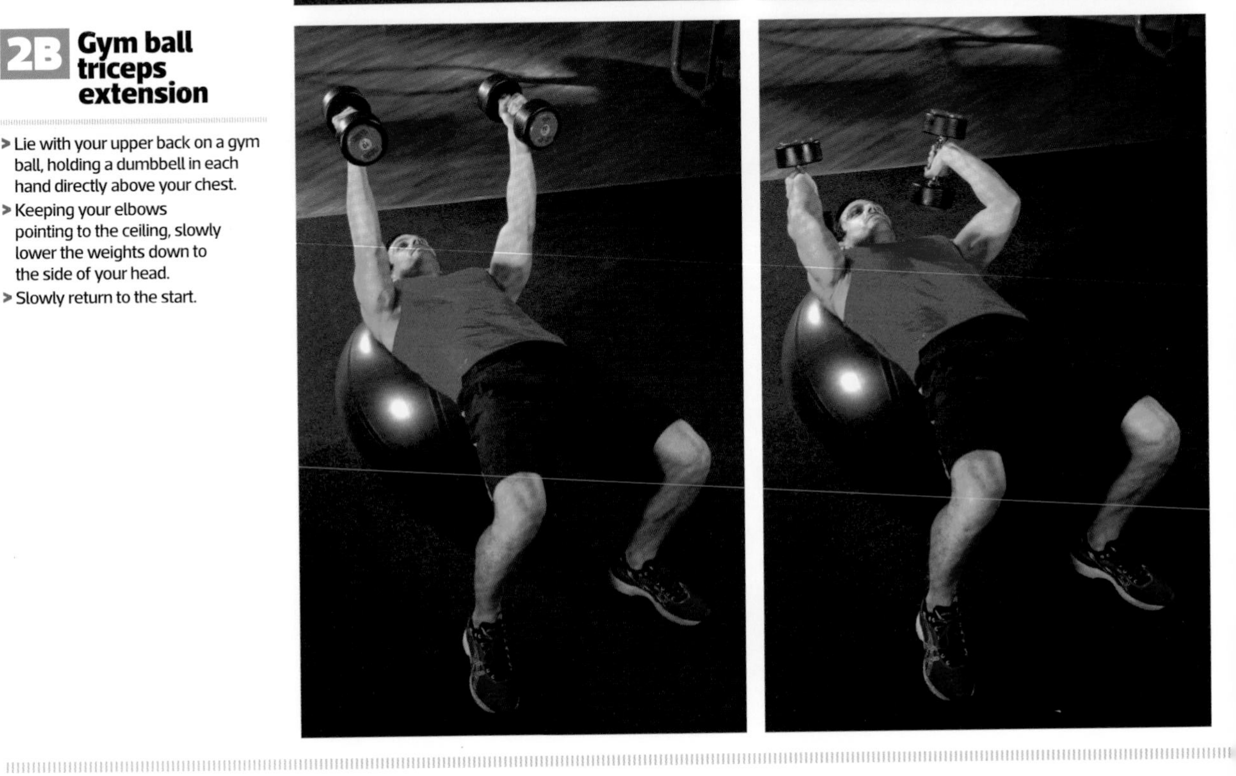

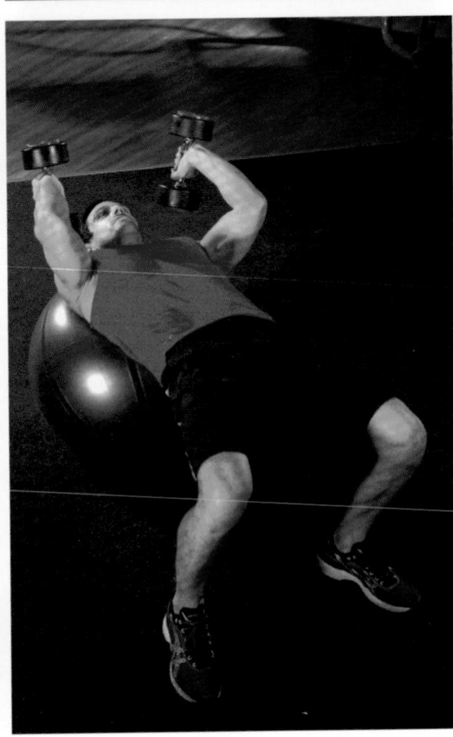

Superset 3

3A Hanging leg raise

- Hang from a pull-up bar or handles.
- Keeping your legs straight and, without swinging, use your abs to raise your legs in front of you until they are parallel to the floor.
- Lower slowly back to the start.

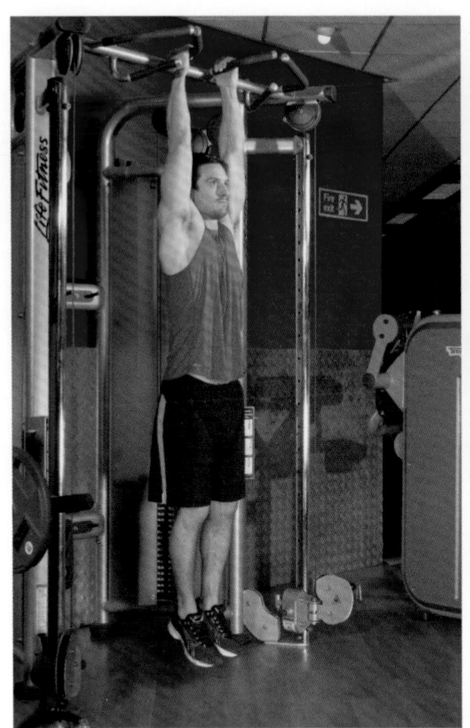

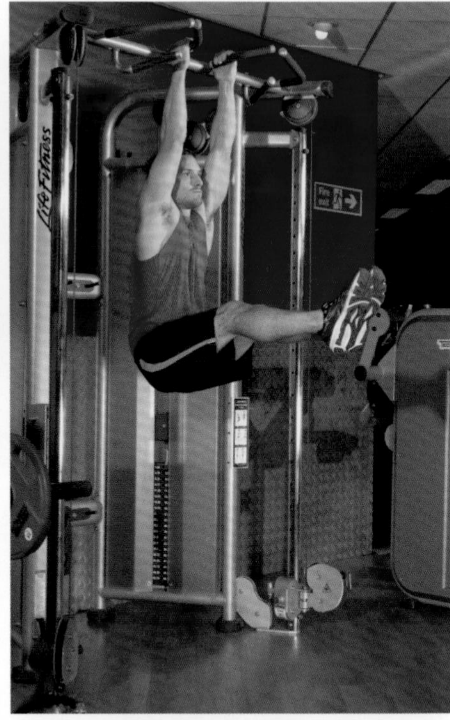

3B Gym ball back extension

- Lie face down on a gym ball with your feet shoulder-width apart and your hands at your temples.
- Engage your core and lift your head and chest off the ball.
- Lower slowly back to the start and repeat.

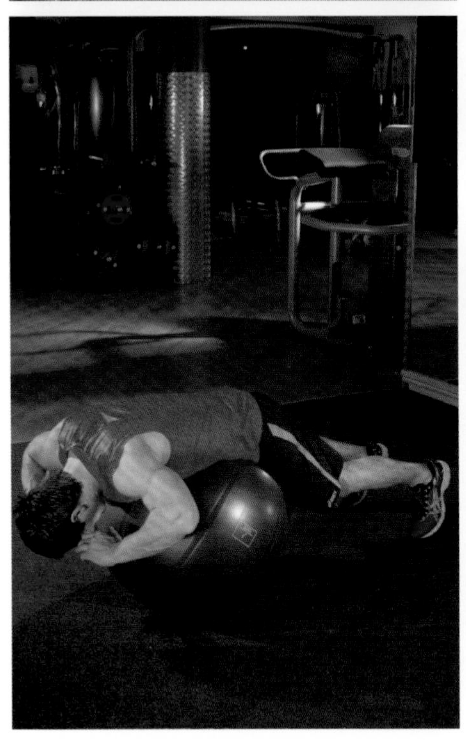

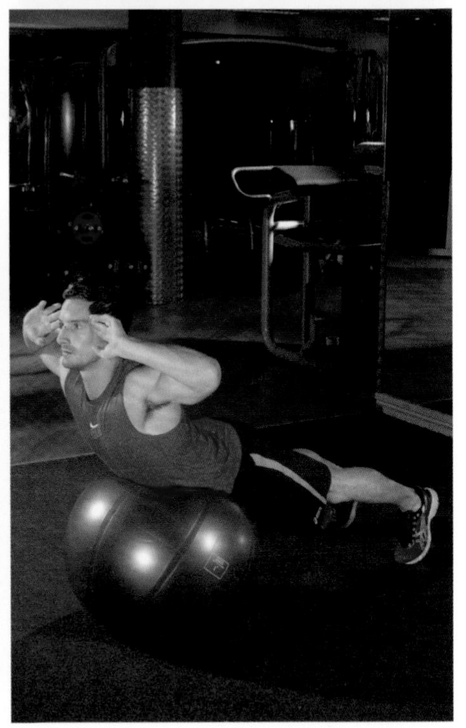

WORKOUT 3

Chest and back

EXERCISE	WEEK	REPS	SETS	TEMPO	REST
SUPERSET 1					
1A Incline bench press	1 2 3 4	10 3 4 5	2 8 6 5	3010 3010 3010 3010	
1B Bent-over row	1 2 3 4	10 8 6 5	2 3 4 5	3010 3010 3010 3010	60sec 60sec 90sec 90sec
SUPERSET 2					
2A Cable pull-over	1 2 3 4	10 12 10 8	2 2 3 4	3010 3010 3010 3010	
2B Fold dip	1 2 3 4	8 10 8 10	2 2 3 3	2010 2010 2010 2010	60sec 60sec 90sec 90sec
SUPERSET 3					
3A Gym ball flye	1 2 3 4	5 5 6 6	4 5 5 5	2010 2010 2010 2010	
3B Lat pull-down	1 2 3 4	10 10 10 10	2 3 3 3	3010 3010 3010 3010	45sec 45sec 60sec 60sec

Superset 1

1A Incline bench press

- Lie on a bench set at a 30-45° angle, holding a barbell with hands just wider than shoulder-width apart.
- Keep your feet flat on the floor and back against the bench.
- Lower the weight down to your chest, flaring your elbows out to the side.
- Press back up powerfully.

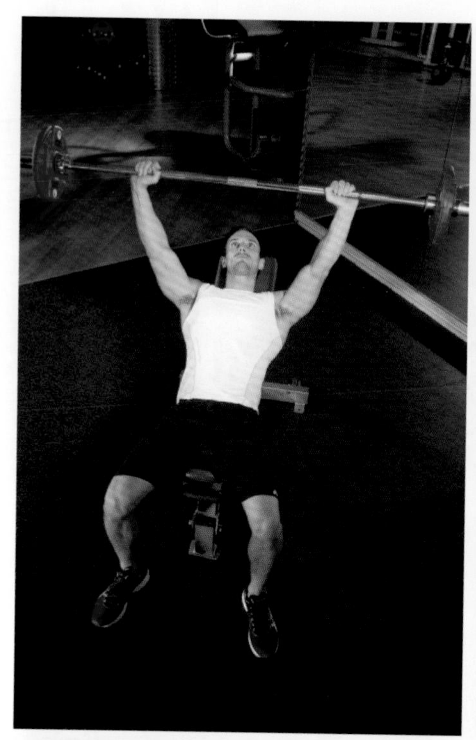

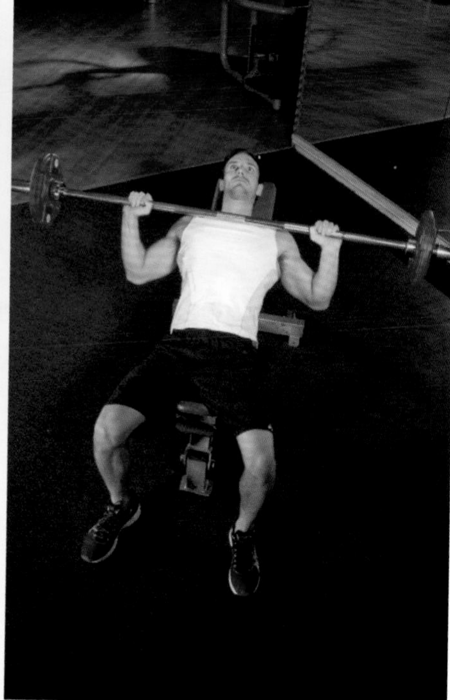

1B Bent-over row

- Start with your core braced, your back straight and your shoulder blades retracted. Bend your knees slightly and lean forward from the hips.
- Grip the bar with your hands just wider than shoulder-width apart, letting it hang at knee level.
- Pull the bar up to your lower sternum, retracting your shoulder blades to allow the bar to come up to the chest, then lower the bar slowly to the start.

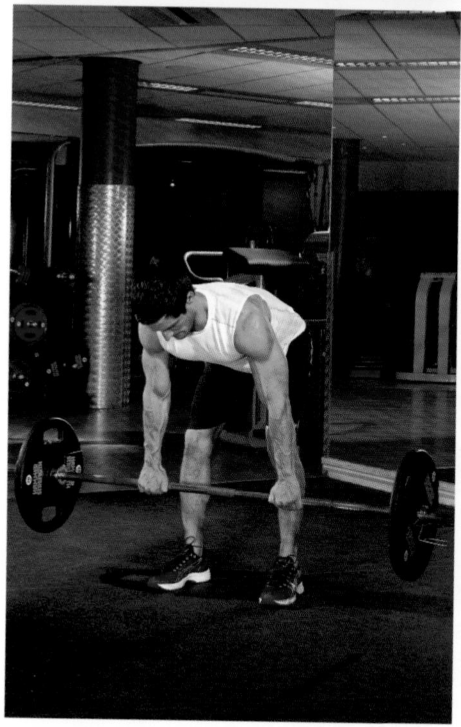

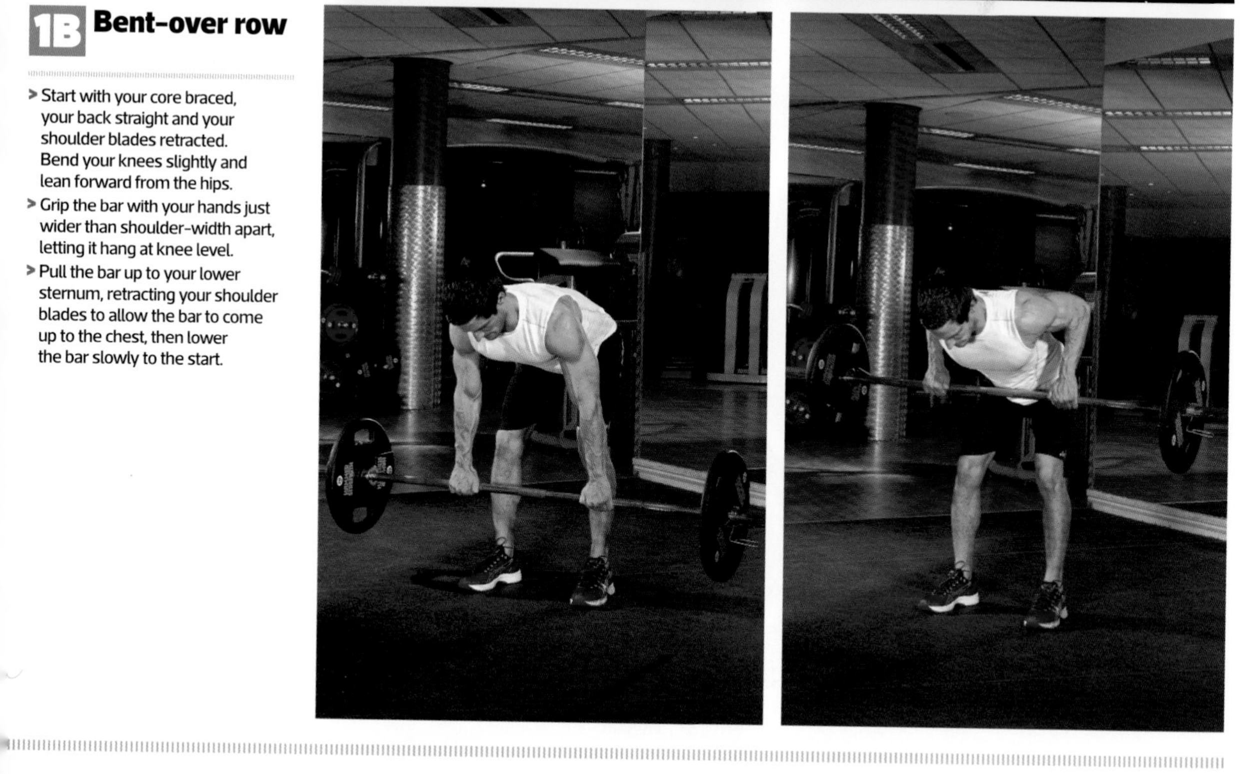

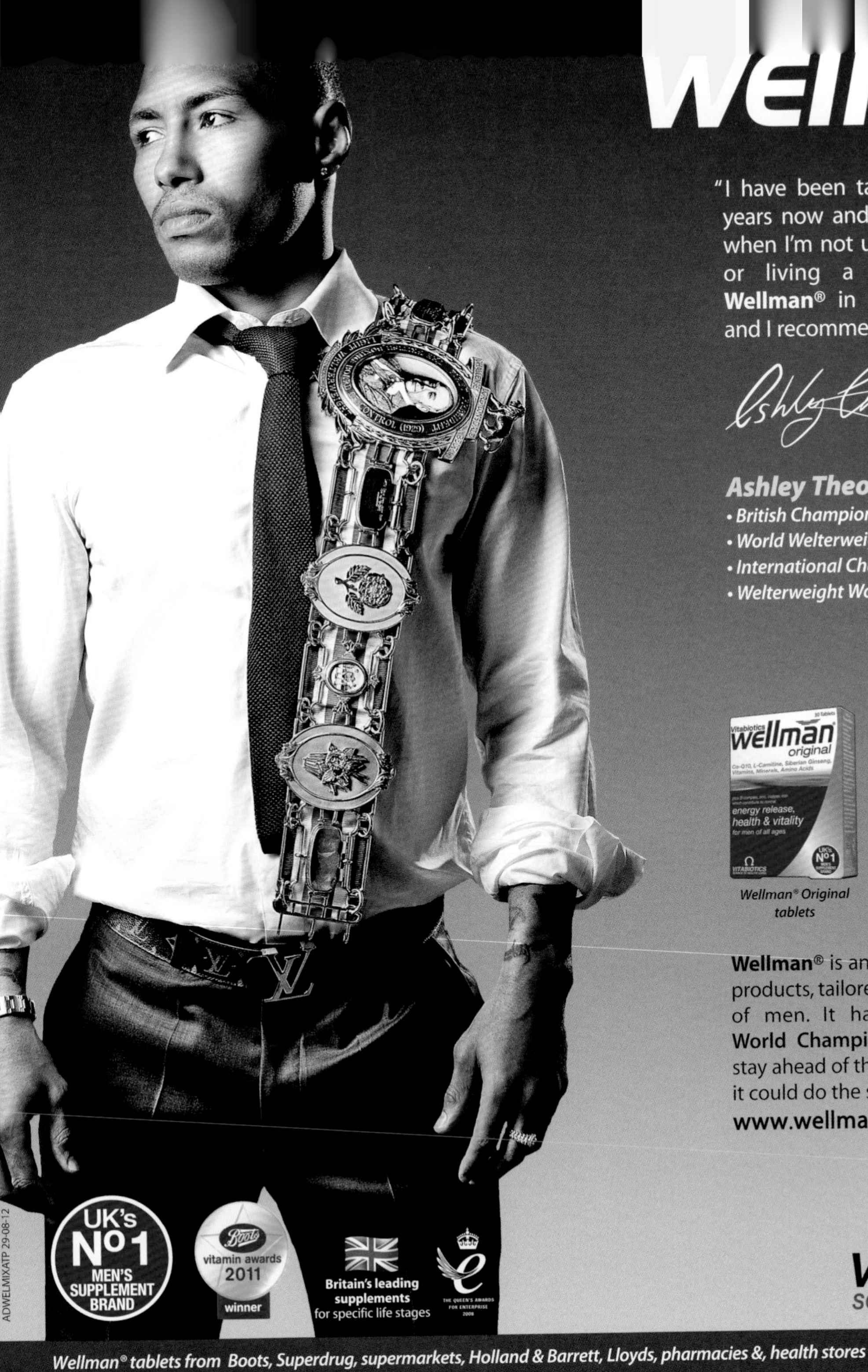
UK's
Nº1
MEN'S
SUPPLEMENT
BRAND
Boots
vitamin awards
2011
winner
Britain's leading
supplements
for specific life stages
ADWELMIXATP 29-08-12

Superset 2

2A Cable pull-over

- Attach a straight bar to the bottom of the cable machine and position a bench next to it by far enough away so that there is tension in the cable throughout the move.
- Lying with your head nearest the cable, pull the bar up and over your torso in a smooth arc before returning slowly to the start.
- Keep a slight bend in your elbows throughout the move.

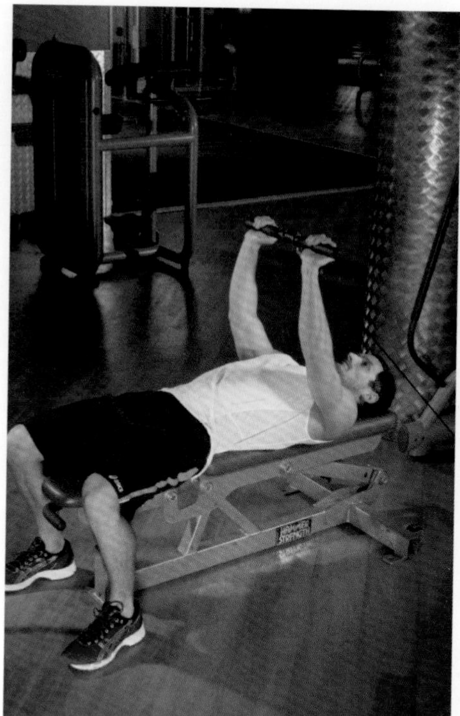

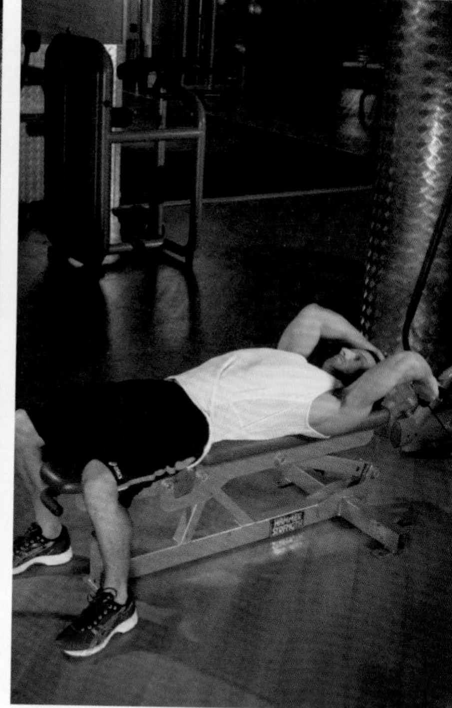

2B Fold dip

- Grasp dip bars either side of your waist.
- Lean forward to take pressure off your shoulders and draw in your knees as you lower your torso until your elbow are bent at 90°.

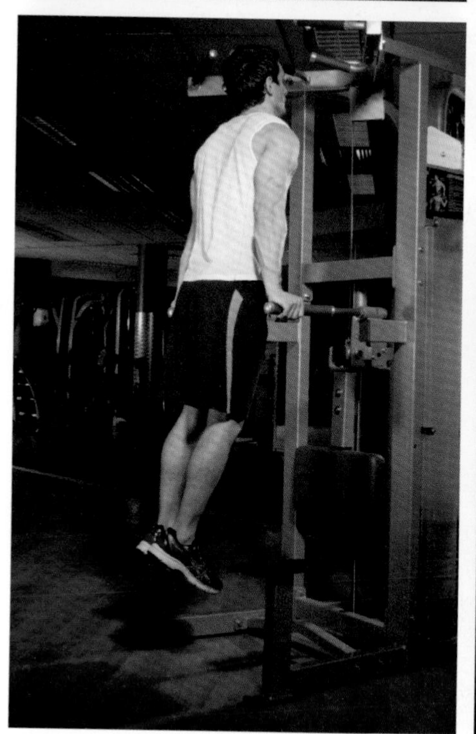

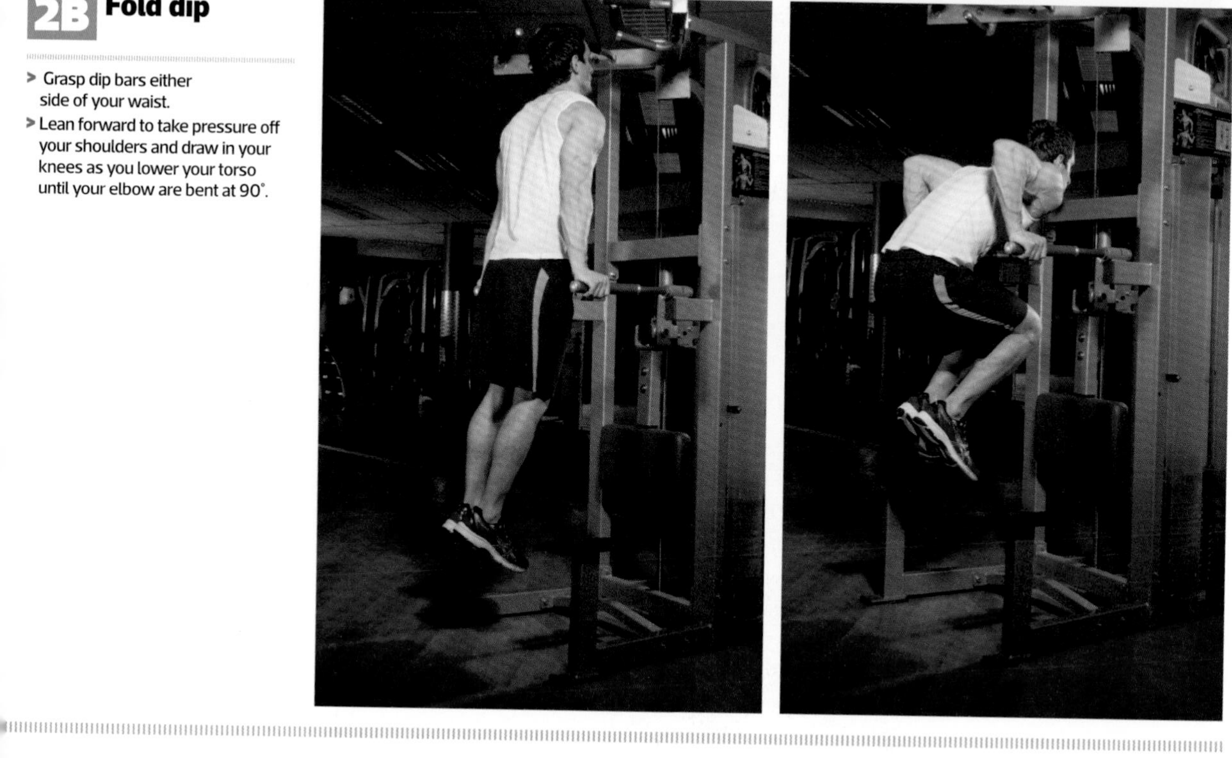

Superset 3

3A Gym ball cable flye

- In the middle of a cable machine with handles attached at the bottom of each weight stack, lie with your head and shoulders supported by the ball with your body horizontal from head to knees, which are bent at 90°.
- Holding a handle in each hand and with your core braced and a slight bend in your elbows, squeeze your pecs to bring the handles up in a smooth arc until they meet over your chest.
- Lower back slowly to the start position.

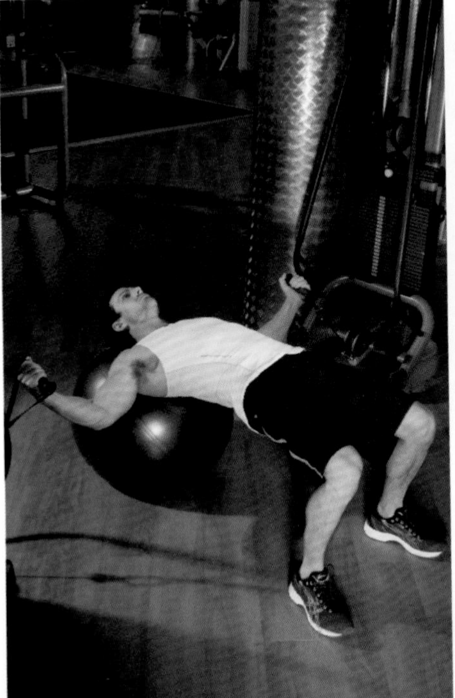

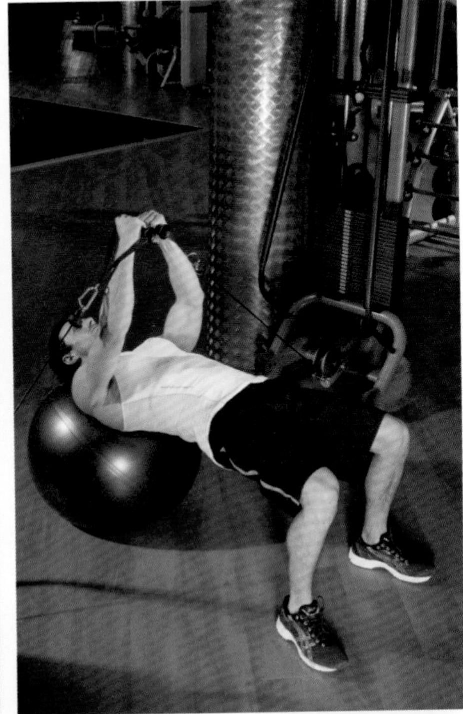

3B Lat pull-down

- Sit on the seat of a lat pull-down machine and take an overhand, wide grip on the bar.
- Look forward, retract your shoulder blades and keep your torso upright.
- Pull the bar down in front of you until it reaches your upper chest. Don't lean back to aid the movement.
- Squeeze your lats at the bottom of the move and return the bar slowly to the top.

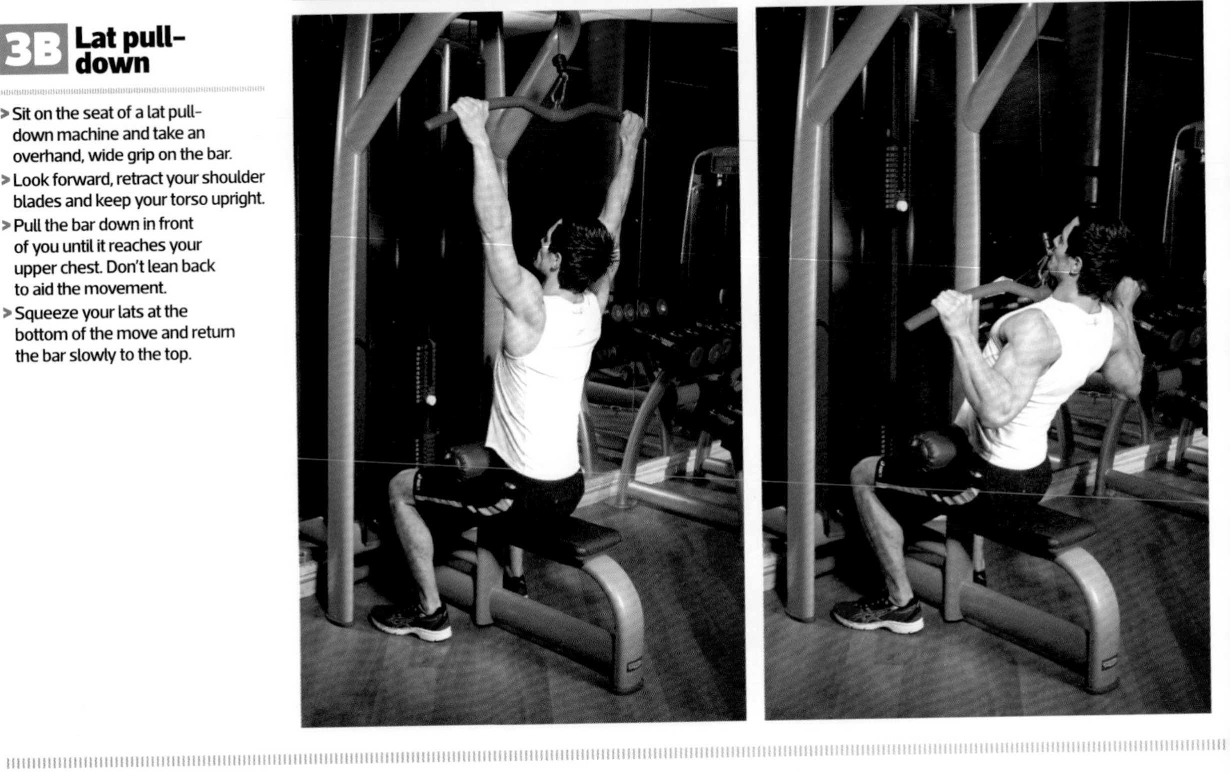

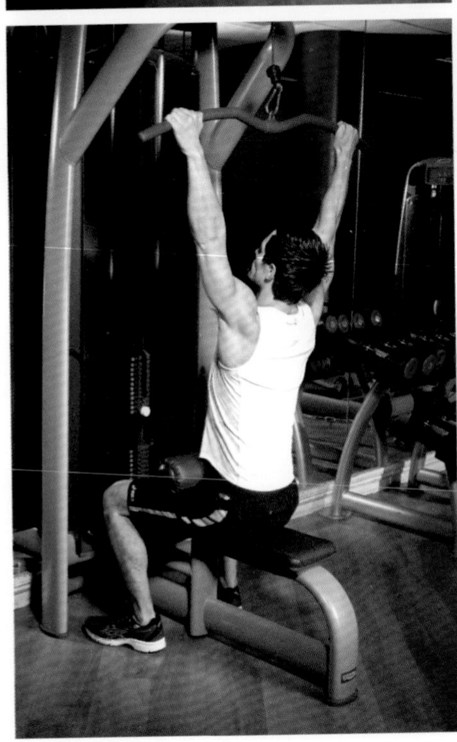

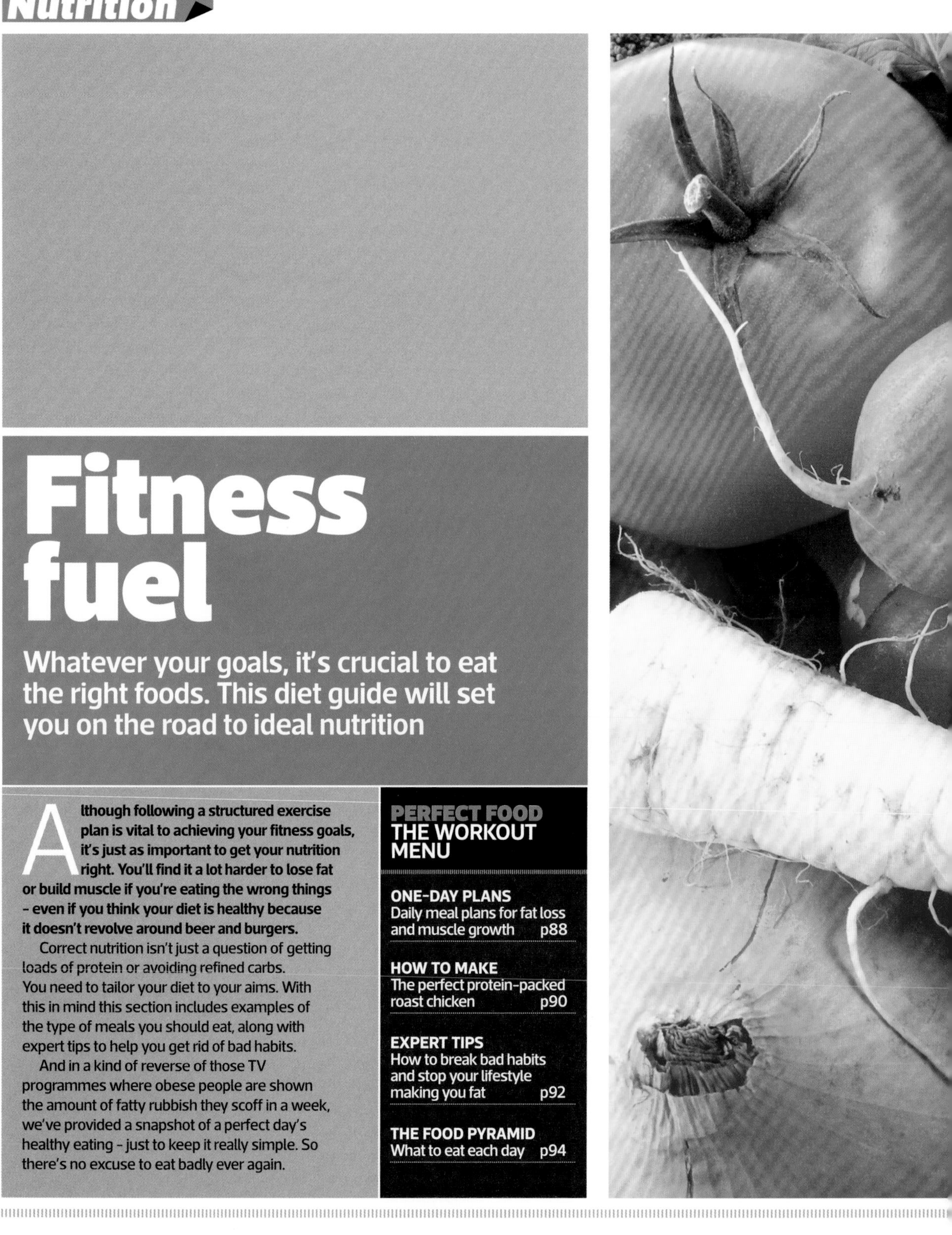

Fitness fuel

Whatever your goals, it's crucial to eat the right foods. This diet guide will set you on the road to ideal nutrition

Although following a structured exercise plan is vital to achieving your fitness goals, it's just as important to get your nutrition right. You'll find it a lot harder to lose fat or build muscle if you're eating the wrong things – even if you think your diet is healthy because it doesn't revolve around beer and burgers.

Correct nutrition isn't just a question of getting loads of protein or avoiding refined carbs. You need to tailor your diet to your aims. With this in mind this section includes examples of the type of meals you should eat, along with expert tips to help you get rid of bad habits.

And in a kind of reverse of those TV programmes where obese people are shown the amount of fatty rubbish they scoff in a week, we've provided a snapshot of a perfect day's healthy eating – just to keep it really simple. So there's no excuse to eat badly ever again.

PERFECT FOOD
THE WORKOUT MENU

ONE-DAY PLANS
Daily meal plans for fat loss and muscle growth p88

HOW TO MAKE
The perfect protein-packed roast chicken p90

EXPERT TIPS
How to break bad habits and stop your lifestyle making you fat p92

THE FOOD PYRAMID
What to eat each day p94

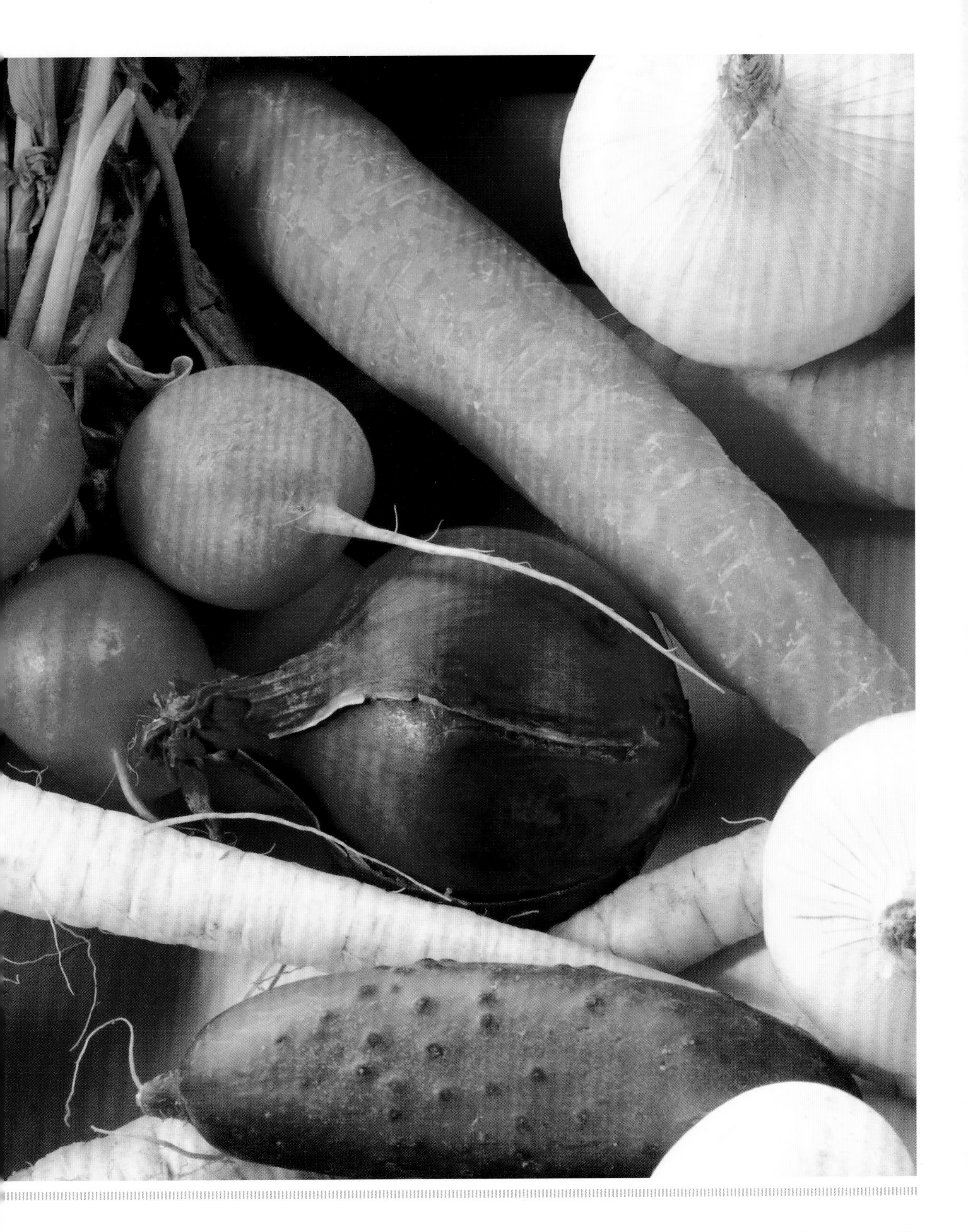

Fat loss menu

Eat like a Stone Age man to hit your fat loss targets with this Paleo plan

Processed foods and refined sugars are relatively recent additions to the human diet, so our bodies tend to store them as fat. This plan is based on the Paleo diet, which includes only foods that man ate in the Stone Age. Replacing processed carbs and sugars with fresh vegetables, healthy fats and animal proteins will help you to build muscle and shed fat.

Almonds are high in heart-healthy monounsaturated, polyunsaturated fats and muscle-soothing magnesium.

Baby spinach is packed with iron, which is vital for the formation of red blood cells, which move oxygen around the body.

Mandarins provide a healthy dose of immunity-boosting vitamin C. They are also a good source of dietary fibre.

Daily totals
1,815 calories
178g carbs
150g protein
73g fat

Breakfast

2 poached eggs contain plenty of muscle-building protein and amino acids.

Lunch

Mandarin and sesame chicken (serves 2)

Ingredients

4tbsp sesame oil | Juice of 1 mandarin | 1 garlic clove, crushed | 1 red chilli, deseeded and chopped | 2tsp freshly grated ginger | 2 chicken breasts | 150g baby spinach | Handful of basil and coriander leaves | ½ red onion, chopped | 5 almonds, chopped | 1tsp sesame seeds | Mandarin segments to garnish

To make

- Mix 2tbsp of sesame oil with the mandarin juice, garlic, chilli and ginger.
- Cut the chicken in several places and marinade in the mandarin mixture for four hours.
- Add the spinach leaves, herbs, onion, almonds and sesame seeds to a bowl.
- Baste the chicken with marinade and grill for 20 minutes, or until juices run clear.
- Chop up the chicken, add to salad and top with mandarin.

Dinner

Grilled pork steak with 1 mashed sweet potato, 50g steamed broccoli and sliced carrots provides protein and good carbs.

Snacks

Berries for antioxidants
Bananas for potassium
Satsumas for vitamin C

Muscle meals

This one-day plan is packed with protein to help you build muscle

If you're serious about putting on muscle, it's important that you get plenty of protein in your daily diet. This plan includes protein with every snack and main meal, ensuring that your muscles are drip-fed a constant supply to fuel growth throughout the day.

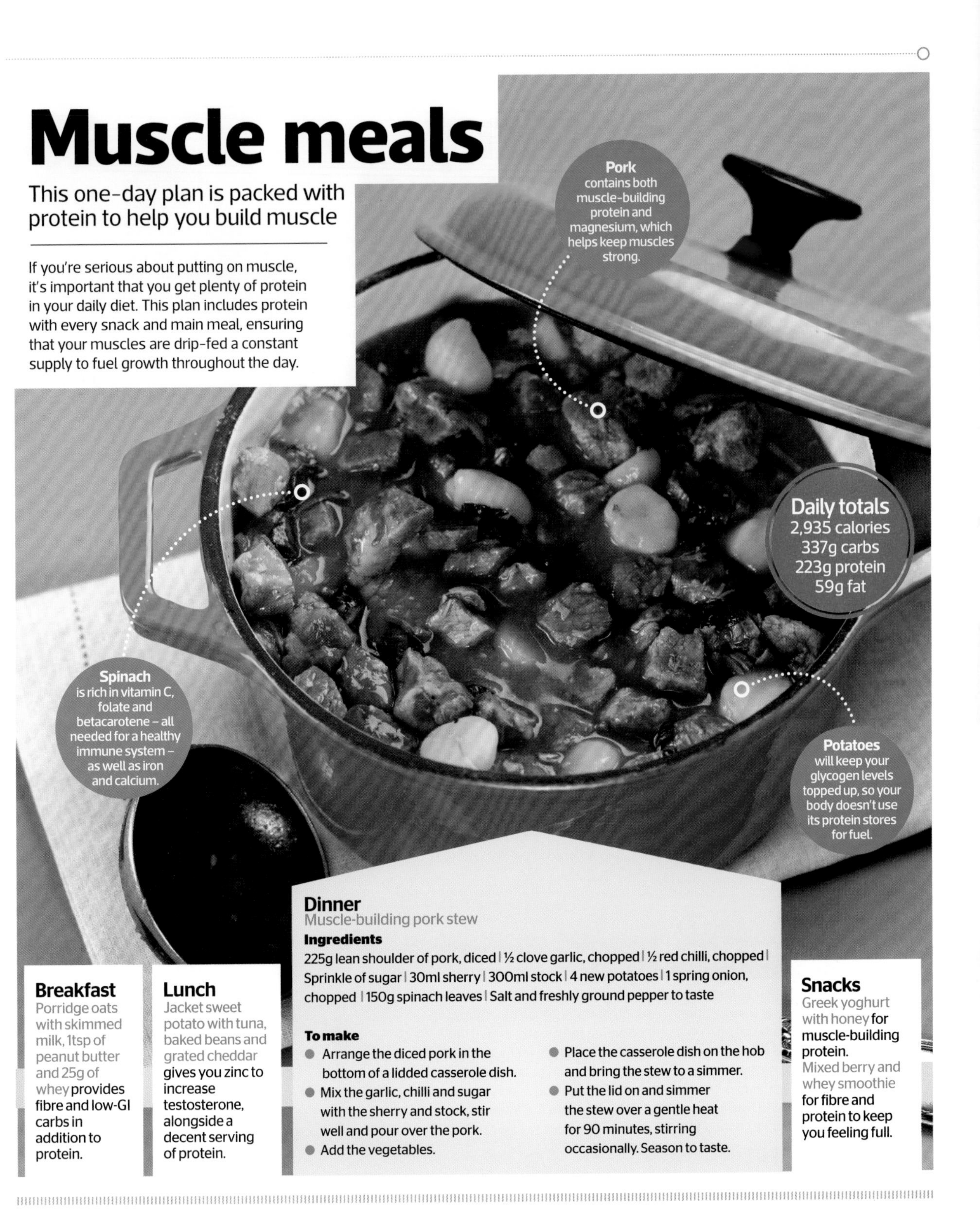

Breakfast

Porridge oats with skimmed milk, 1tsp of peanut butter and 25g of whey provides fibre and low-GI carbs in addition to protein.

Lunch

Jacket sweet potato with tuna, baked beans and grated cheddar gives you zinc to increase testosterone, alongside a decent serving of protein.

Dinner

Muscle-building pork stew

Ingredients

225g lean shoulder of pork, diced | ½ clove garlic, chopped | ½ red chilli, chopped | Sprinkle of sugar | 30ml sherry | 300ml stock | 4 new potatoes | 1 spring onion, chopped | 150g spinach leaves | Salt and freshly ground pepper to taste

To make

- Arrange the diced pork in the bottom of a lidded casserole dish.
- Mix the garlic, chilli and sugar with the sherry and stock, stir well and pour over the pork.
- Add the vegetables.
- Place the casserole dish on the hob and bring the stew to a simmer.
- Put the lid on and simmer the stew over a gentle heat for 90 minutes, stirring occasionally. Season to taste.

Snacks

Greek yoghurt with honey for muscle-building protein.

Mixed berry and whey smoothie for fibre and protein to keep you feeling full.

Perfect poultry

Prepare a flawless roast chicken with our expert guide

Few things in life are as satisfying as a really good Sunday roast. And luckily chicken, that staple of many a man's weekend roasting tin, happens to be one of the leanest, healthiest meats you can eat. If you cook it right, that is.

Packed with muscle-building protein, roast chicken contains far less saturated fat than other meats, such as beef or pork, making it an excellent option for anyone who wants to lose weight. Chicken also provides plenty of vitamin B3, which helps prevent the body from storing fat. Lee Streeton, executive chef at the Waldorf Astoria Syon Park (londonsyonpark.com), explains how to make a masterful roast chicken.

Quick tip

'People often overcook chicken,' says Streeton. 'The legs take longest to cook, so make an incision on the inside of one after 1hr 10min to check its progress. If clear juices run out rather than blood, it's ready to eat.'

How to make it Your perfect roast

Preheat the oven to 180°C. Remove the wishbone from the chicken, then place the chicken in a terracotta roasting dish. Baste the chicken with a little butter and season it with salt and black pepper. Add a little rapeseed oil to the dish, then place it in the oven and leave it to roast for between 1hr 10min and 1hr 30min. Once the juices run clear (rather than bloody) when you pierce the meat, remove the chicken from the oven and place it on a large chopping board. Pull the legs away from the body and separate the drumsticks from the thighs. Slice down the breasts to carve.

Do the aftermath

Make the most of your leftover chicken with one of these healthy dishes

Quick tip
'Chicken can easily turn out dry and flavourless,' says Streeton. 'Avoid this by basting it all over and adding plenty of seasoning before cooking.'

Chicken soup

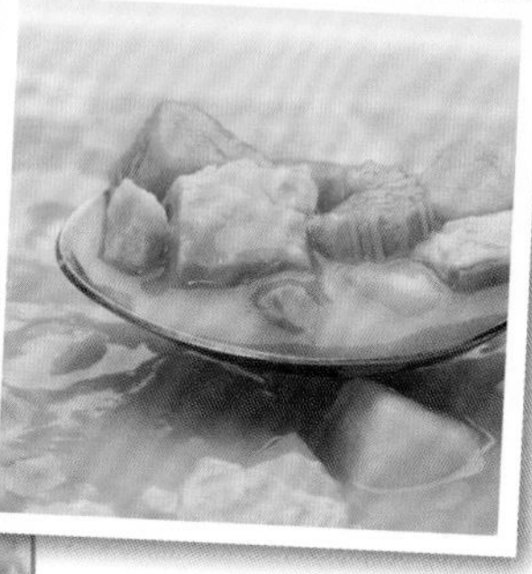

Carrots provide plenty of calcium pectate, which helps to reduce cholesterol.

Onions offer a healthy dose of quercetin, which helps to reduce muscle inflammation, and sulphur, which improves blood flow.

Potatoes contain starch, which can help to improve blood sugar control.

Celery lowers cholesterol by increasing bile acid secretion.

Chicken salad

Olive oil is full of heart-healthy oleic acid.

Spinach contains plenty of bone-strengthening vitamin K.

Rocket is a source of B vitamins, which are essential for metabolic function, and cancer-fighting phytochemicals.

Cherry tomatoes are packed with immunity-boosting vitamin C.

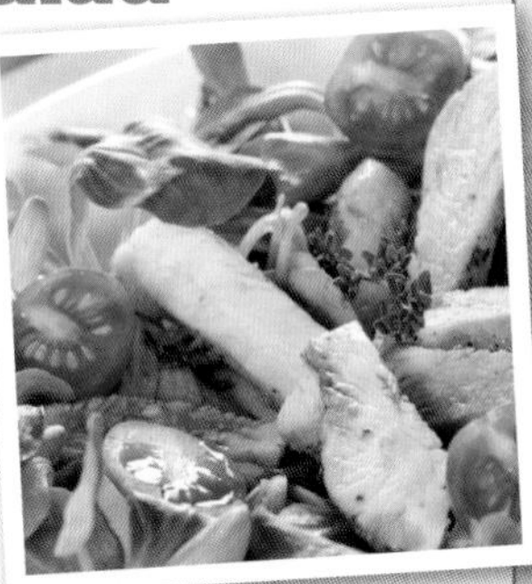

Chicken sandwich

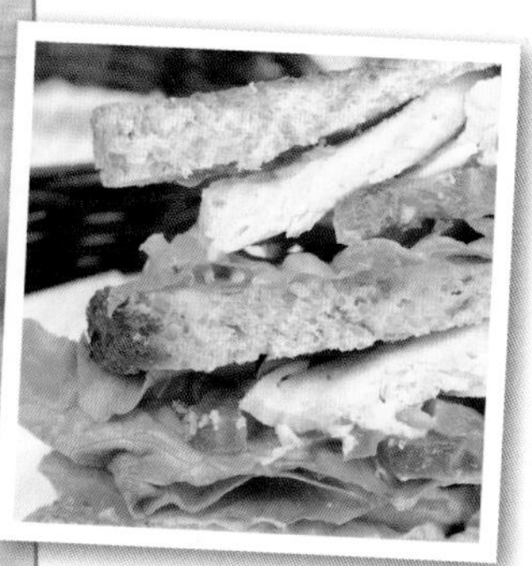

Tomatoes are full of the powerful antioxidant lycopene, which is also thought to boost bone health.

Wholemeal bread contains plenty of fibre to keep you feeling full.

Lettuce is packed with immunity-boosting vitamin C.

Cheddar cheese is a great source of casein, a high-quality muscle-building protein.

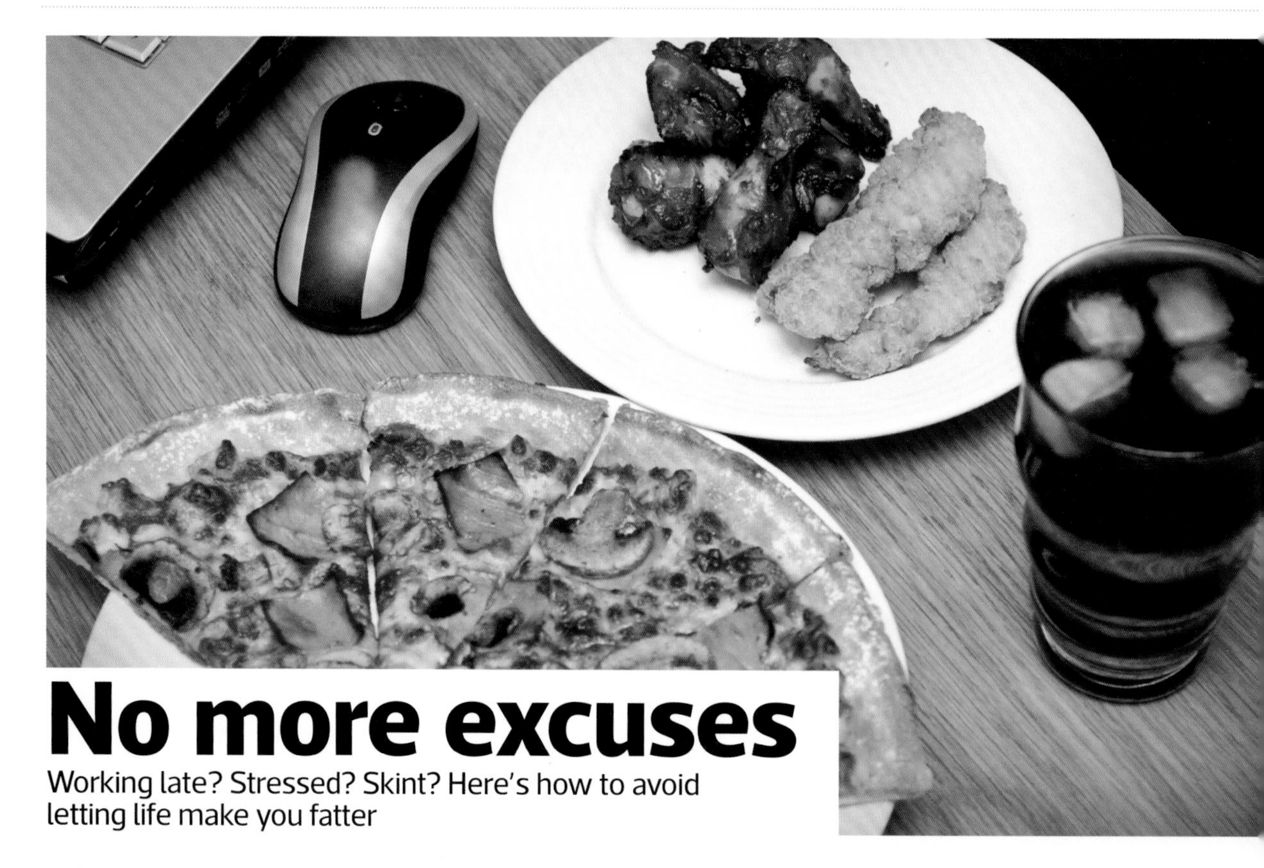

No more excuses

Working late? Stressed? Skint? Here's how to avoid letting life make you fatter

I'm too busy

THE EXCUSE **I've got a busy life, leaving no time to cook.**

FIX IT Preparing food quickly doesn't mean it's unhealthy. 'Grilling a chicken breast, seasoned with pepper and lemon, while steaming some veggies can be done in the time it takes to order a takeaway,' says nutrition consultant Lynn Clay. It provides high-quality protein to keep you full, and you get a shot of vitamins and minerals from the veg.

It's too expensive

THE EXCUSE **Healthy meals drain my wallet. Ready meals are cheap.**

FIX IT 'You pay a premium for ready meals,' says Clay. 'Cook from scratch and you'll not only reduce your intake of salt and added preservatives but also save a small fortune.' Tuna, eggs and lentils are cheap and should be cupboard staples, while seasonal fruit and veg, beans and salads are very cheap ways of getting your daily vitamin needs.

I'm stressed

THE EXCUSE **When work is hectic I crave sugary, fatty comfort foods.**

FIX IT You're better off with a carb-based snack. 'Carbohydrate-rich meals increase levels of serotonin, a hormone known to induce a feeling of calm,' says Elisabeth Weichselbaum of the British Nutrition Foundation (nutrition.org.uk). Try a slice of wholemeal bread with peanut butter and some fruit. Still not working? Hit the gym. A study from the University of Missouri shows high-intensity exercise reduces stress.

I've got no willpower

THE EXCUSE **I can't resist sweets, chips and other unhealthy foods.**

FIX IT Prevention is key. If you never fill your cupboards with sugary snacks, you're not constantly testing your willpower. 'But eating healthily doesn't mean avoiding your favourite foods,' says Weichselbaum. 'If you're a pizza addict, use a thin, wholemeal base, go easy on the cheese and add veg.'

I'm too tired

THE EXCUSE **It's 4pm and I'm fading – I need a chocolate bar.**

FIX IT You may initially enjoy that sugar rush but it always leads to a crash. 'A protein-rich snack will release energy over a longer period, while chocolate and crisps will only give you energy for a short time before your blood sugar comes crashing down,' says nutritional therapist Henrietta Bailey (puresportsmed.com). Get through your afternoon slump with a handful of unsalted nuts. They'll keep you full and provide vital vitamins and minerals.

I'm eating out

THE EXCUSE **In a restaurant I have no control over what's available.**

FIX IT You can't change the amount of salt in your meal but there are a few tricks to keep you on track. 'Look on the menu for sources of lean protein, such as white meat or fish, and choose a tomato-based sauce rather than a cream-based one,' says Clay.

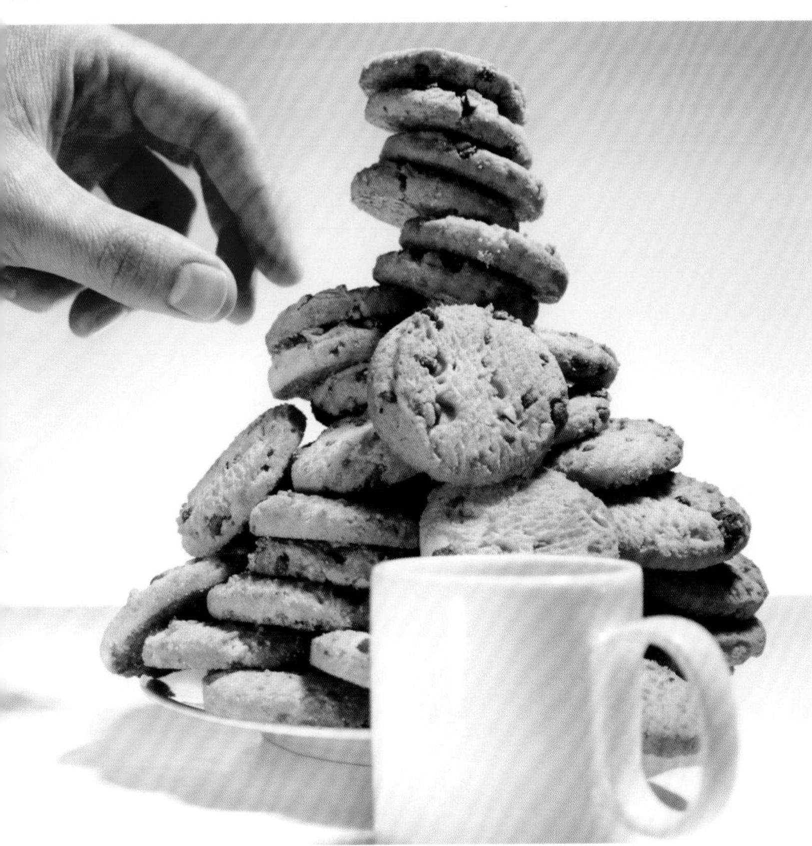

Mind over fatter

Find yourself snacking mindlessly? Here's how you can break your bad eating habits and get slim

1 Don't make it easy

Easy access to snack foods invariably leads to munching, so do what you can to minimise temptation. 'Put in some interruption that will make you think twice before snacking,' says Professor Brian Wansink, author of *Mindless Eating: Why We Eat More Than We Think*. 'If there's a packet of sweets on your desk, you won't think twice about eating them because they're right in front of you, but if you put barriers in the way, it'll test how much you want them.' Wansink found that office workers ate 125 fewer calories a day when the sweets were placed two metres away from their desk than when they were sitting within reach.

2 Forward planning

'Think ahead and be prepared for all outcomes,' says nutritionist Lucy-Ann Prideaux (simply-nutrition.co.uk). 'Take a moment to think about how you would like to eat and, more importantly, how you would like to feel at the end of the day.' Preparing healthy meals and snacks to take with you to work may be time-consuming, but your body will thank you for it in the long run. 'Your day won't always go to plan, however, so make sure you give yourself a degree of flexibility in your food choices,' Prideaux adds. 'Always try to assess whether or not the food that's available to you is a good option to fuel and nourish your body.'

3 Drink more water

'It's very easy to confuse dehydration with hunger,' says Wansink. 'We know our body is craving something and we just assume that it's food – but frequently it's liquids, especially in active people. I would guess that seven times out of ten what people think of as hunger is really just a mild case of dehydration.' You don't necessarily have to drink water, but make sure the beverage you choose is low in caffeine and sodium. 'Caffeine and sodium dehydrate you even more, giving your mouth a feeling of thirst that can encourage you to snack,' Wansink says.

4 Use the hunger/fullness scale

'Recognising and working with your body's physiological hunger and fullness cues can really help to control snacking,' says Prideaux. 'Imagine your hunger on a scale of one to ten. You're starving at level 1, mildly hungry at level 3 or 4, comfortably full at level 7 or 8 and completely stuffed at level 10. If you train yourself to eat as soon as you reach level 3 or 4 and to stop eating as soon as you reach level 7 or 8 – between which points your blood sugar levels will be at their most stable – then over time you'll become much more aware of your body's hunger and fullness signals, and you'll be far less inclined to indulge in mindless snacking, boredom eating or comfort eating, all of which are common causes of weight gain.'

5 Develop new habits

One great way to reduce snacking is to invent some sort of condition every time you have cravings – and we don't mean a made-up disease that can be cured with peanut M&Ms. 'Tell yourself you can have anything you want from the vending machine if you are going to work out that day, or if you have a light dinner, or some sort of trade-off,' says Wansink. 'If you regularly stop by the shops on your way home from work and buy a chocolate bar, take an alternative route to reduce that temptation or tell yourself, "You can only have the chocolate if you go for a run when you get home". That way, either you break the habit or you alter it so you're getting something positive out of your snack.'

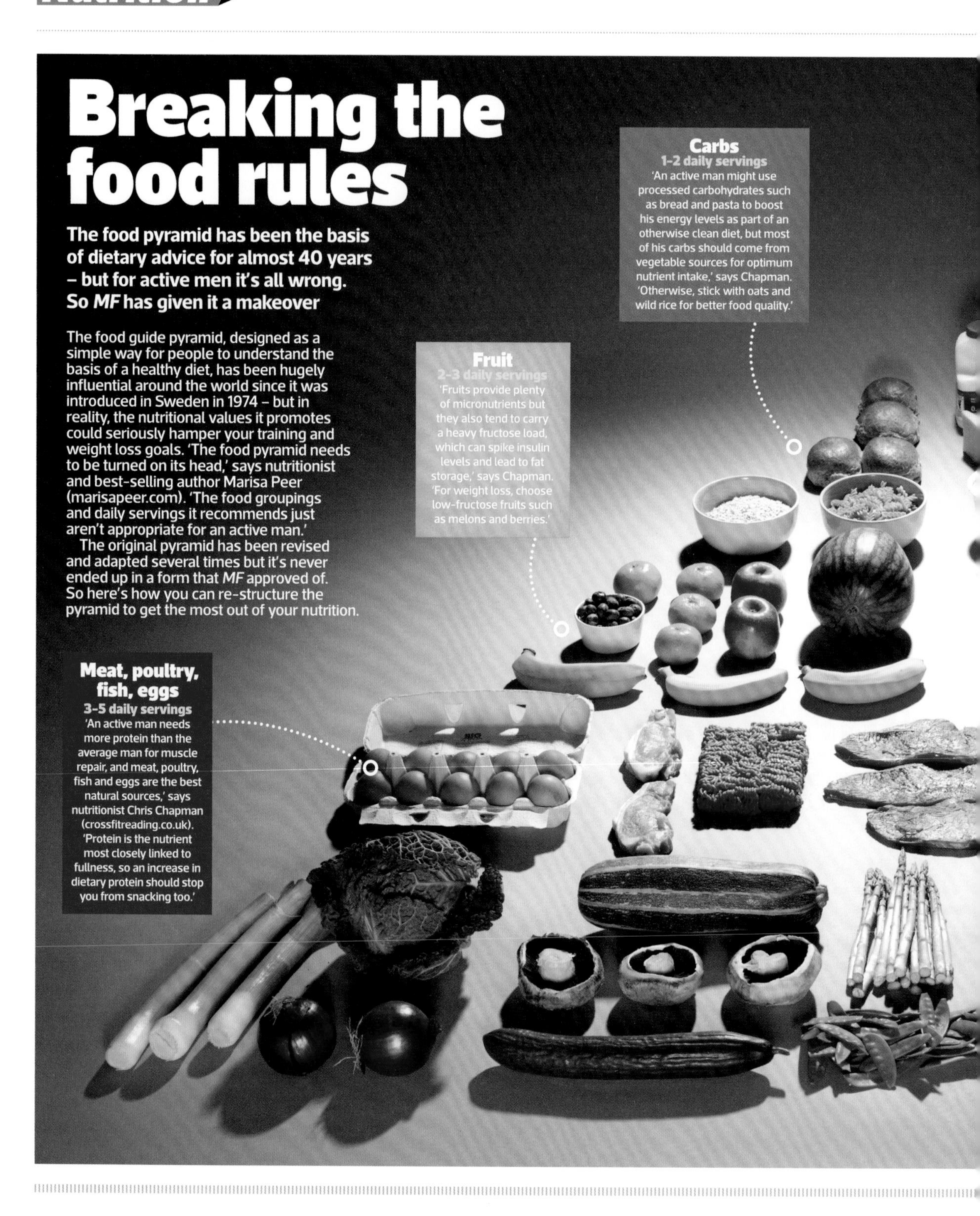

Breaking the food rules

The food pyramid has been the basis of dietary advice for almost 40 years – but for active men it's all wrong. So *MF* has given it a makeover

The food guide pyramid, designed as a simple way for people to understand the basis of a healthy diet, has been hugely influential around the world since it was introduced in Sweden in 1974 – but in reality, the nutritional values it promotes could seriously hamper your training and weight loss goals. 'The food pyramid needs to be turned on its head,' says nutritionist and best-selling author Marisa Peer (marisapeer.com). 'The food groupings and daily servings it recommends just aren't appropriate for an active man.'

The original pyramid has been revised and adapted several times but it's never ended up in a form that *MF* approved of. So here's how you can re-structure the pyramid to get the most out of your nutrition.

Carbs

1-2 daily servings

'An active man might use processed carbohydrates such as bread and pasta to boost his energy levels as part of an otherwise clean diet, but most of his carbs should come from vegetable sources for optimum nutrient intake,' says Chapman. 'Otherwise, stick with oats and wild rice for better food quality.'

Fruit

2-3 daily servings

'Fruits provide plenty of micronutrients but they also tend to carry a heavy fructose load, which can spike insulin levels and lead to fat storage,' says Chapman. 'For weight loss, choose low-fructose fruits such as melons and berries.'

Meat, poultry, fish, eggs

3-5 daily servings

'An active man needs more protein than the average man for muscle repair, and meat, poultry, fish and eggs are the best natural sources,' says nutritionist Chris Chapman (crossfitreading.co.uk). 'Protein is the nutrient most closely linked to fullness, so an increase in dietary protein should stop you from snacking too.'

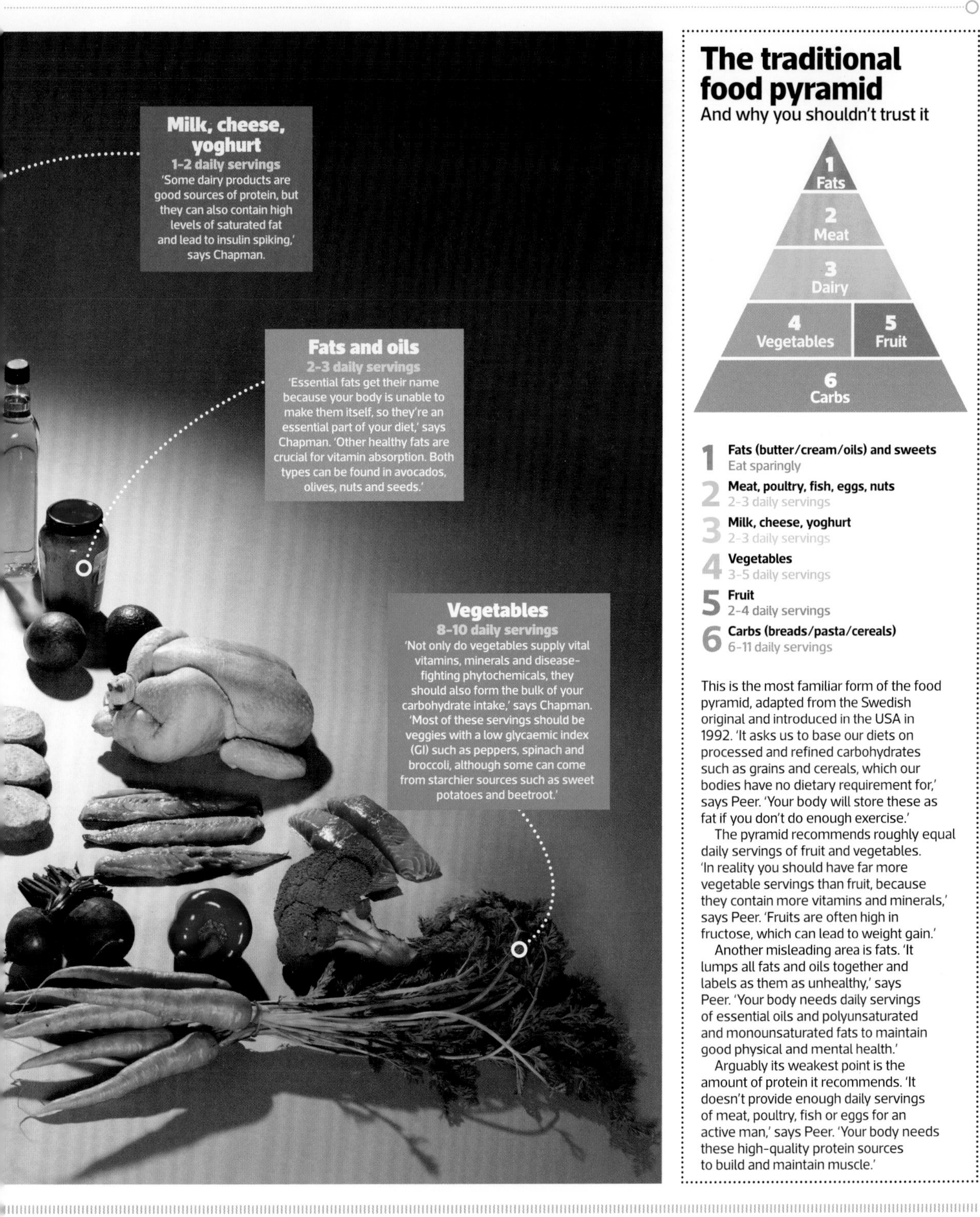

The traditional food pyramid

And why you shouldn't trust it

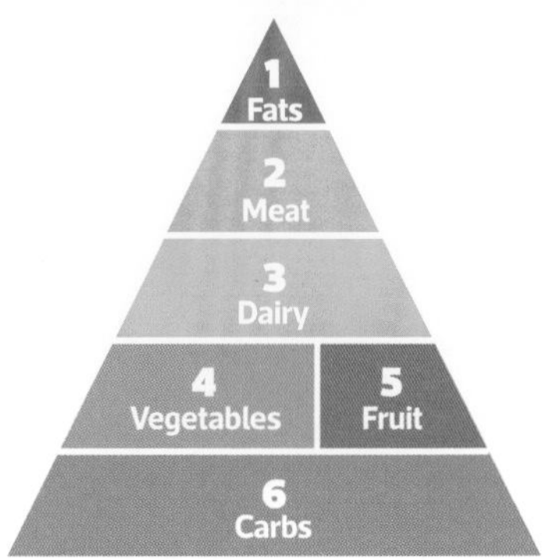

1. **Fats (butter/cream/oils) and sweets**
   Eat sparingly
2. **Meat, poultry, fish, eggs, nuts**
   2-3 daily servings
3. **Milk, cheese, yoghurt**
   2-3 daily servings
4. **Vegetables**
   3-5 daily servings
5. **Fruit**
   2-4 daily servings
6. **Carbs (breads/pasta/cereals)**
   6-11 daily servings

This is the most familiar form of the food pyramid, adapted from the Swedish original and introduced in the USA in 1992. 'It asks us to base our diets on processed and refined carbohydrates such as grains and cereals, which our bodies have no dietary requirement for,' says Peer. 'Your body will store these as fat if you don't do enough exercise.'

The pyramid recommends roughly equal daily servings of fruit and vegetables. 'In reality you should have far more vegetable servings than fruit, because they contain more vitamins and minerals,' says Peer. 'Fruits are often high in fructose, which can lead to weight gain.'

Another misleading area is fats. 'It lumps all fats and oils together and labels as them as unhealthy,' says Peer. 'Your body needs daily servings of essential oils and polyunsaturated and monounsaturated fats to maintain good physical and mental health.'

Arguably its weakest point is the amount of protein it recommends. 'It doesn't provide enough daily servings of meat, poultry, fish or eggs for an active man,' says Peer. 'Your body needs these high-quality protein sources to build and maintain muscle.'

Train like a sports pro

Follow the training advice from sports professionals to build elite levels of fitness

You might think that you lack the skills to perform like an elite athlete. In fact, the biggest thing that's likely to hold you back is not having adequate strength and conditioning, the two main areas that sports fitness coaches aim to develop.

When you're strong and you don't tire easily you have greater control over your body and can execute your sporting skills more easily. That's why there's a popular belief in the strength and conditioning community that says 'strongest always wins'.

Of course, the pro sportsmen in this section, such as the England rugby player Ben Foden and UFC star Rashad Evans, also have bodies that any gym-goer would envy, so doing their workouts will make you look good as well as helping you to perform when it matters.

WINNING SPORTS WORKOUTS

RUGBY
Ben Foden p98

MMA
Rashad Evans p102

DISCUS
Lawrence Okoye p106

LONG JUMP
Chris Tomlinson p110

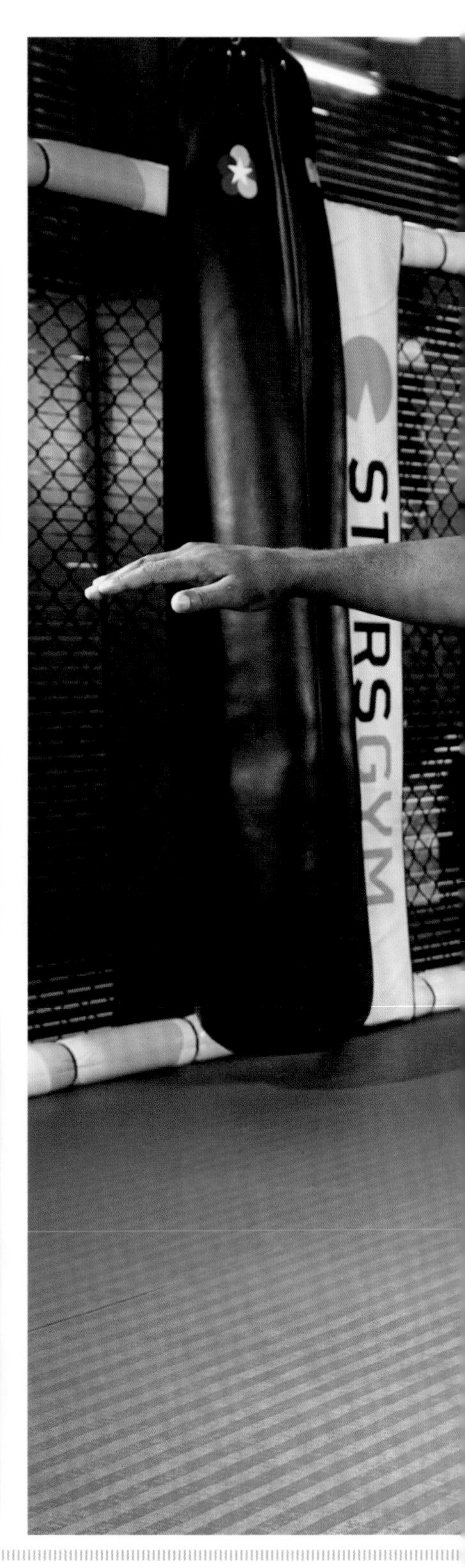

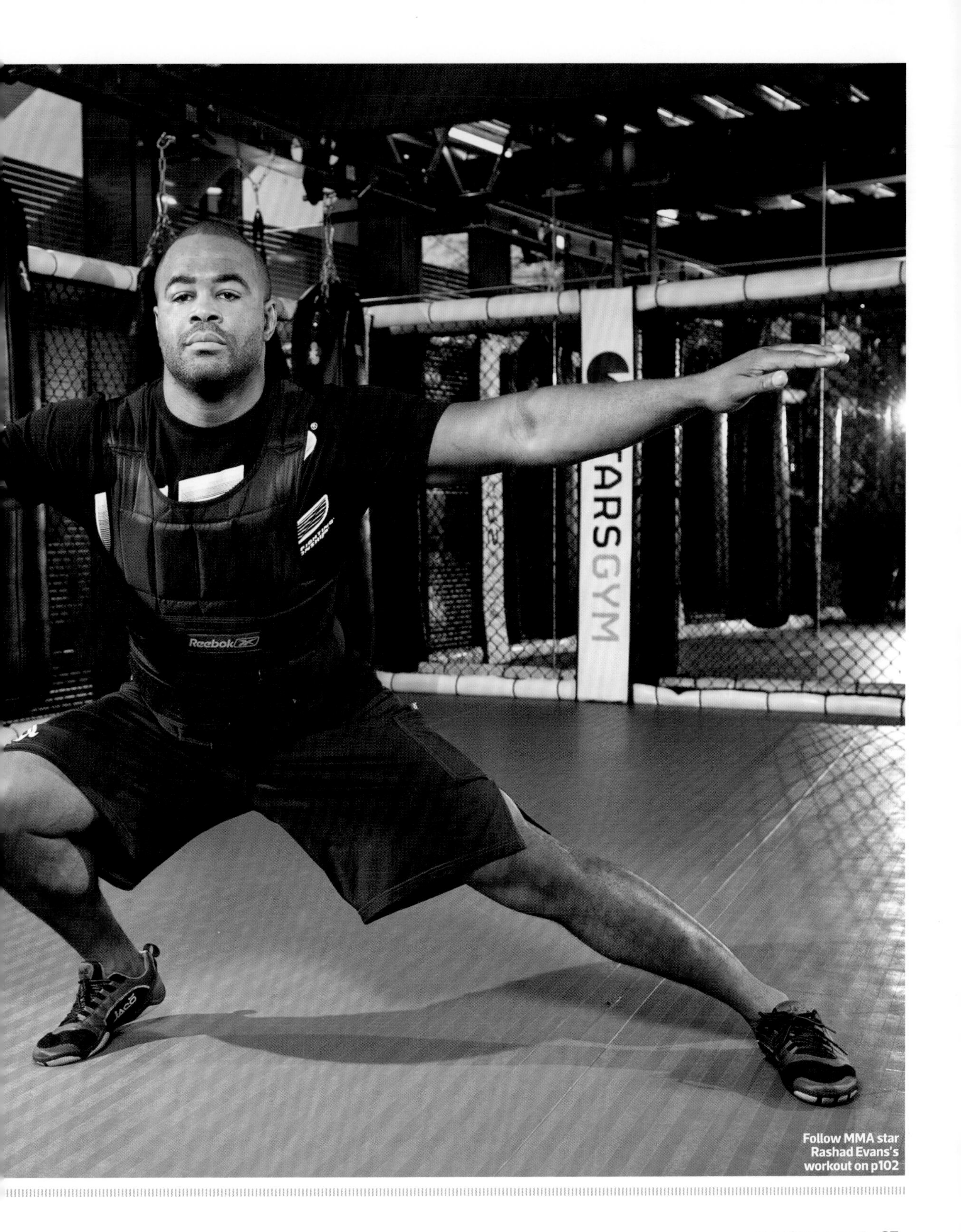

Follow MMA star Rashad Evans's workout on p102

FULL SPEED AHEAD

England full-back Ben Foden tells *MF* how to build the explosive power to make breaks and blast through tackles

Ben Foden started his rugby career at scrum-half, but it's as a full-back that he's achieved his most striking success both with Northampton Saints and the senior England team. In 2011 he started every game of the Six Nations and World Cup campaigns, adding three tries to the two he recorded in 2010. At club level he won the Premiership and European Challenge Cup with his previous club, Sale Sharks, and won the Challenge Cup again in 2009 with Northampton before reaching the final of the Heineken Cup in 2011. Here he talks about his career and how he trains to build the power and explosive speed he needs to succeed in top-level rugby union.

Has your role with England changed now you're one of the most capped backs in the squad?
I've had to step up into more of a leadership role. I can use the experiences I've gained to mentor a few of the guys coming through. It's exciting times for England. A lot of faith is being put in the young guys and they'll be hungry to prove to the world that they're ready for international rugby. Hopefully we'll see a few new stars.

How does your training help you on the field?
I've always tried to be explosive in the way I play. I've needed acceleration, strong hand-offs, aimed to get around the outside of the opposition. You need fast feet and the ability to change direction quickly. You need to be explosive in one quick, fluid movement.

> 'The back-row players need to make sure that every kilo is lean muscle'

How do you develop that?
For me there's an emphasis on power. In the preseason you can focus on building strength, but in the season I'll work on my power. That involves big lifts of heavy weights with low numbers of high-tempo reps. With England we'll do lots of SAQ [speed, agility

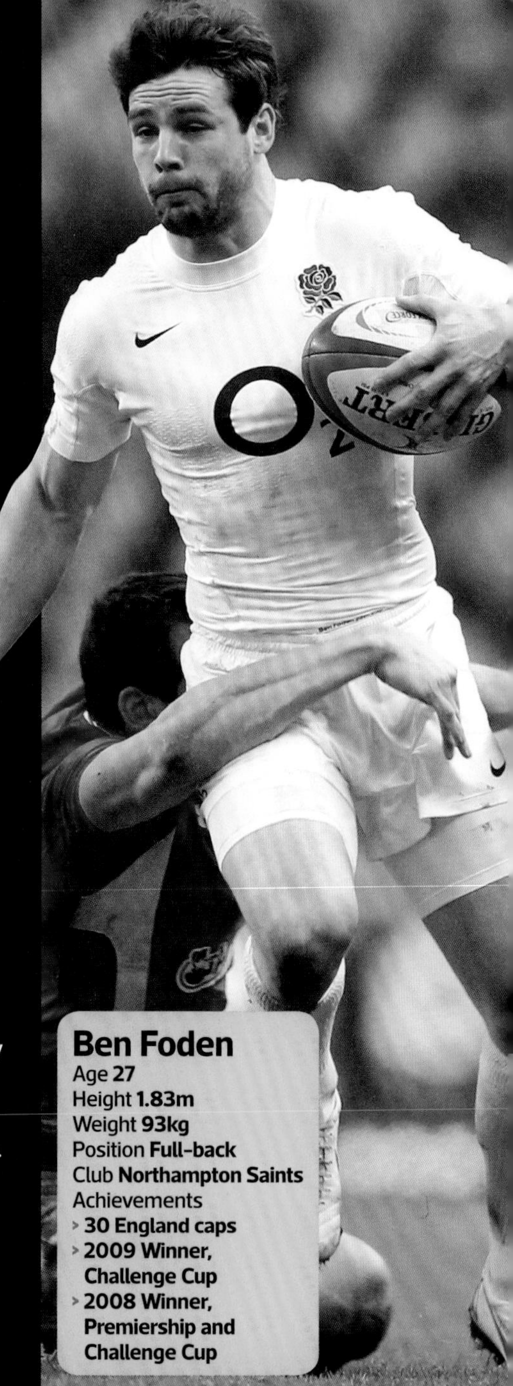

Ben Foden
Age **27**
Height **1.83m**
Weight **93kg**
Position **Full-back**
Club **Northampton Saints**
Achievements
- **30 England caps**
- **2009 Winner, Challenge Cup**
- **2008 Winner, Premiership and Challenge Cup**

Statistics correct at 24th September 2012

nd quickness] training with ladder work and cones for quick feet and hen a short sprint over 40m.

What do players do to build muscle?
'm lucky that my weight never really luctuates. I stay around 93-95kg. Others tend to struggle. The back-row players need to make sure that every kilo of weight is lean muscle so they can get around the park. The ypical bruiser of old now needs to be agile as well as powerful. If you ook at Olympic lifters they'll be only 75kg but be able to power clean wice their weight. Power ratio is so mportant. You have to be strong but athletic. The front row need to keep heir weight on for the big hits when hey're scrummaging so they'll focus on muscle growth. Others struggle o keep the weight on. Lee Dickson, he Saints and England scrum-half, eats what he wants but never puts a gram on. So they keep him on hypertrophy work to put muscle on.

What do your own sessions involve?
'll usually do weights first, with a core complex between each exercise, then drag a weighted sled and finish with bungee sprints. Everything leads up o the most explosive movement and hen sprints at the end of a session.

How do you cope with doing hard gym sessions and playing matches?
At the end of the 2011 season we had three weeks off before meeting with the England squad so it felt as if we'd just rolled into another season. But because of that the coaches got us straight into ball work rather than itness training. In the tournament I didn't feel out of shape but there's a difference between feeling fit and being fit – look at what the Welsh eam did in preparation [doing cryotherapy sessions to increase heir ability to train harder]. I felt that we could have been pushed harder.

Ben Foden uses Multipower Sportsfood. For nutrition tailored to your needs visit multipower.com/uk.

Ben Foden's POWER WORKOUT

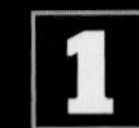

1 Box squat

Sets 4 **Reps** 4

- Set a box or bench behind you and with the weight supported across your shoulders, lower until you're sitting.
- Make sure you keep your back straight and your core braced before you explode up through your legs until standing.

Foden says
'The focus is on the concentric, powerful phase of a squat. This is essential for sprinting where channelling your energy upwards will get you moving forward faster. I'll work up to sets where I'm squatting 150kg.'

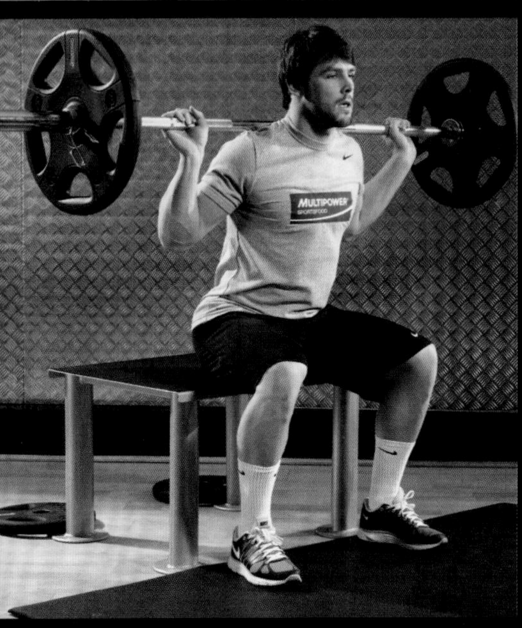

2 Bent-over row

Sets 5 **Reps** 3

- Hold a barbell at shin level, legs slightly bent and back straight.
- Pull the bar to your sternum, squeeze your shoulder blades together at the top then lower under control.
- An alternating grip (pictured) helps you to lift a heavy load. Switch hands and do an even number both ways

Foden says
'Tempo is key here. Raise quickly and lower slowly to work your biceps and upper back.'

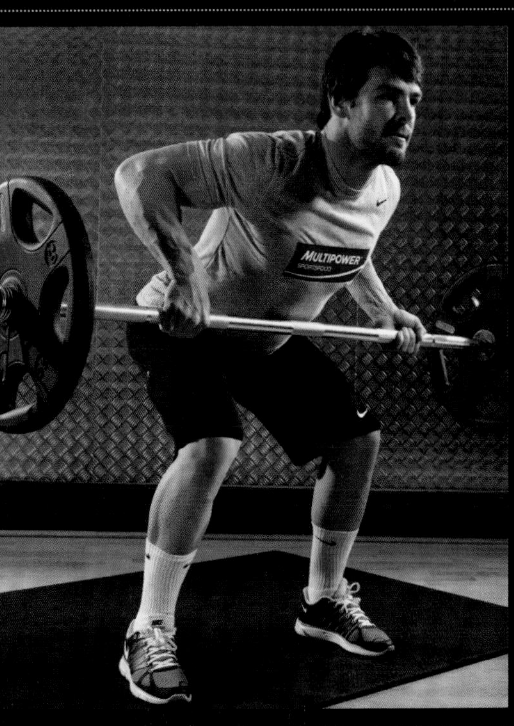

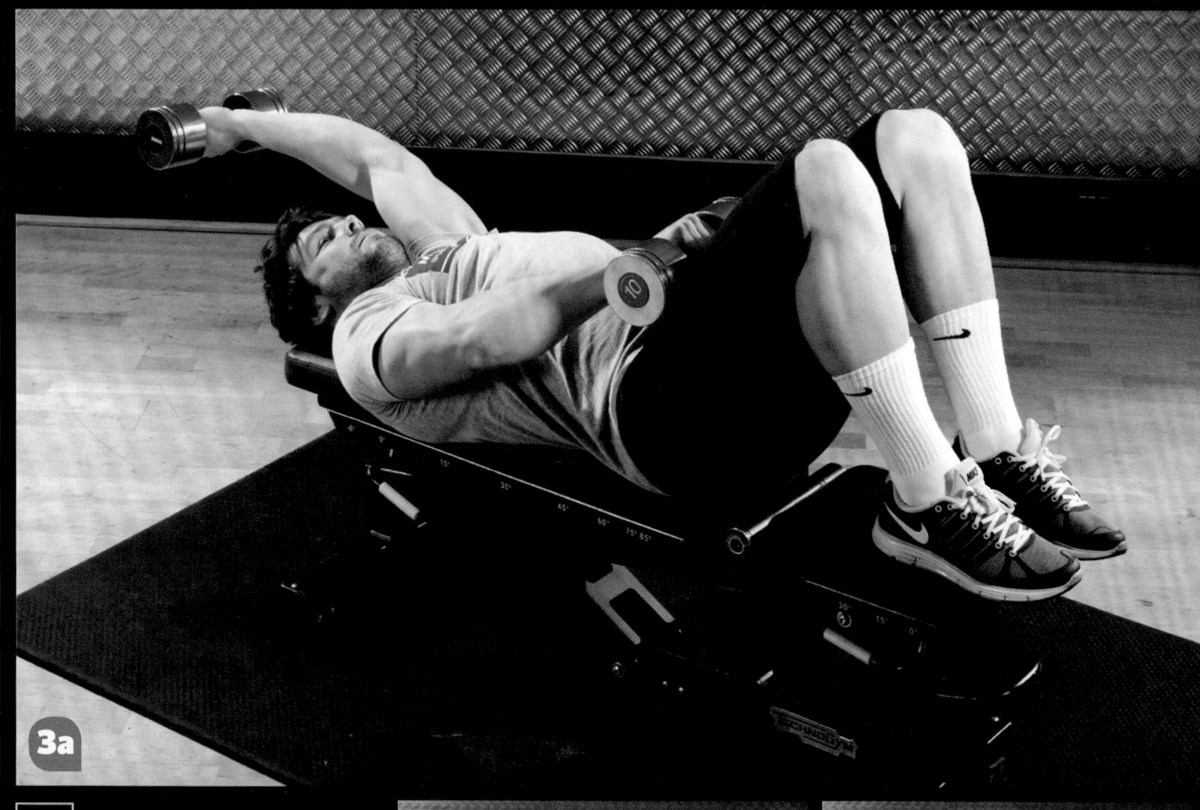

3 Shoulder complex

Sets 4 **Reps** 6 each move

3a One-arm alternating dumbbell pull-over
- Lie on a bench holding dumbbells straight above you. Bring one arm forward and the other backwards, then switch to complete one rep.

3b Deep flye
- Slowly lower the weights as far as you can before returning them to the middle to complete one rep.

3c Chest press
- Finish with six reps of a standard dumbbell chest press.

Foden says
'I wouldn't use dumbbells heavier than 10kg because these moves are designed to increase stability rather than strength. This combination works the shoulder joint through different ranges of movement. Putting my legs on the bench stops me cheating and ensures that all the effort required to remain stable comes from my shoulders.'

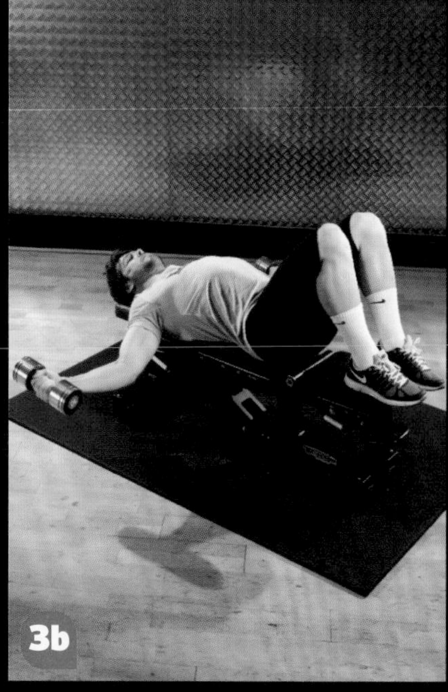

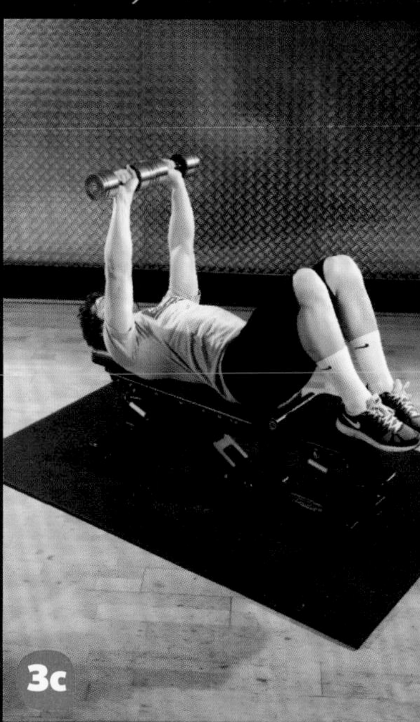

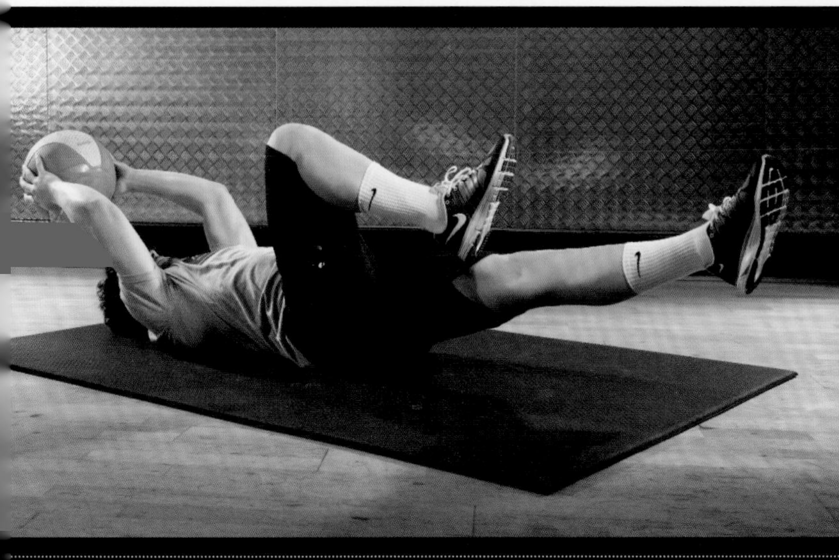

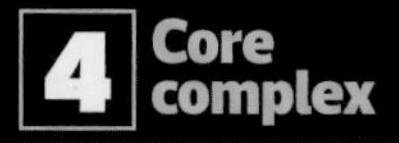

4 Core complex

Sets 4 **Reps** 20 each side

> Hold a medicine ball just off the floor behind your head throughout the move.
> Contract your core to bring one leg in towards you with the other straight but off the floor, alternating legs each time.
> Avoid arching your back during the move and make sure your heel follows the line of your legs.

Foden says

'I'll include this abs move between each main exercise to build a solid core, which is vital for harnessing your power and taking big hits. The exercise also mimics the sprinting action to improve that.'

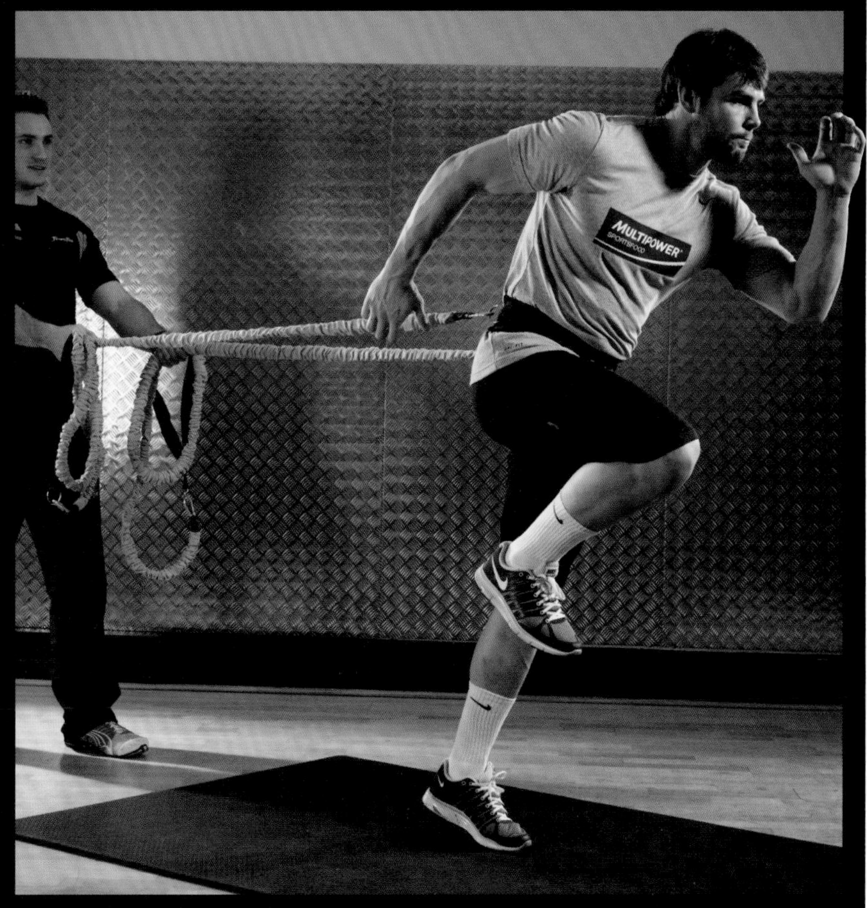

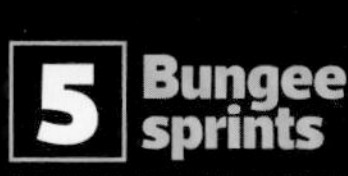

5 Bungee sprints

Sets 4 **Reps** 20m

> Attach bungee ropes around your waist and get a partner to hold them tight.
> Tension will build as you move forward, making each stride harder so you work with greater intensity.
> Train with a partner so one of you is always working while the other is assisting them, but resting.

Foden says

'I'll aim to start slowly, focusing on perfecting my sprinting technique, but build until I'm going all out at the end. The further I go the more tension there is in the rope and the more powerfully I have to pump my legs before it throws me back. It's tremendous for building acceleration.'

POWER CAGE

Former UFC champion Rashad Evans explains how to train your lower body for one-punch knockout strength

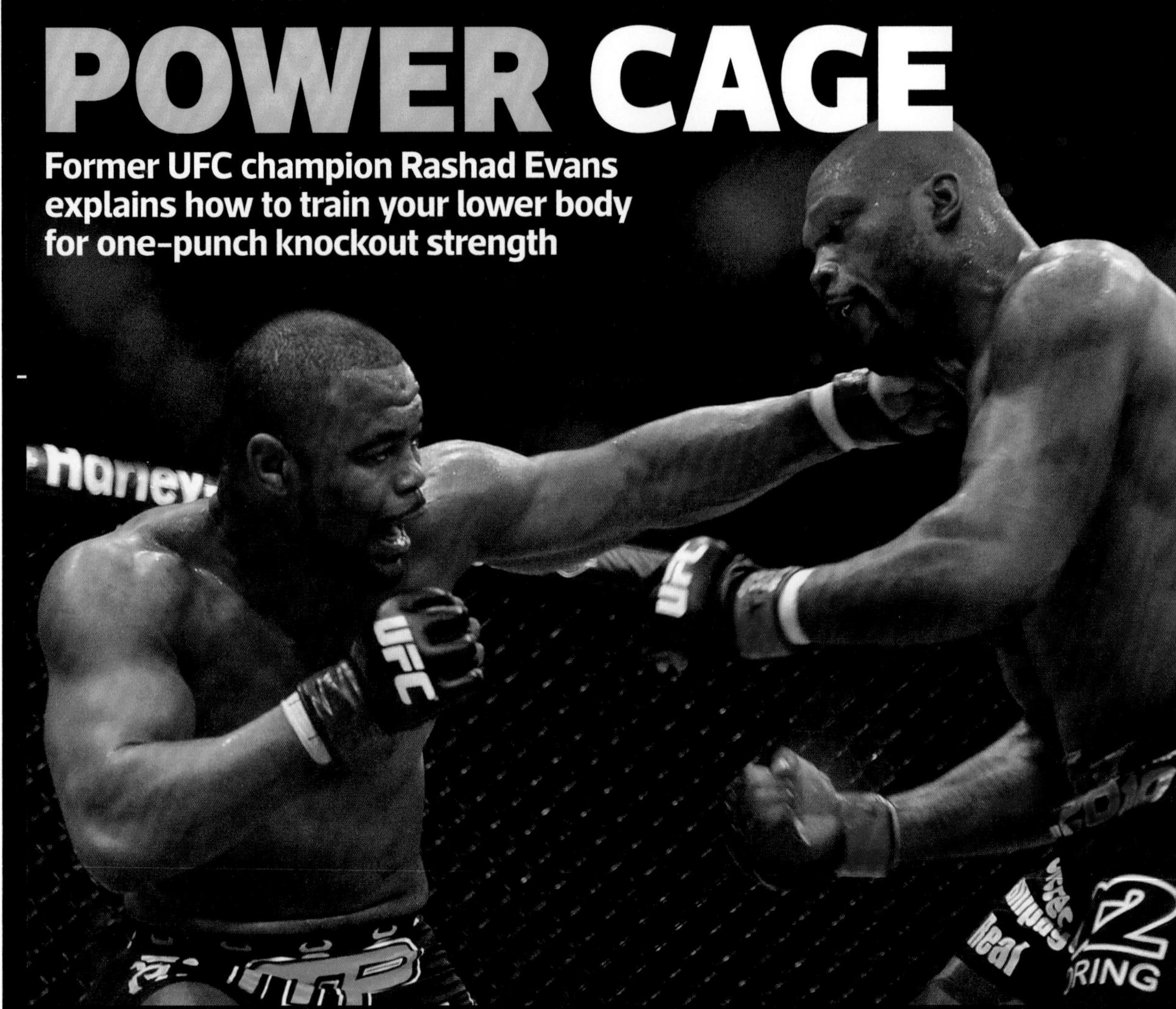

The sport of MMA has evolved considerably since Rashad Evans made his UFC debut in 2005, and Evans's ability to evolve with it has played a massive part in his continued success in the Octagon. With a college wrestling background, Evans spent the early part of his MMA career using his wrestling skills to dominate opponents in the cage, while working diligently to develop his striking capabilities outside it. He announced his arrival as a fully rounded mixed martial artist in 2008 by knocking out former UFC light heavyweight champion Chuck Liddell with a single punch. He went on to win the title from Forrest Griffin later that year, although he subsequently lost it to Lyoto Machida.

> 'I make sure that my workout has the same work-to-rest ratio as an actual fight'

Asked what the key factor is in his punching power, Evans's answer is instant. 'It's all about your legs. If you've got strong legs and a strong base, everything else can be developed from there.' The next three pages present six simple exercises that will help you build knockout punching power.

How often do you do strength and conditioning workouts in the gym?
When I'm training for a fight I do specific strength and conditioning

Statistics correct at 24th September 2012

Rashad Evans

Age **32**
Height **1.80m**
Weight **93kg**
MMA Record
17 wins 1 draw 2 defeats
Achievements
- **Former UFC light heavyweight champion**
- **NCAA Division 1 wrestler**

workouts three times a week to supplement my MMA sessions.

What does a typical conditioning workout entail?
I do a lot of sprint drills and explosive moves like tyre flips and box jumps because they help to mimic the movements you make during a fight. I try to stick to low-impact moves, so I can do them again and again to strengthen my ligaments and tendons.

What specific qualities are you trying to develop in your workouts?
Explosiveness is very important and so is functional strength. I also have to work on my endurance by making sure that my workout is based around the same work-to-rest ratio as an actual fight. For example, I'll do 15 seconds of sprinting with five seconds of rest and keep repeating that for five minutes to replicate the conditions of a five-minute round.

Does your fight conditioning come predominantly from sparring or from your workouts?
I get most of my conditioning from the sparring, but the specific conditioning stuff that I do in the gym is crucial. It's the thread that weaves everything together and simulates the transitions between striking and grappling that take place during a fight.

Rashad Evans's LEGS WORKOUT

'Perform two circuits of the following five exercises with no rest between reps or sets,' says Evans's strength and conditioning coach Mike van Arsdale. 'Ride the exercise bike for three minutes at 55rpm after the first circuit, then for a further ten minutes at 55rpm after the second circuit. Wear a weighted vest for the first circuit and then take it off for the rest of the workout.'

1 Squat

Reps 16

- Stand with your feet shoulder-width apart and your toes pointing out slightly.
- Brace your core and lower yourself by bending at the knees until your thighs are parallel to the floor.
- Maintain a natural arch in your back and keep your knees in line with your feet.
- Push back up through your heels to return to the starting position, looking forward throughout.

Van Arsdale says
'The squat is a fundamental strength move that should be a key part of any legs workout.'

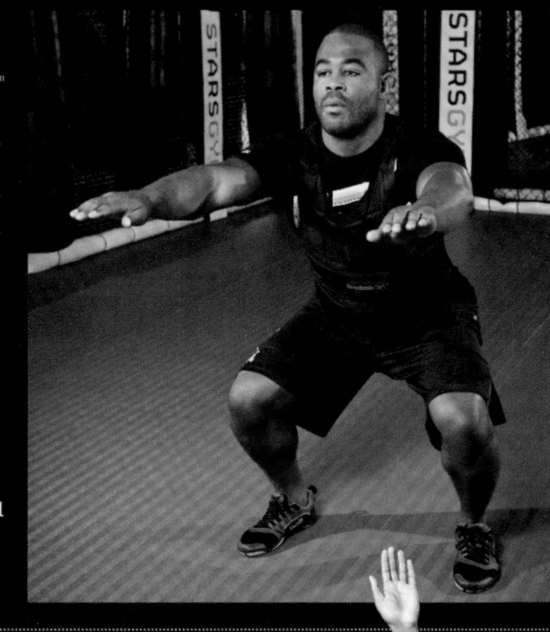

2 Alternating forward lunge

Reps 8 each side

- Stand looking forward with your feet apart.
- Take a big step forward with your right foot and lower your left knee until it almost touches the floor, ensuring that both your feet are pointing forward and your right knee is over your right foot but does not go beyond it.
- As you lower your left knee, raise your left arm vertically upwards.
- Push up off your front foot to return to the starting position and then repeat on the opposite side.
- Keep your torso upright and keep looking forward throughout.

Van Arsdale says
'Alternating forward lunges are great for building unilateral strength, which is useful for MMA because you hardly ever push off from both your feet at the same time.'

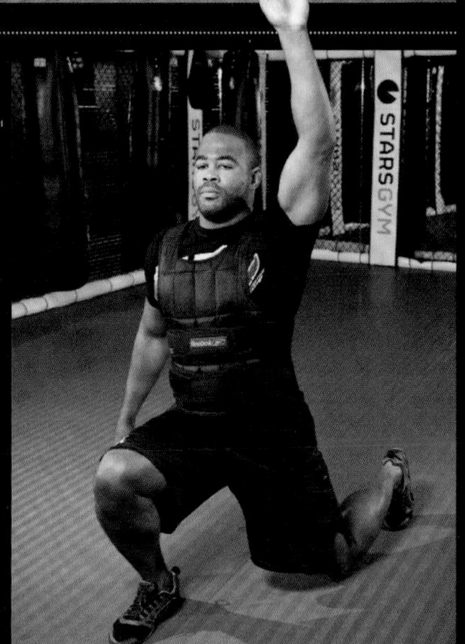

3 Alternating lateral lunge

Reps 8 each side

- Begin with your feet close together and your torso upright, looking forward.
- Take a big step to your right, keeping your left knee in line with your left foot with both feet pointing forward.
- As you step out, raise your arms to a horizontal position.
- Step back to the starting position and repeat on the opposite side, ensuring that your torso is upright and your head is up, looking forward throughout.

Van Arsdale says
'You can find yourself in some unusual positions during an MMA fight, so this move is great for building the ankle stability you need in those positions to reduce the risk of injury.'

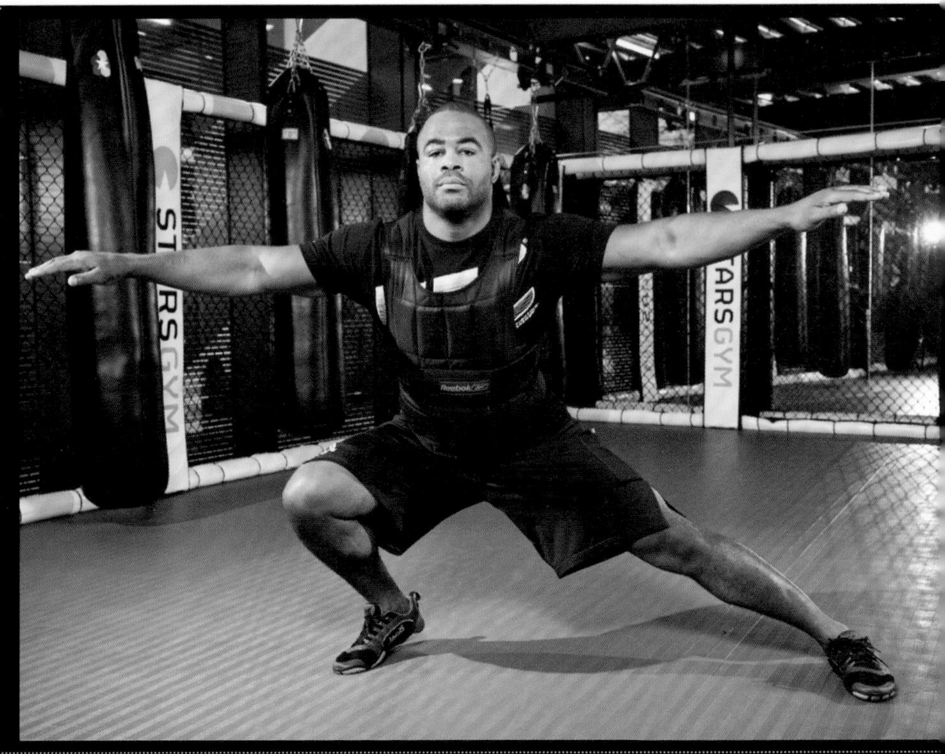

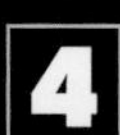

4 Jumping lunge

Reps 8 each side

- Start in a split stance with your right foot forward.
- Bend both knees, keeping them in line with your feet.
- Jump up and swap leg positions in mid-air, landing in a split stance with your left foot forward.
- Repeat the squat.

Van Arsdale says
'Jumping lunges will help to build up your cardio, allowing you to fight hard for a full five-minute round.'

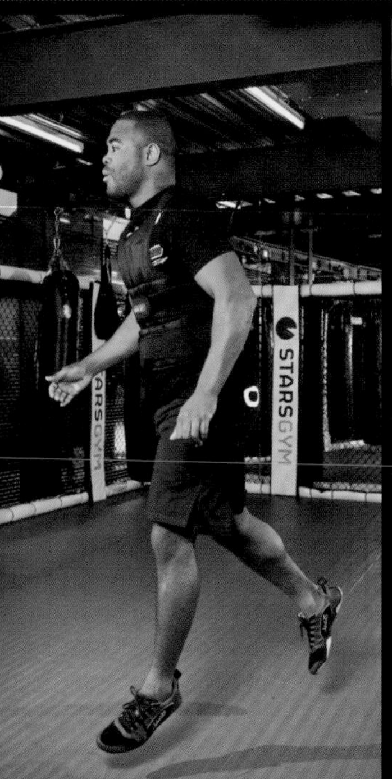

5 Jump squat

Reps 16

- Squat down as in exercise 1.
- Push up explosively to jump off the ground before returning to the starting position.

Van Arsdale says
'Jump squats build explosive power, which will help to improve both your punching and your wrestling.'

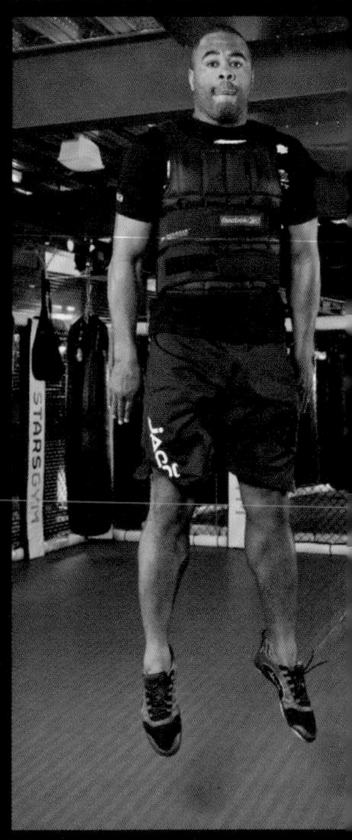

MMA skills

HEADHUNTER

Practise these technique moves alongside your leg-strength workouts and you'll deliver a knockout blow with your hands or feet

1 Overhand right

- With your feet planted, spin your right heel and drive your right knee down.
- Rotate your hips and wind up your right hand.
- Use the power generated by your hips to swing your right hand over your shoulder and down onto your opponent's chin, while keeping your left hand up to protect your chin from a counter-attack.

Evans says

'You have to sit down on your punch and use your hips to generate power. You can't be bouncing around – your legs have to be rooted.' Evans knocked out Chuck Liddell with an overhand right at UFC 88.

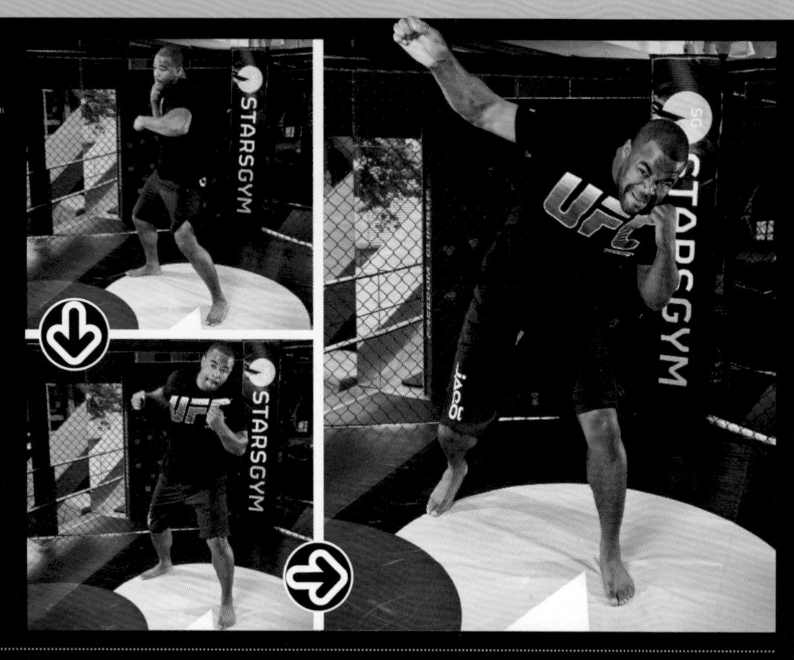

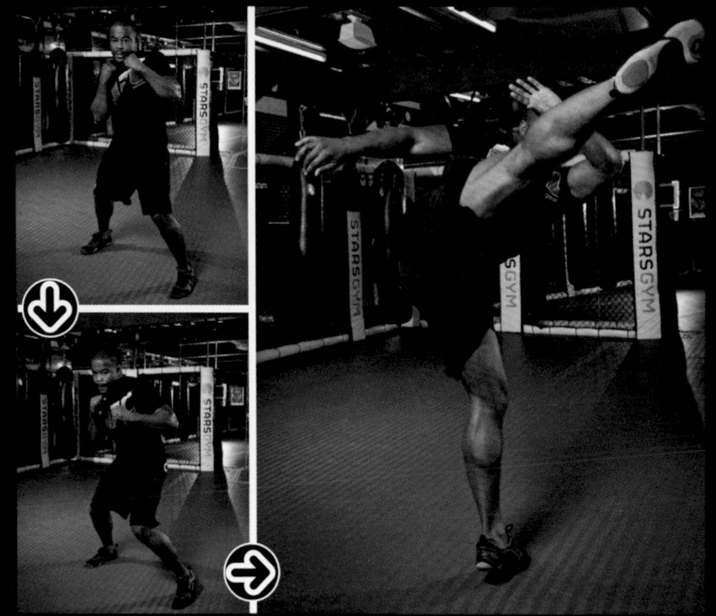

2 Right roundhouse kick to the head

- Stand in a fighting stance with your feet shoulder-width apart and your hands up to protect your face.
- Shift your weight onto your front leg and kick your right leg in an arched motion from the floor to the target, while whipping your right hand past your hip for momentum.
- Lead with your shin and, when the leg is nearing its target, turn your hip to create more speed and leverage. Make sure you pivot on the ball of your left foot to allow your body to turn with the kick, and engage your core throughout.

Evans says

'Keep your left hand up as you throw it and bring your right back up again straight afterwards in case you miss.' Evans used a right roundhouse kick to the head to knock out Sean Salmon at UFC Fight Night: Evans vs Salmon in 2007.

THROW YOUR WEIGHT

British discus record holder Lawrence Okoye on mastering the discus throw and how playing rugby on the wing has helped

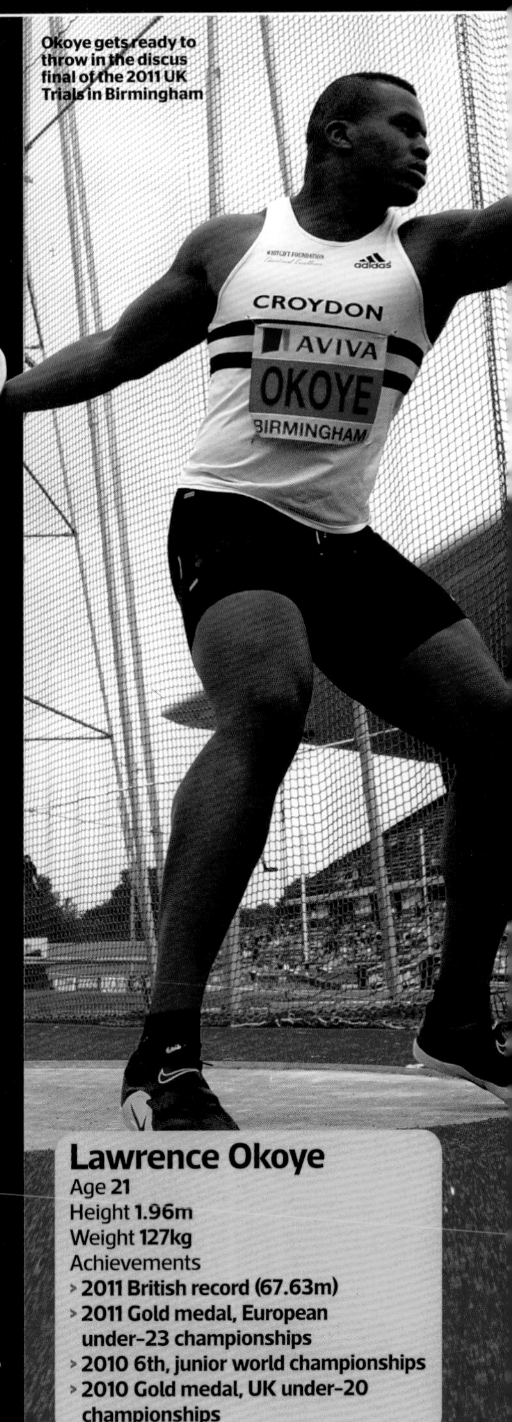

Okoye gets ready to throw in the discus final of the 2011 UK Trials in Birmingham

As record-breakers go, Lawrence Okoye is something of a phenomenon. In July 2011, aged 19, he broke the 13-year-old British discus record with a mammoth throw of 67.63m, and in doing so caught the attention of the athletics world. That's because it was the longest throw recorded by a teenager in the ancient sport's long history and propelled Okoye to ninth in the world rankings.

The former rugby union player – who declined an offer to join the Premiership's London Irish to focus on the discus – only began full-time discus training in September 2010. Given the technical difficulty of the sport, many of the world's top throwers have a couple of decades' training under their belt.

'The best throwers in the world will be throwing from the age of eight or nine, especially in Germany,' says Okoye. 'But I started seriously when I was 18. I'm far behind in that sense but I've made up for it quite quickly and done pretty well. The average age of an Olympic finalist is 30 so to make the final at an Olympics at 20 is very unusual.'

He was unfortunate to miss out on selection for the GB team competing at the 2011 world championships in South Korea but was able to compete on the world stage at the London Olympics, where he reached the final. *MF* joined him at Lee Valley.

What made you choose the discus and start training full-time in 2010?
I'd thrown previously but not seriously at all. I'd do one or two competitions a year just for fun. Then in 2010 my friend Zane Duquemin [who Okoye now trains with] threw really far. I asked him how he did that and he put me in touch with his trainer John Hillier [himself a former international discus thrower]. Four weeks later I had thrown the second furthest for my age group. That's how it started for me. I just went on from there.

What qualities make a good discus thrower?
You need to be powerful. It's an advantage to have long levers – so long arms, long legs. You need to be flexible and have a strong core. Physio after each session helps me

Lawrence Okoye

Age **21**
Height **1.96m**
Weight **127kg**
Achievements
- **2011 British record (67.63m)**
- **2011 Gold medal, European under-23 championships**
- **2010 6th, junior world championships**
- **2010 Gold medal, UK under-20 championships**

Statistics correct at 24th September 2012

maintain my flexibility. The top guys are really strong, stronger than any rugby player, but speed and power are crucial too. Those who can move quickly with strength and power in that way are really impressive.

Have any skills you learned on the rugby field transferred to the discus?
Playing rugby has been great for this discipline because I need to be able to move my body quickly. I played on the wing so speed and acceleration were essential. The last thing you want is to be slow. I was already naturally powerful before I started throwing and lifting for the sport and that's why I'd say rugby has helped me get to where I am in the discus.

Is the upper or lower body more important?
The lower body is definitely more essential to the discus but the upper body is important because it's where you finish the throw. Everything starts with your lower body – that's where you get most of your power. The bench press is not as important as my squat or clean. The only upper-body training I do is in the gym and I get the strength from the bench, incline bench, flyes and lateral raises. I don't do much for the arms because they don't really contribute much for the throw. I don't need to do biceps curls at all; if I do, I do them just for the beach [laughs].

Do you need to do any endurance work?
No. There is minimal cardio work so it's very important that I look after my nutrition to keep on top of my body fat. But I will do some anaerobic fitness such as interval sprinting.

Lawrence Okoye uses products from Maximuscle to optimise his sporting performance. For more information visit maximuscle.com.

Lawrence Okoye's WORKOUT

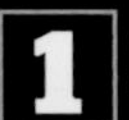

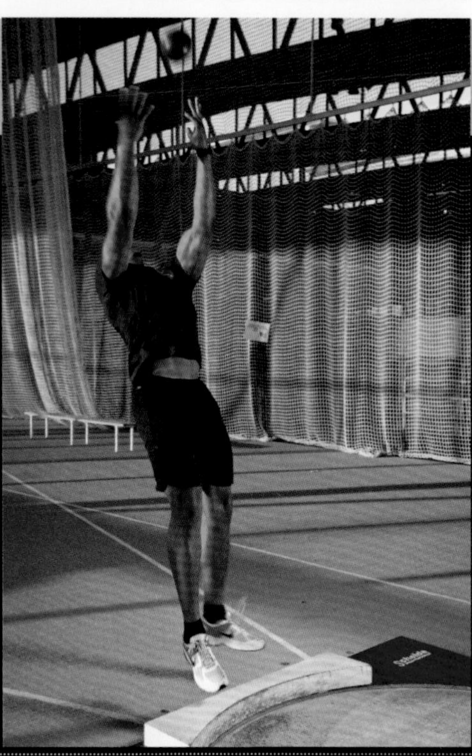

1 Overhead throw

Sets 1 **Reps** 10

- Stand on a slightly raised platform holding a standard 7.26kg rubber shot put or medicine ball with straight arms.
- Squat down and drive your hips forward and yourself up and back off the floor to launch the weight behind you.

Okoye says
'Overheads are an explosive move upwards, involving your hips and lower back. Powerful hips are vital to get distance in your throw.'

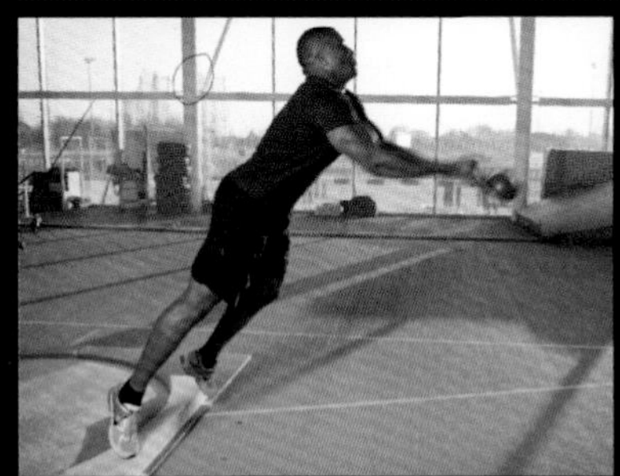

2 Underarm throw

Sets 1 **Reps** 6

- Face the opposite way from the overheads and this time use your hips to accelerate yourself up and forwards.
- Drive from your heels all the way through to the release.

Okoye says
'These are more quad-based but they help develop explosive power in the hips and legs. All the power should come from the lower body to mimic the discus throw.'

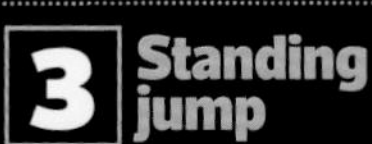

3 Standing jump

Sets 1 **Reps** 10

- Use your arms to generate momentum and drive forwards with your hips as you push off your feet.
- A variation is to combine three standing jumps as one rep, aiming to maintain the energy and momentum throughout.

Okoye says
'This will transfer the motion from my arms all the way through to my leg drive. My PB is 3.31m.'

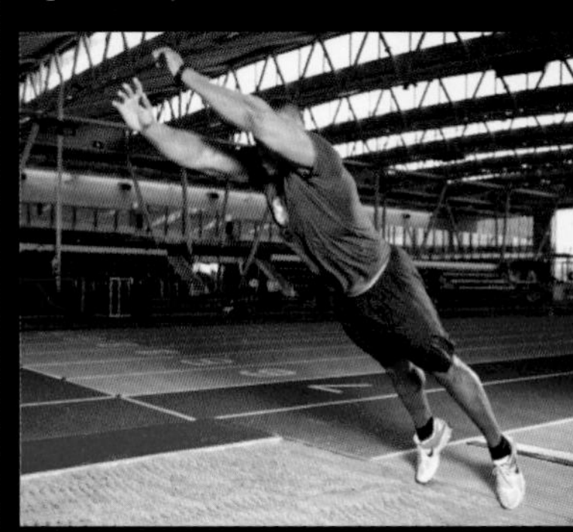

Discus

4 Power clean

Sets 5 **Reps** 3-5

- Hold a bar level with your thighs with your hands shoulder-width apart.
- Explode upwards with your hips, bringing the bar up to shoulder height and then back down. Your arms should do as little of the work as possible.

Okoye says

'I do normal cleans as well but this technique, where you don't "catch" the bar at the top, means I can go heavier with the weight and emphasises the power I can generate from my hips. I'll usually hit around 140kg for three.'

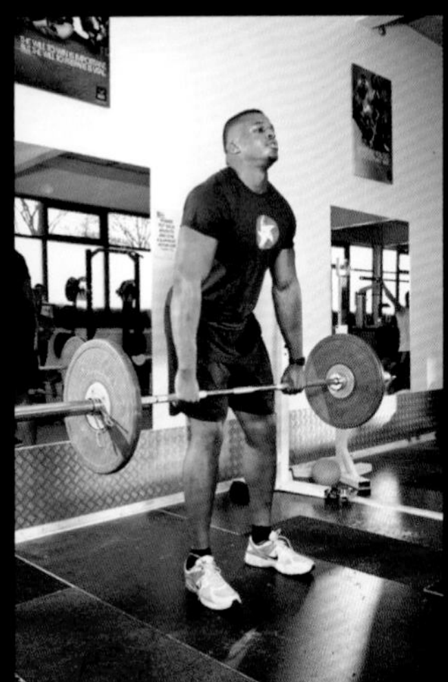

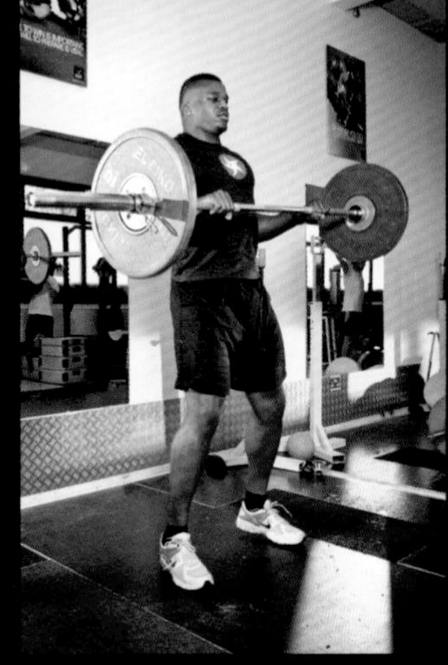

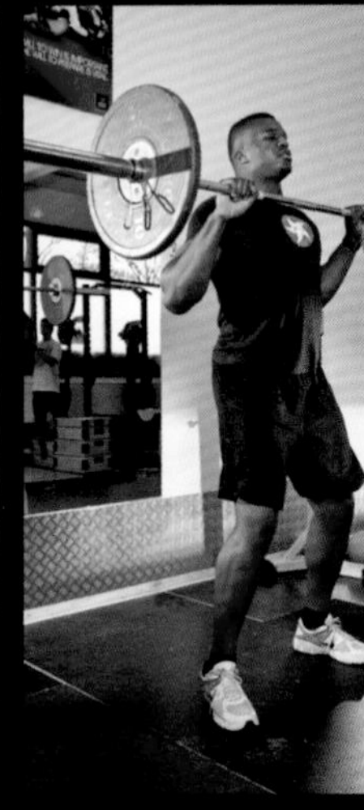

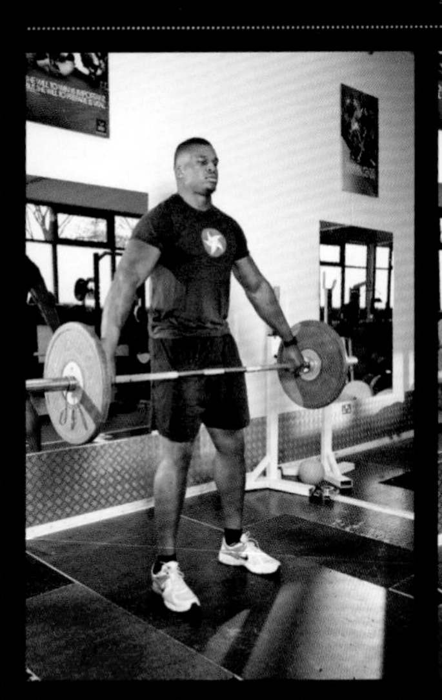

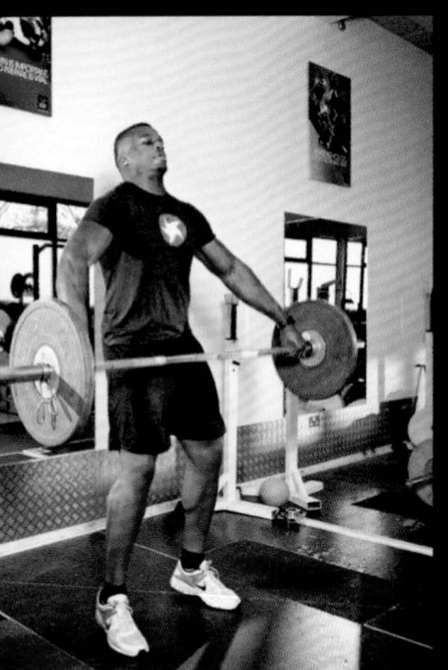

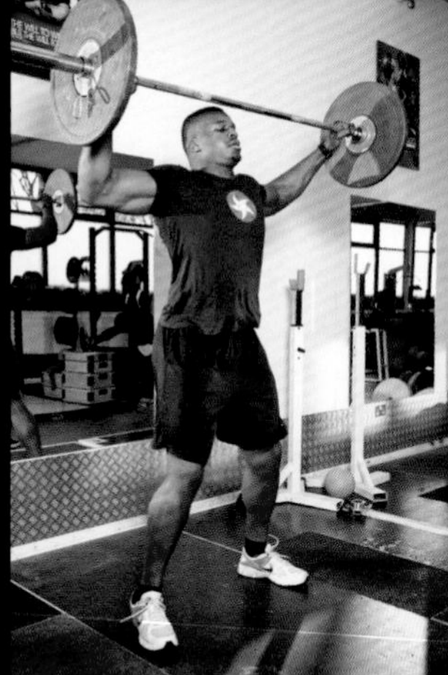

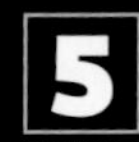

5 Power snatch

Sets 5 **Reps** 3-5

- Hold a bar with your hands double shoulder-width apar
- Drive your hips forwards and accelerate the bar upwards to around head height before lowering it.

Okoye says

'I perform the snatch usir the same principles as th clean. It's all about intens and dynamic movement keep the reps low but the weight high. I'll normally around 100kg for three.'

Anatomy of a discus throw

Lawrence Okoye explains how his workout produces his 67m-plus discus throw

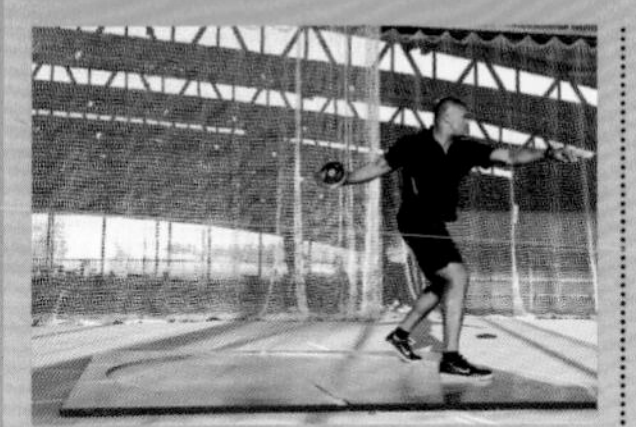

'Stand tall at the back of the circle with your hips forward and knees slightly bent. Relax and wind up by twisting from side to side. The core work helps maintain energy transfer throughout the throw.'

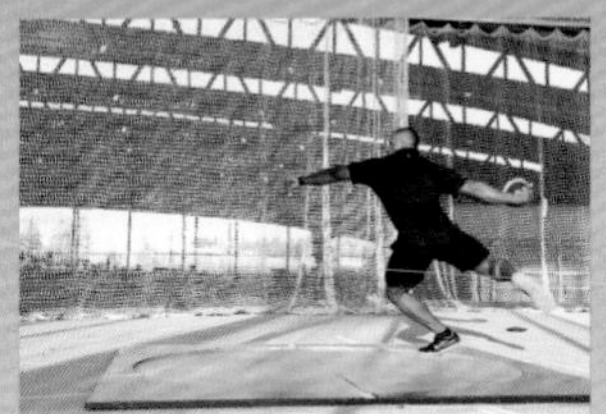

'Pivot on the ball of your left foot, getting your bodyweight outside the circle with a long sweep of your right leg.'

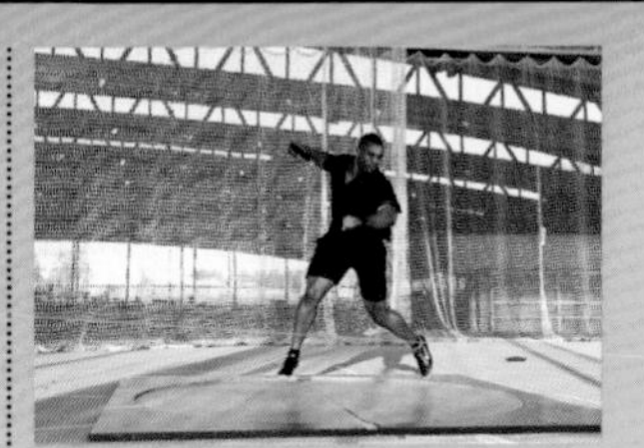

'Turning back into the circle, drive hard off your left leg, jumping towards the front. This is where the shot put and standing jump work come in.'

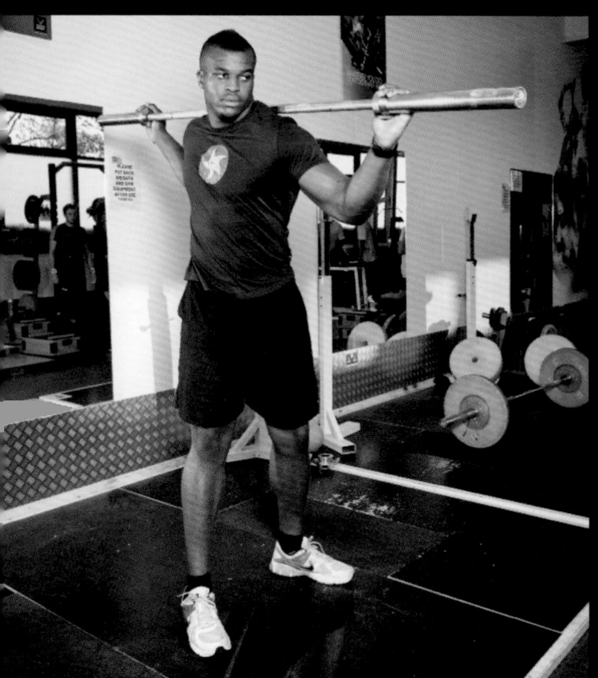

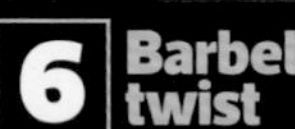

6 Barbell twist

Sets 3 **Reps** 10-15

- Stand holding a barbell across your shoulders.
- Bracing your core, twist from side to side slowly, keeping your head looking forwards.

Okoye says
'This helps mirror the rotation required for the discus. It is all about getting the midsection and obliques strong because they take a battering when you throw.'

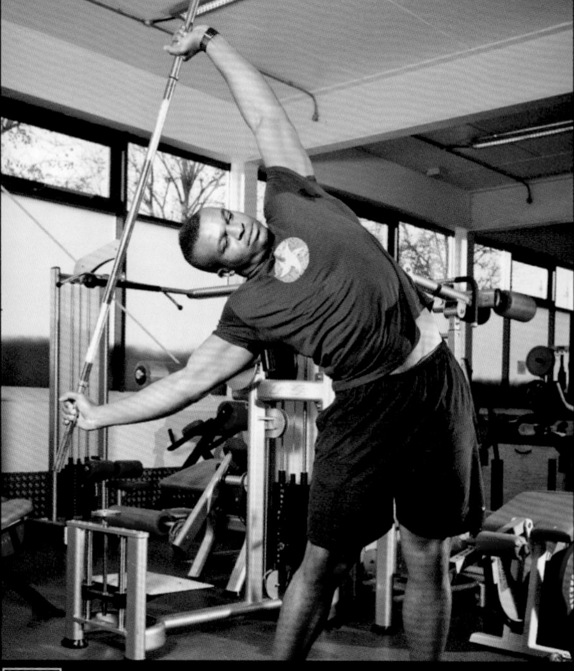

7 Barbell side bend

Sets 3 **Reps** 5 each side

- Hold an empty bar with your hands twice shoulder-width apart and your arms straight.
- Contracting your core, slowly bend to one side. Alternate sides.

Okoye says
'Make sure the movement is slow and controlled. Contract your obliques as hard as possible to work the core. Doing them quicker defeats the purpose. I normally use an empty 20kg barbell.'

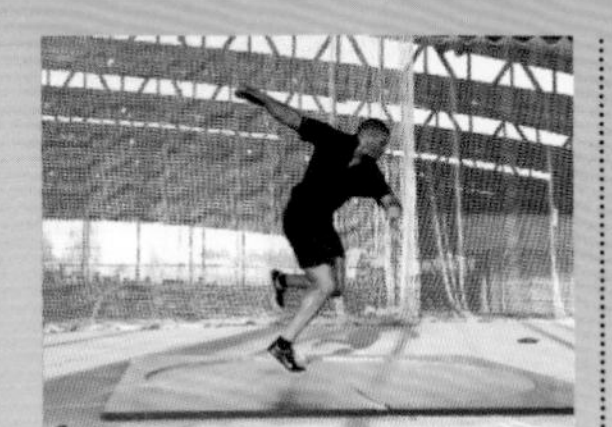

'Sweeping your right leg back in, aim to land in the middle of the circle. Get your left foot down at the front of the circle quickly, keeping your upper body as "wrapped" as possible.'

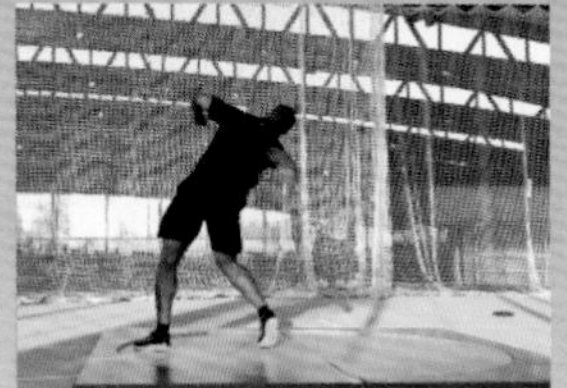

'There are two ways of throwing at this point: feet down or reverse. People who reverse leave the ground when they deliver and their right foot replaces the left.'

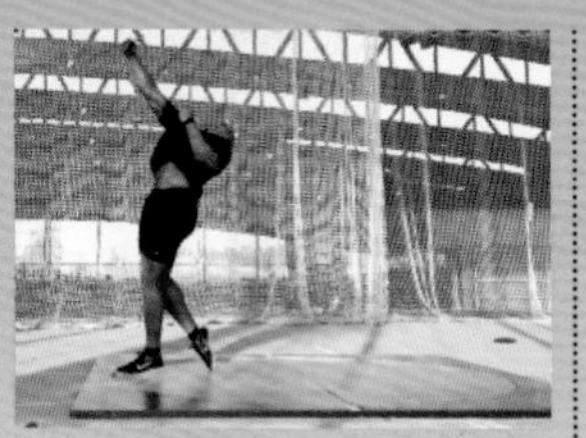

'I throw feet down. For this, as you turn your right foot, knee and hip inwards your right leg hits your left but both stay on the floor. It makes the delivery more like a punch and triggers your right arm to whip through as you throw.'

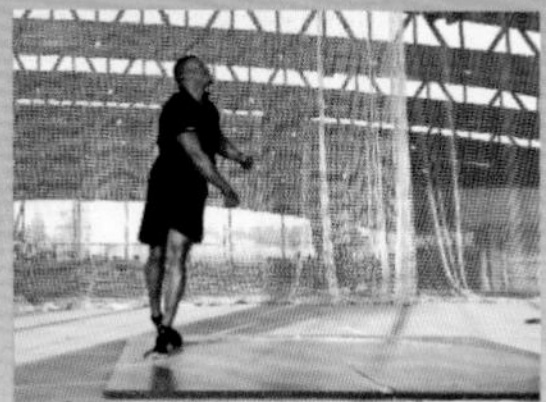

'Good balance, and ensuring you put the generated force through the discus, will keep you within the circle so you don't foul.'

OFF TO A FLYER

British long jump record holder Chris Tomlinson on how to power into the sandpit – and why he doesn't bench press

Like most of Britain's elite athletes, long jumper Chris Tomlinson is no stranger to hard work. In 2002 he broke both wrists going for a personal best in the power clean, but was back to training (in casts) within days and broke the British record three months later – a record he recently extended to 8.35m. And, as MF found out when we joined him at Lee Valley, he thinks he can go even further, given the right preparation. 'Having stepping stones to success is important,' says Tomlinson, who's friendly in the gym but all business when it's time to hit the field. 'My stepping stones are technique, discipline and diet. You work on improving them and eventually it comes together.'

What's the key to a good long jump?
Power and explosiveness. Technique's important, but technique won't give you the difference between a 6.20m and an 8.20m – it'll give you the difference between an 8.30m and an 8.35m. It'll get you a record, but you need the leg strength to get close to it in the first place.

So you do squats rather than bench presses?
Yeah. We're trying to defy gravity, and any weight we have on our upper body is pulling us down. I'd probably have trouble bench pressing my bodyweight, but I power clean about 140kg and I can one-leg snatch 90kg. You also need a lot of flexibility – I'll do a lot of yoga poses, especially before I get on a flight.

> 'We're trying to defy gravity, and upper-body weight will pull us down'

Do you do a lot of single-leg work?
Well, everything has to be as transferable as possible. Some guys might be able to standing long jump or vertical jump half a metre further than me, but I'll beat them in a running long jump. I do quite a lot of full jumps compared with other people – you need to make sure that what you're doing is training the full approach. I'll generally do two sessions jumping maximally in a week, and I might do three to seven jumps in a session. You're practising running, take-offs, plyometrics, the leg chute... it's like putting together a jigsaw and every piece counts.

What else do you have to work on?
I do a few yoga poses, I do a lot of flexibility work. I'll do a lot of it

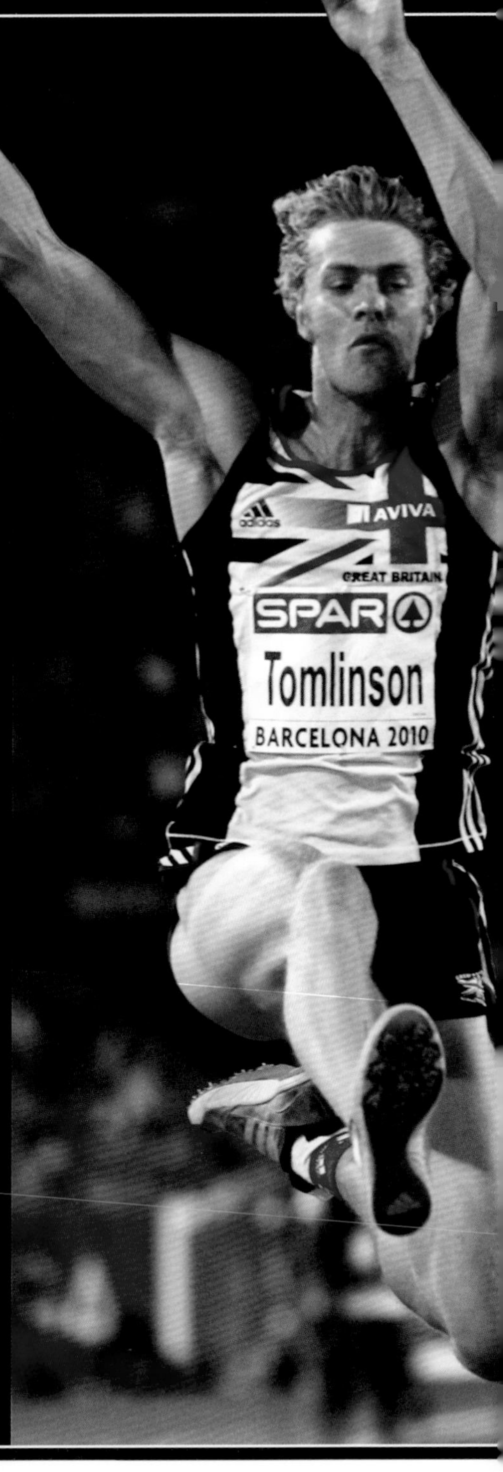

Statistics correct at 24th September 2012

when I go on a flight – it's especially important in international competitions, when you're stiffening up from cramming yourself into a seat.

Chris Tomlinson

Age **31**
Height **1.98m**
Weight **85kg**
Achievements
- **2011 British record (8.35m)**
- **2010 Bronze medal, European championships**
- **2008 Silver medal, world indoor championships**

Are you happy with how your training is going?
At the moment I'm on a pretty good high. [In 2001] I had my most successful start to a season ever and broke the British record. I'm doing some world-class long jumping.

Breaking both wrists sounds like a bad injury. How did you do it and how badly did it affect your training?
I was going for my power clean max at the time, 107kg. As I went to catch the bar, I got underneath it, lost my balance and one wrist went, then the other one. In terms of injuries, it's probably one of the less significant ones I've had because so much of what I do is with my legs. I ran with my casts on, I did squats with them on – there were plenty of other things I could do.

Chris Tomlinson's WORKOUT

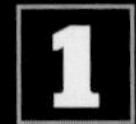

1 One-leg snatch

Sets 3 **Reps** 3

- Hold a bar with your hands double shoulder-width apart, with one leg raised slightly off the floor.
- Drive your hips forward and accelerate the bar upwards.

Tomlinson says
'Holding the top position of the snatch reinforces the position you want for the "hang" part of a long jump. I'll warm up with this.'

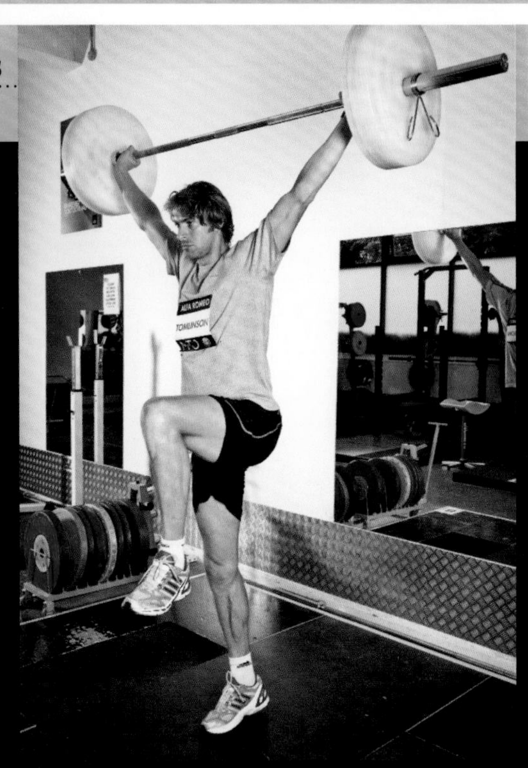

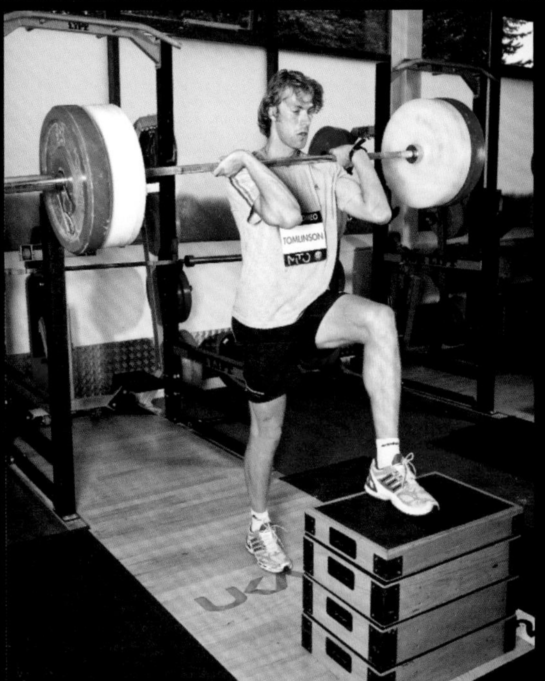

2 One-leg clean

Sets 3 **Reps** 3

- Hold a bar with your hands roughly shoulder-width apart, with one leg raised slightly off the floor and a box at knee height in front of you.
- Explode upwards with your hips and 'catch' the bar in a normal clean position, planting your leg on the box. Your arms should do as little of the work as possible.

Tomlinson says
'I do normal cleans as well, but these really emphasise driving off a single leg, which is very sport-specific.'

Long jump

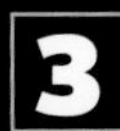

Bulgarian split squat

Sets 3 **Reps** 5

- Hold a bar across your shoulders and put one foot on a box set to roughly knee height.
- Squat down until your lead thigh is parallel to the floor. Push back up through your heel.

Tomlinson says
'These are more about strength than power. I'll do them after I've done my snatches and cleans – and not in the same session as jumping.'

'You practise running, take-offs, plyometrics, the leg chute… it's like putting together a jigsaw and every piece counts'

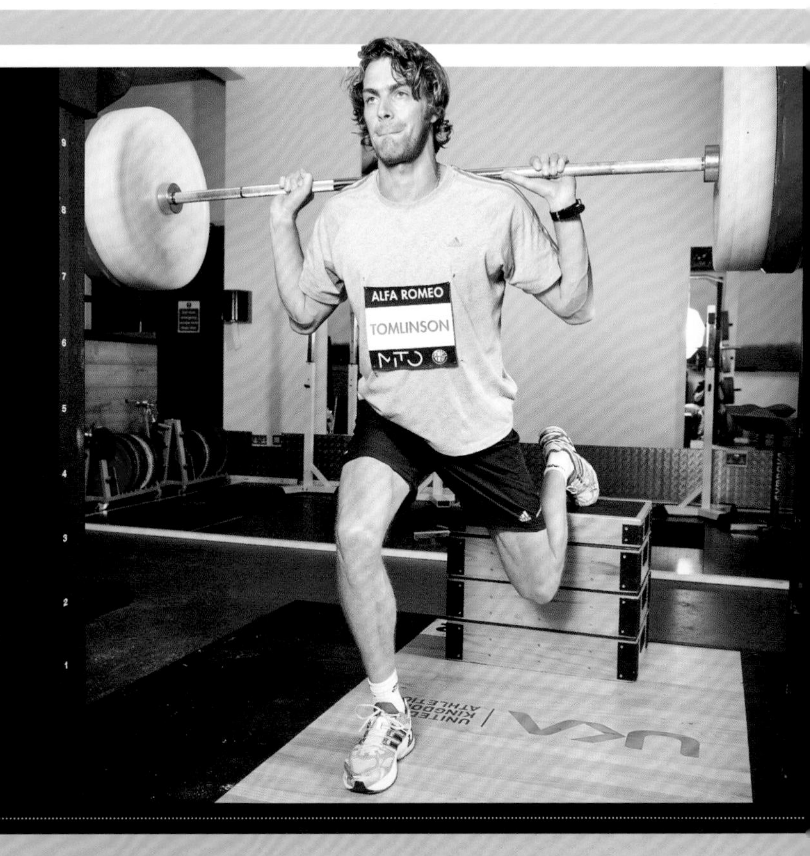

Anatomy of a jump

Chris Tomlinson explains how his workout builds to an 8m-plus leap

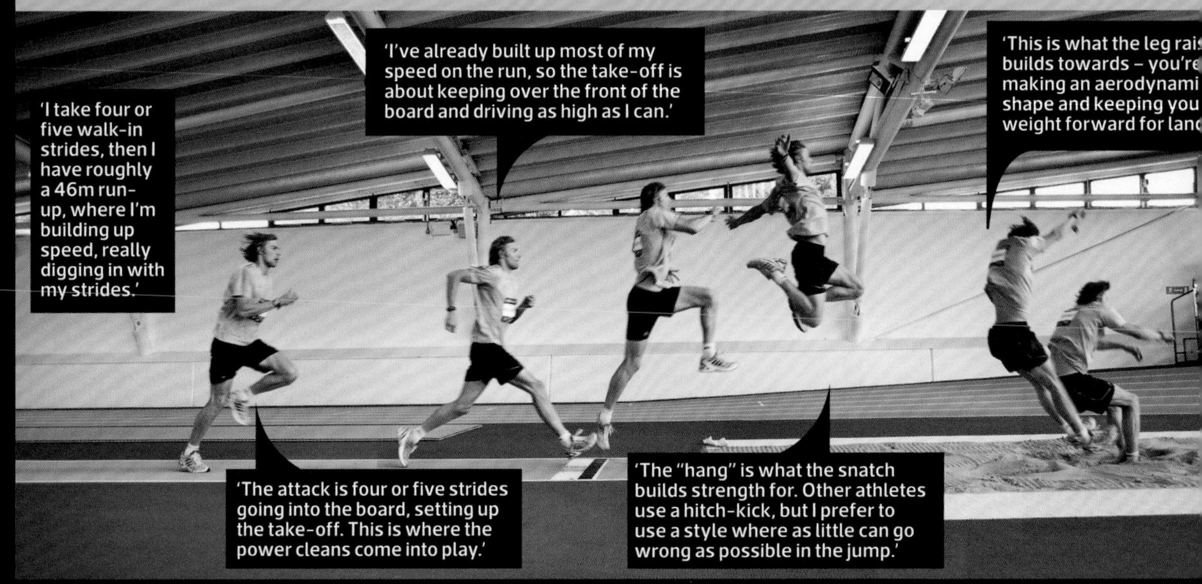

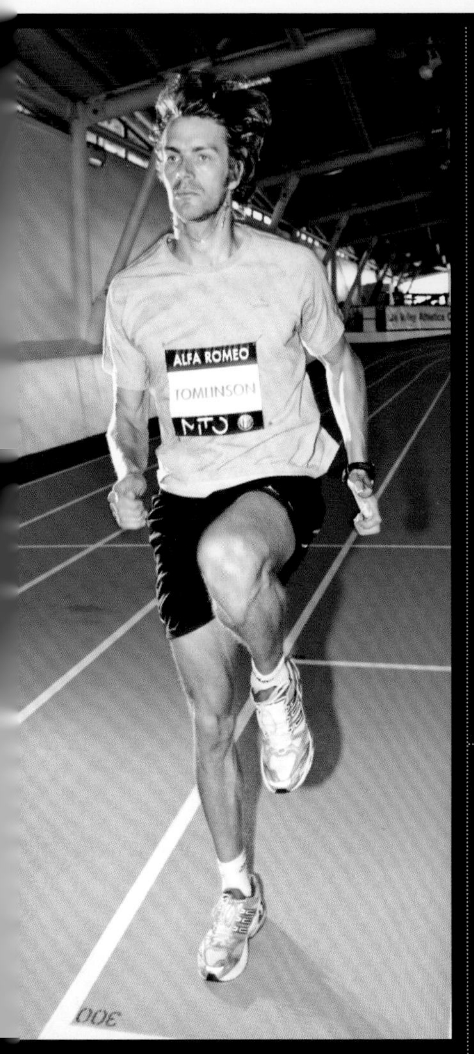

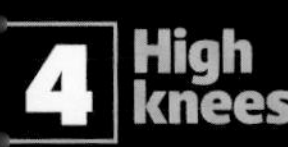

4 High knees

Sets 5 **Reps** 20m

- Run while bringing your knees high – your thighs should be at least parallel to the floor at the top of each stride.
- Keep your arms bent at a roughly 90° angle. Your thumbs should go from hip to lip – if you extend any further, you're losing power.

Tomlinson says

This drill is a great foundation for running. If you get it right, your top-end running mechanics will be pretty decent. Stay light on your feet.'

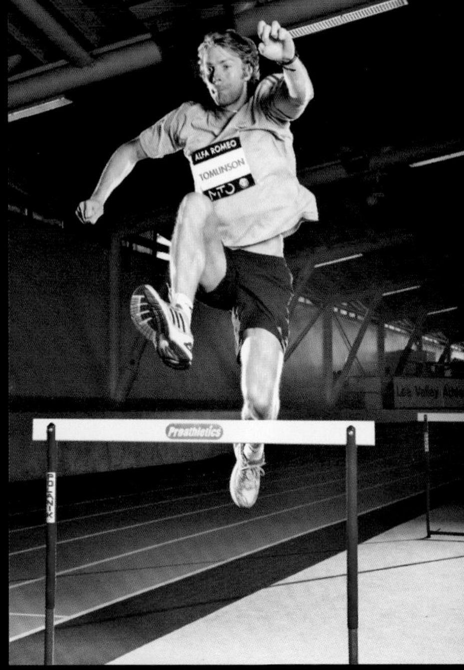

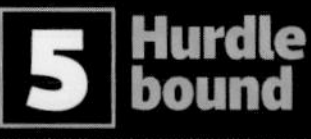

5 Hurdle bound

Sets 3 **Reps** 2

- Set two hurdles at a height that's just about manageable, roughly 5m apart.
- Bound over them as if you're taking off for a long jump. Emphasise height rather than speed.

Tomlinson says

'Single-leg explosiveness is really important. There are plenty of guys who'll beat me on a two-footed vertical or broad jump, but they can't beat me in the long jump.'

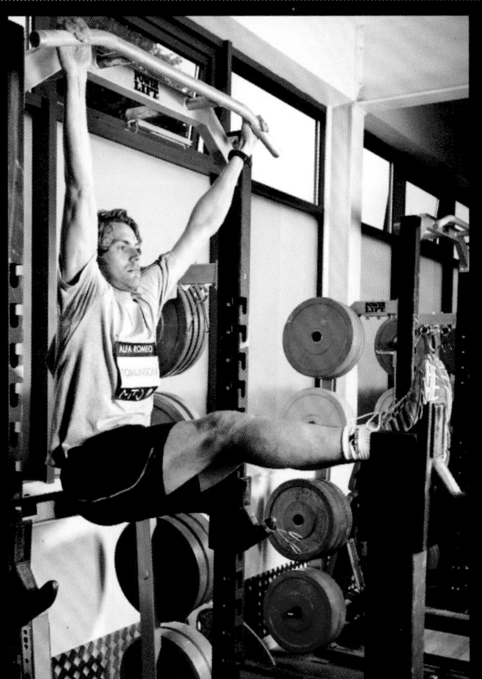

6 Hanging leg raise

Sets 3 **Reps** 30sec

- Hang from a bar with your palms facing forward. Raise your legs until they're parallel to the floor, then hold.
- If it's too difficult at first, start out doing it with your knees bent and build up to the straight-leg version.

Tomlinson says

'I use this to help me hold the leg chute position at the end of the jump. It's good for your hip flexors, too.'

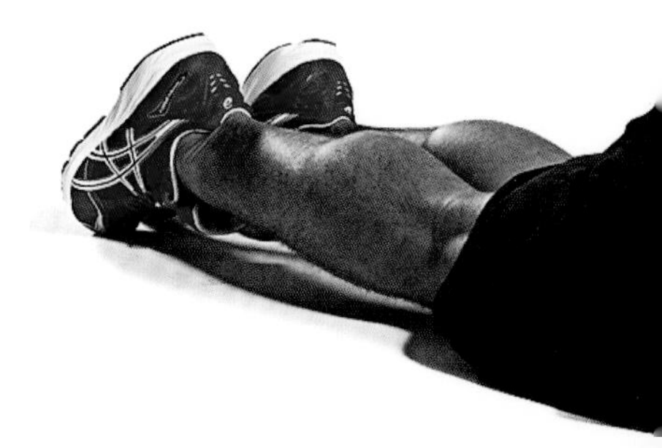

Carve rock hard abs

Do these moves to sculpt a solid six-pack

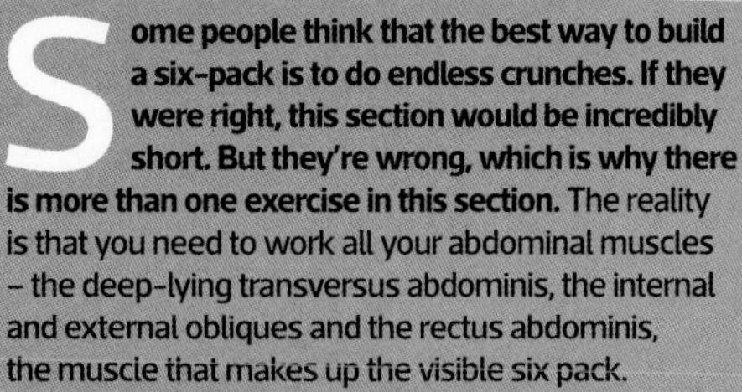

Some people think that the best way to build a six-pack is to do endless crunches. If they were right, this section would be incredibly short. But they're wrong, which is why there is more than one exercise in this section. The reality is that you need to work all your abdominal muscles – the deep-lying transversus abdominis, the internal and external obliques and the rectus abdominis, the muscle that makes up the visible six pack.

Of course, if your body fat levels are too high, you won't be able to see your six-pack, so you also need to do programmes such as the 12-week body plan. Doing direct abs work as well as the main training programme is the best way of adding real size to your abs so that they stand out.

SIX-PACK MOVES

YOUR ROUTE TO KILLER ABS

Barbell rollout	p116
Modified V-sit	p117
Reverse crunch	p118
Dumbbell crunch	p119
Star side plank	p120
Medicine ball crunch and throw	p121
Gym ball jackknife twist	p122
Hand walkout	p123

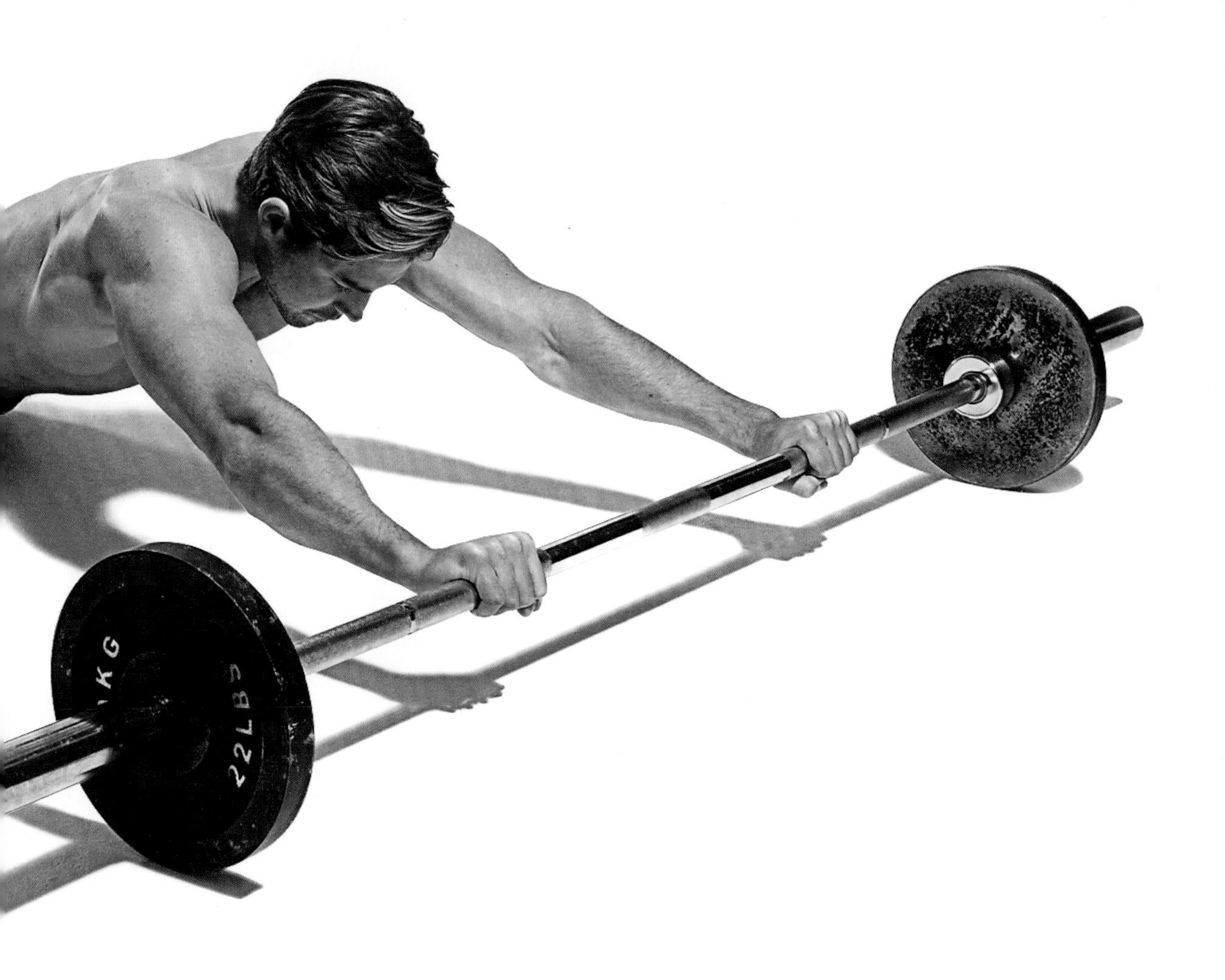
22LBS

Barbell rollout

Sets 4
Reps 4-

Do the barbell rollout to get better at sport and bag a six-pack

When it comes to abs training, sports and conditioning coaches don't see eye to eye with physique-focused trainers. Sports coaches are wary of isolation moves and conventional abs exercises that have little application on the field. One of the few abs exercises that both camps love, however, is the rollout. This is beacuse it packs a lot into one moves – it works the whole kinetic chain (your muscles, bones and nerves), requires stability at the end of the range of movement and strength to get back to the start position.

Why do it

- This exercise is ideal for the end of your workout because it will exhaust your abs.

How to do it

- Start by kneeling on the floor with your hands on the bar, below your shoulders and just wider than shoulder-width apart.
- Your spine should remain in a neutral position throughout the move.
- Contract your abs and slowly roll the bar away from you, making sure you don't let your hips drop and your back hyperextend.
- When you can't go any further without compromising good form, roll the bar back to the start.

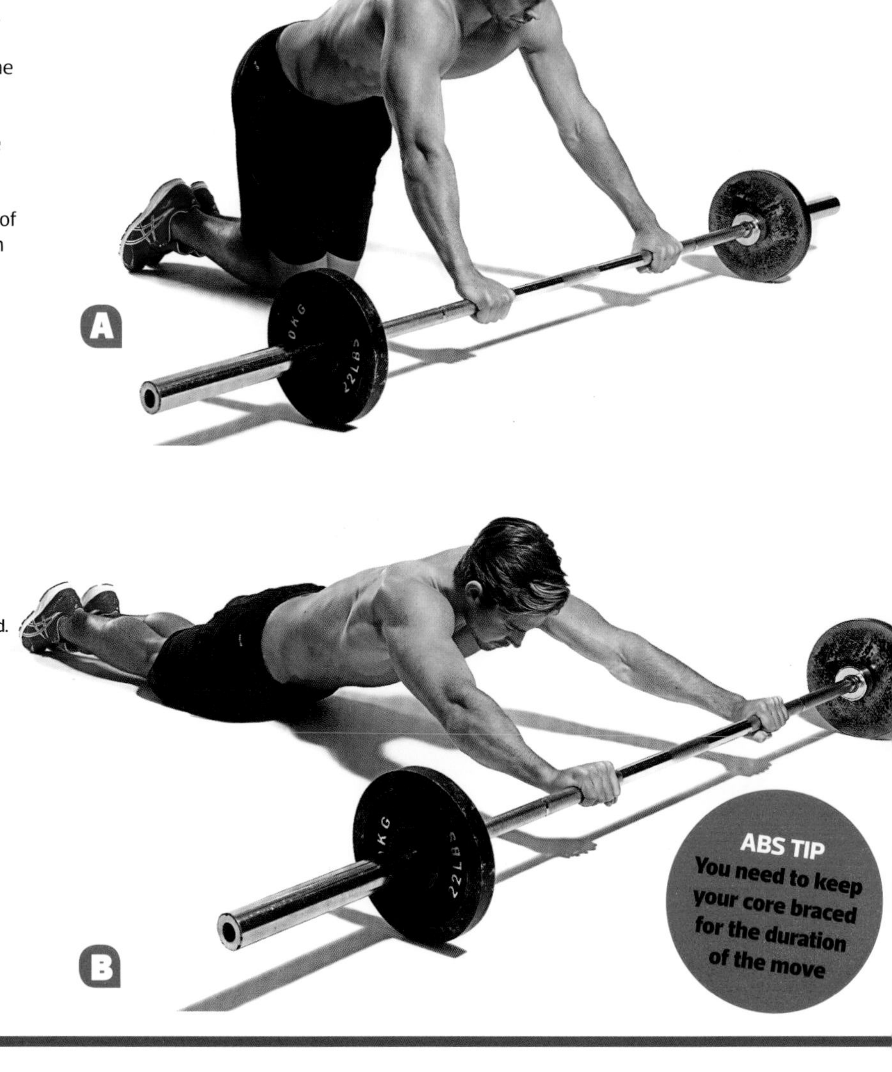

ABS TIP
You need to keep your core braced for the duration of the move

Modified V-sit

Sets 4
Reps 12

:ulpting a solid six-pack doesn't 'ways require heavy weights

Time under tension is important for building muscle, and there's no better way to keep ır abs under pressure for an ended period than with a ıtrolled V-sit. The full version uires good hip flexibility, this modified version can done by anyone and works ır obliques, hip extensors balance as well as the lominals. Stay fractionally the ground between reps s tough, but you'll see benefits in the mirror.

ıy do it

ıis exercise hits your upper ıd lower abs in one go.

w to do it

ɘ flat with your arms by your sides ıd your feet together just off the floor. t up and extend your arms forward hile at the same time bringing ur knees in to your chest. owly return to the starting position.

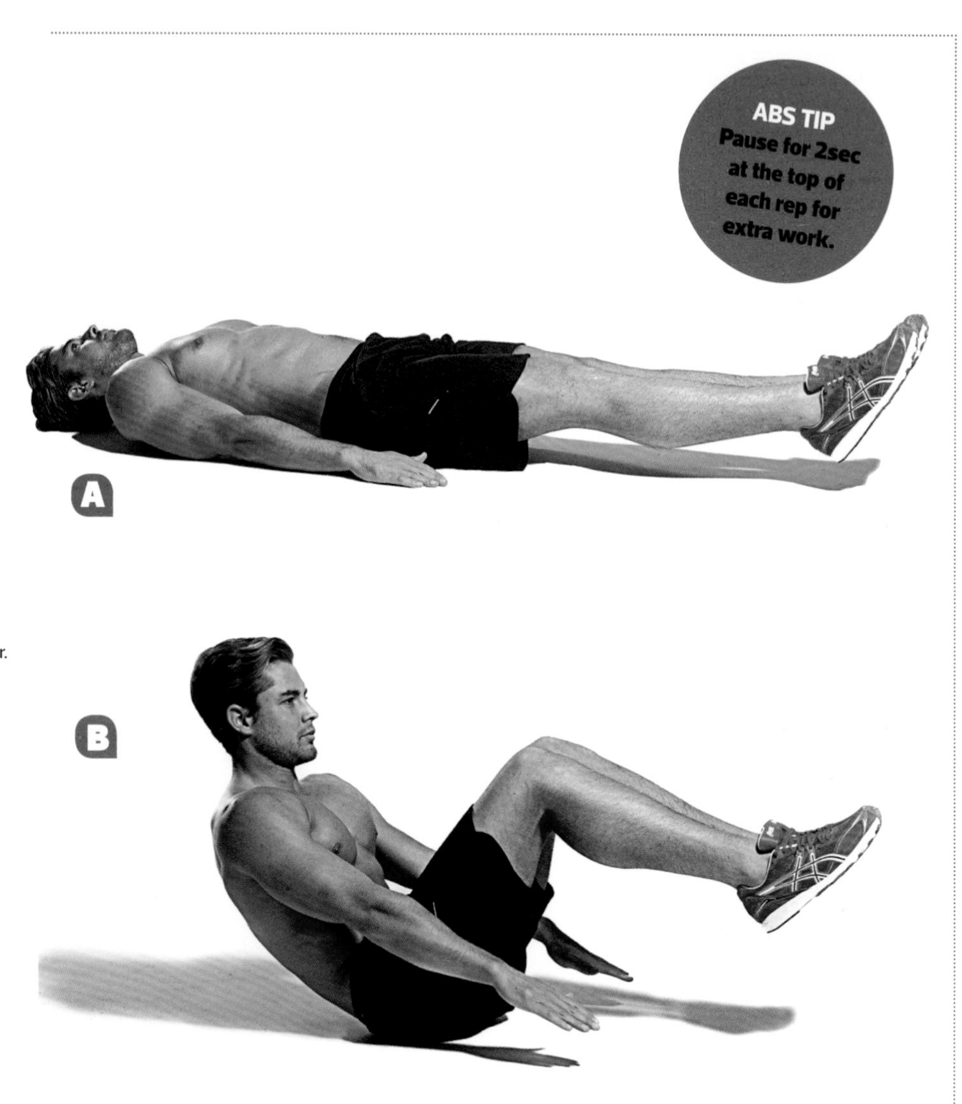

Reverse crunch

Sets 4
Reps 12

Working your lower abs is the only way to get a proper six-pack

If you've been training your abs hard with crunches, you've probably already built a two-pack. But if you fail to include any lower abs exercises into your workout regime, all you're doing is ensuring that this two-pack never spreads south and turns into a solid six-pack that you could grate cheese on. This specifically targets your lower abs so you can complete your rock-hard core.

Why do it

> It works the muscles that the standard crunch can't reach.

How to do it

> Start with your head and shoulders flat on the floor with your fingertips at your temples, your knees bent at 90° and your feet flat on the floor.
> Contract your abs to lift your hips, then curl your knees towards your chest, keeping them bent at 90°. Pause at the top, squeezing your abs, then lower your legs slowly back to the start.

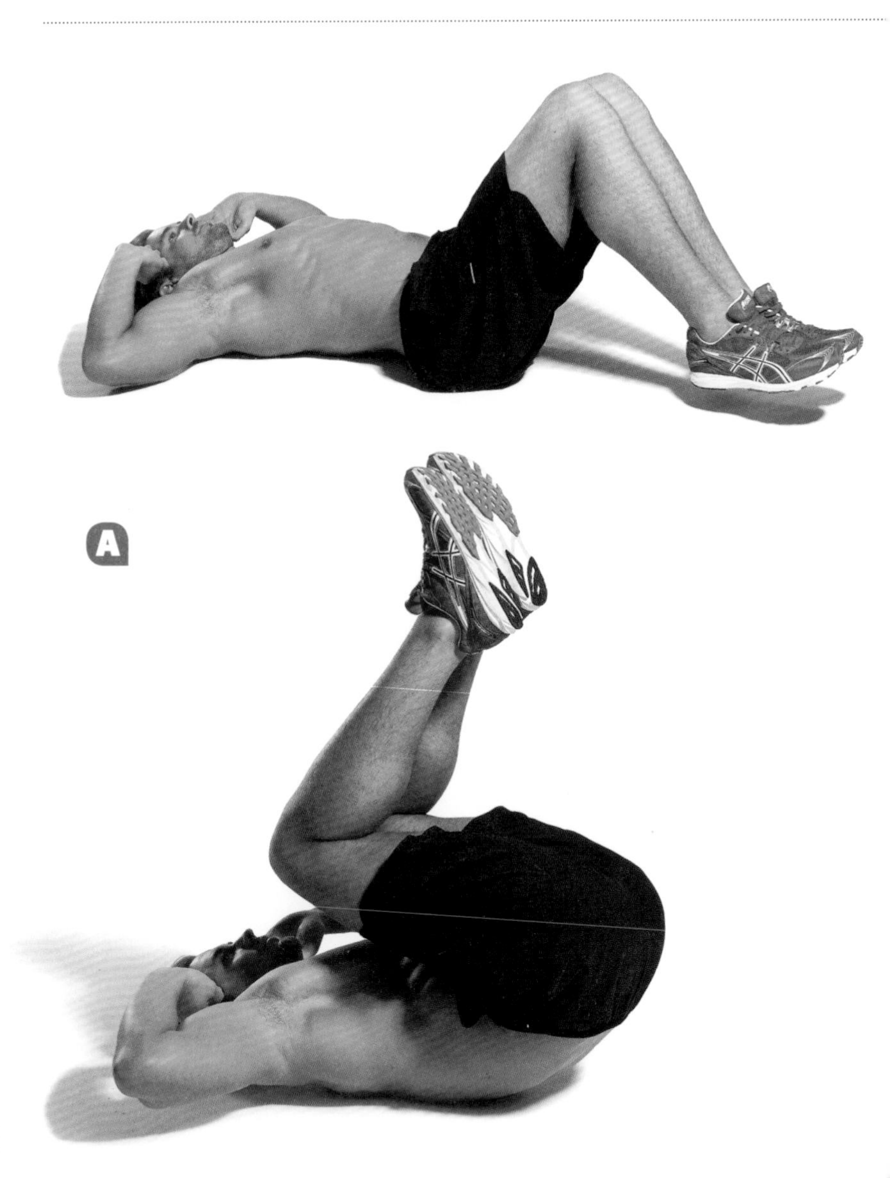

ABS TIP
Lowering your legs under control will increase this move's effect

Dumbbell crunch

ɑake the classic abs move harder ɑnd get a six-pack quicker

Sets 4
Reps 12

Are you doing crunches until the cows come home but still finding you haven't sculpted the ·rfect six-pack? The chances are ·u're not working your abs hard ·ough. Like every other muscle ·oup, they need increasingly heavy ·ads to keep growing. The fix is ·mple: start adding extra weight the crunch to force your abs out their comfort zone so they have · choice but to grow back bigger.

·hy do it

Endless crunches won't work forever – adding weight forces your muscles to adapt and grow.

·ow to do it

·ie on your back with knees ·ent, holding a dumbbell in each ·and with bent elbows.
·ontract your abs to lift your torso ·p, straightening your arms as your ·hest rises towards your knees to ·ake the weights towards your feet.
·ause at the top of the move before ·owering slowly back to the start.

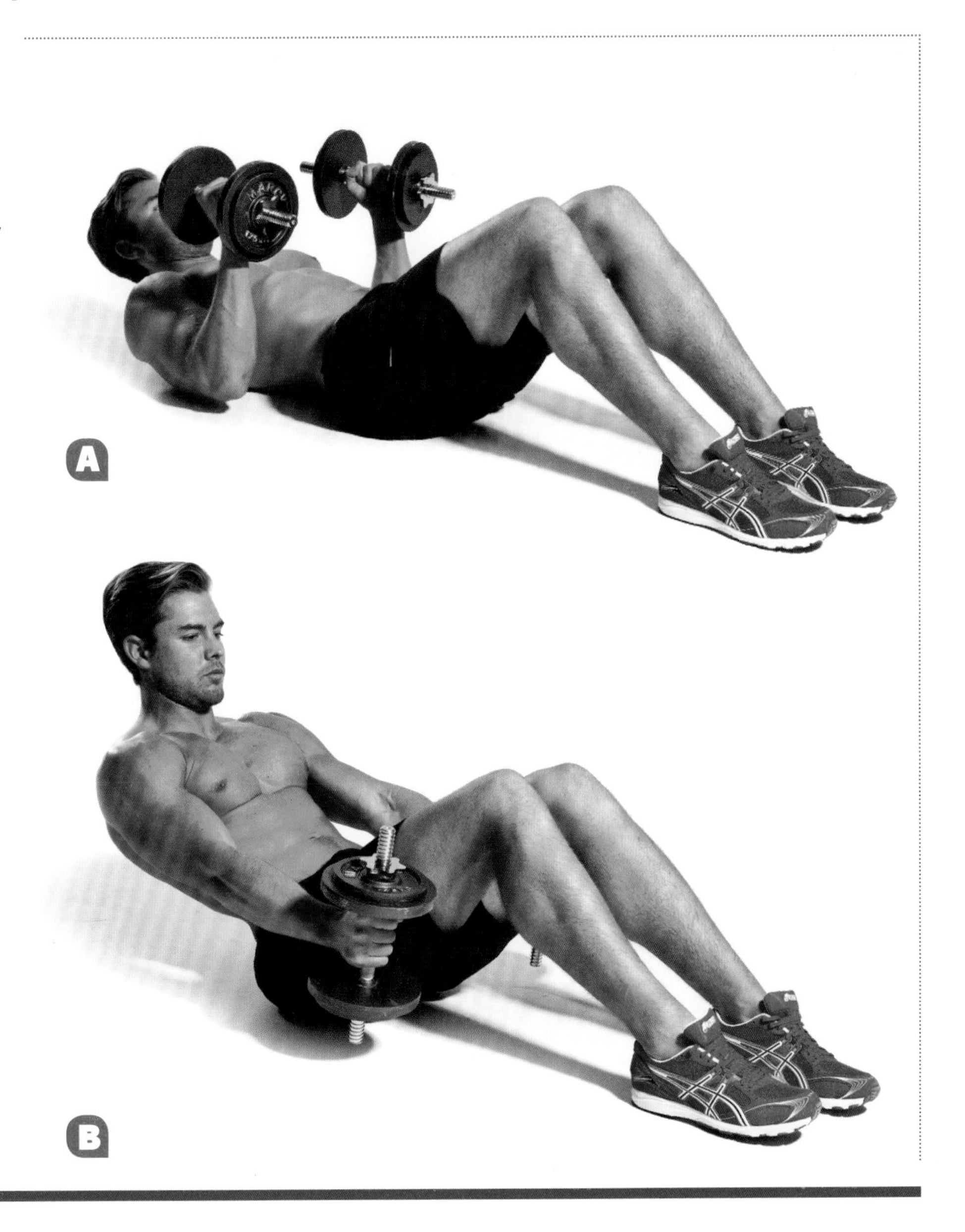

Star side plank

Get better core control with this super-effective static move

Sets 6
Time
10-15sec
each side

You can't underestimate the importance of having a solid core. Not only will it allow you to lift heavier in all the major lifts and move more effectively on the sports pitch, you'll also have the foundations to build an impressive six-pack. This upgrade on the plank will work your core and obliques – those muscles either side of your abs – really hard, as well as recruiting muscles in your shoulders and quads as you raise and straighten your arm and legs to form a star shape. It's a great (and strangely under-used) move to build stability and strength across your body.

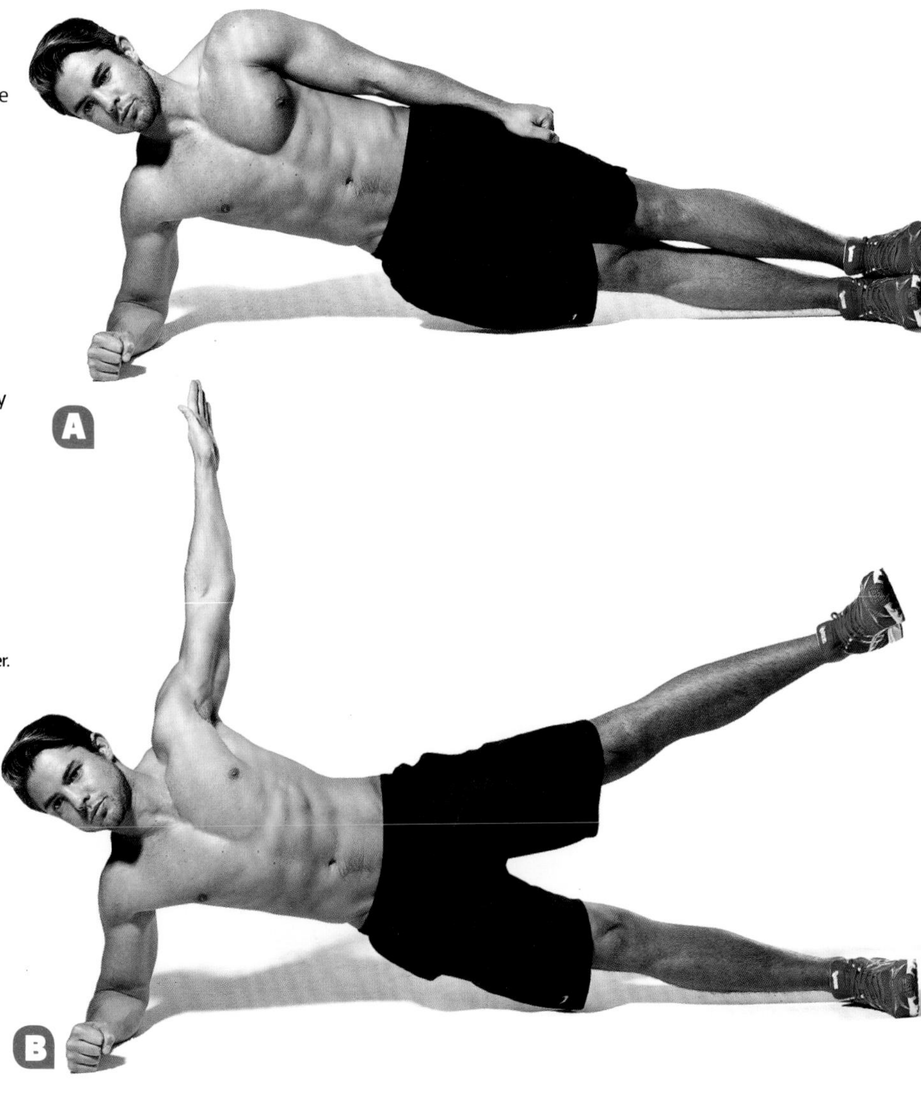

Why do it

> It's a variation on the classic plank that'll blitz your obliques.

How to do it

> Lie on your side, supported on one forearm with your elbow under your shoulder and one leg on top of the other.
> Raise your hips off the ground to form a straight line from head to heels, then raise and straighten your arm and leg and hold.

ABS TIP
Once you can hold it for 15sec, try it with a light dumbbell in your raised hand

Medicine ball crunch and throw

Sets 4
Reps 12

dd a medicine ball throw to our crunch for a solid six-pack

Doing cunches is a good start if you're trying to build an impressive six-pack. But adding weight d explosive power to the move th the medicine ball crunch and ow makes for a tough and highly ective abs builder. Not only are ur abs forced to work harder crunch your torso up with the tra resistance from the med ll and generate enough force to pel the ball forward, but they o need to keep your torso up so at you can receive the ball back.

hy do it

Holding the ball forces you to control our core throughout the move.

ow to do it

tart flat on your back with knees ent at 90°, holding a medicine ball vith both hands against your chest. runch up and powerfully push e medicine ball away from you wards a partner. Hold at the top of e move as he passes the ball back, en lower back down and repeat.

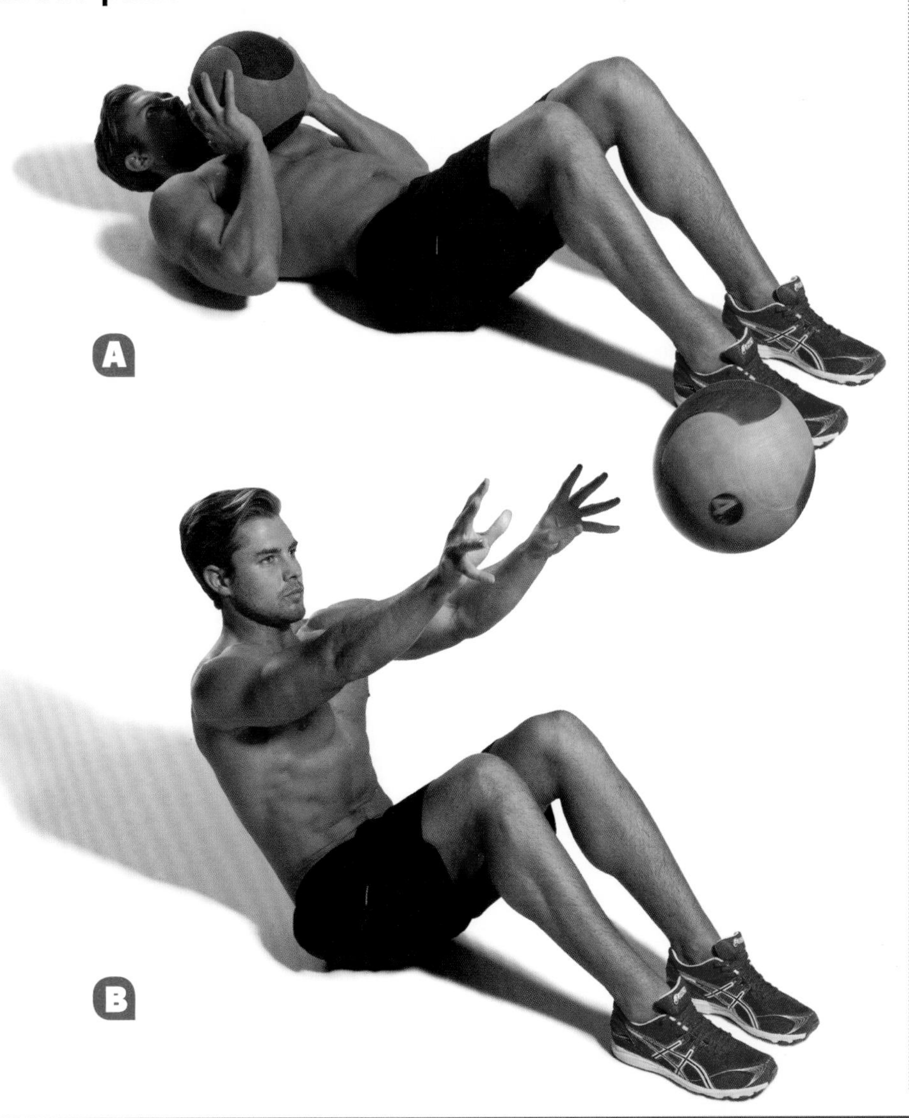

ABS TIP
If you don't have a training partner, throw the ball, fetch it and repeat

Gym ball jackknife twist

Sets 4
Reps 8
each side

This twisting move works multiple muscles at once to help you build an impressive six-pack

Most abs exercises target just a small part of your six-pack, but the gym ball jackknife twist is different. Not only does it work the top, middle and lower abs, it also works the deep core muscles beneath your six-pack and your obliques, which run down each side of it. And because this is a complex move that requires you to draw in your knees and then twist to the side, it keeps the target muscles under tension for far longer than most abs exercises. This makes the move highly effective at sculpting a solid core.

Why do it

- The added instability of the ball will force your stabiliser muscles to work, building a strong core.

How to do it

- Start in a press-up position with your shins resting on a gym ball and your body in a straight line from head to heels.
- Contract your abs to draw your knees in towards your chest, then twist to the side. Reverse the move back to the start then repeat, twisting to the other side.

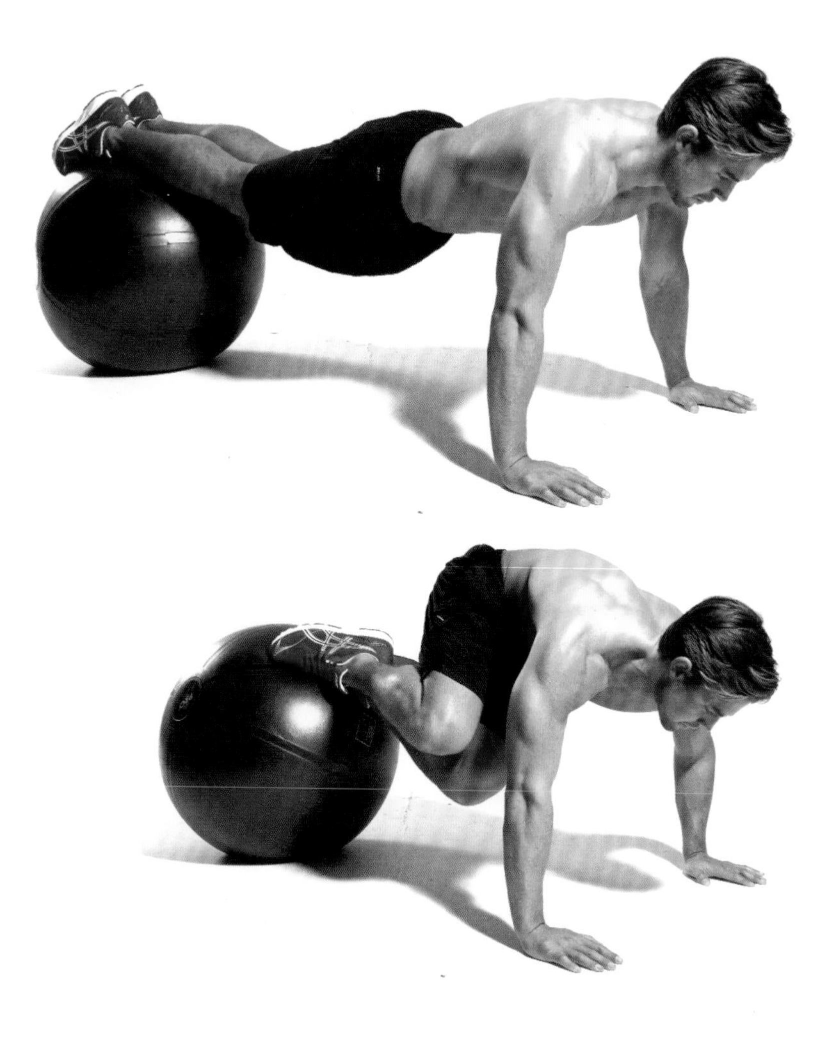

ABS TIP
Get better at this move by doing planks with your feet on the ball

Hand walkout

Sets 4
Reps 6-8

Work your entire core with this surprisingly tough move

Being able to walk on your hands provides far more benefits that just being able to join the circus. This surprisingly tough abs move works your entire core region, as well as your shoulders, lats, chest and arms, making it a great exercise to build a strong, V-shaped upper body complete with six-pack. The key to the move is to not rush it: the slower you can do it, the longer you place these target muscles under tension so they have a great stimulus to grow back bigger and stronger. The beauty is you can make the move harder by holding a plank or doing press-ups at the bottom before walking back up to the start position.

Why do it

- It's a kit-free version of the barbell rollout, one of the best six-pack builders in existence.

How to do it

- Bend from your hips so that your hands and feet are close together on the floor.
- With your feet rooted to the spot, slowly walk your hands forward until your body forms a straight line from head to heels, then walk back to the start position.

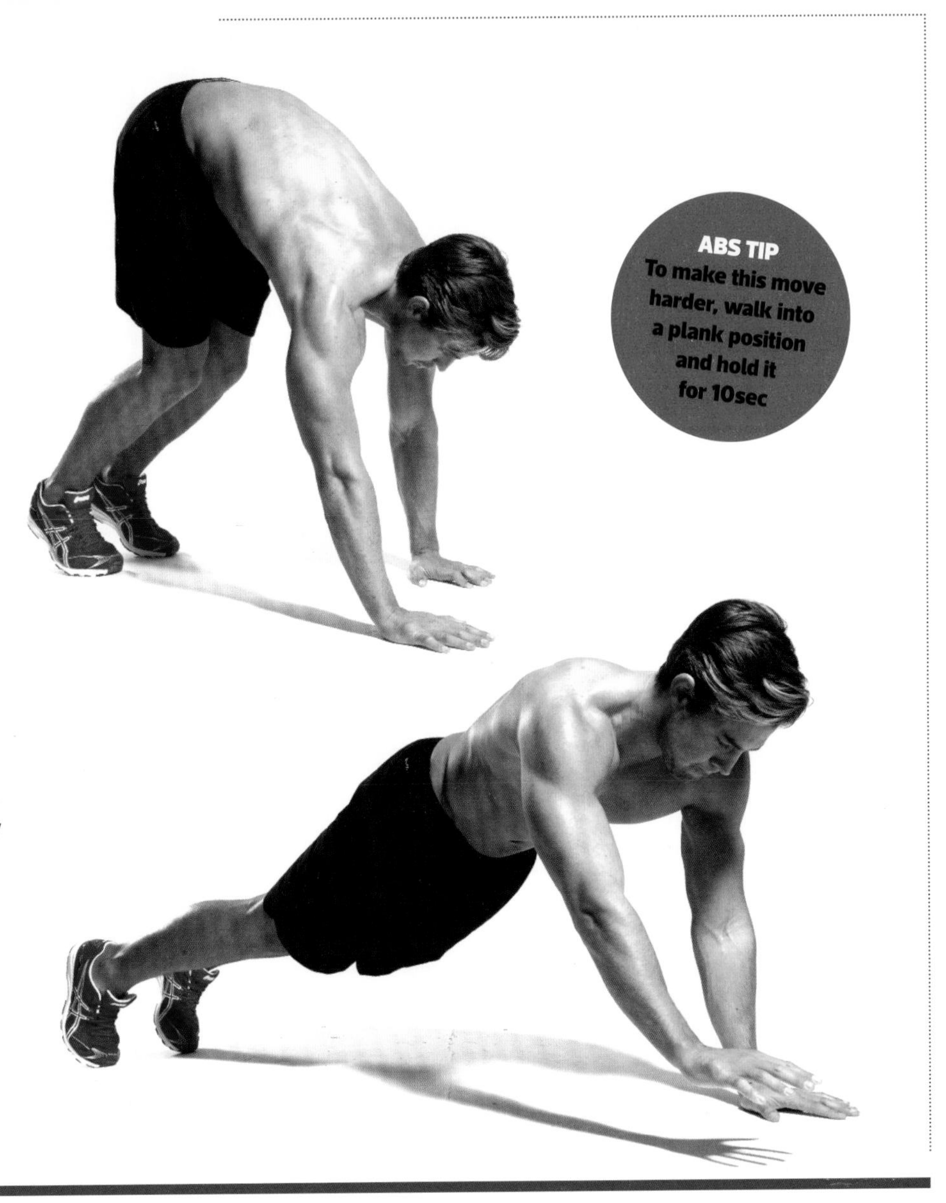

ABS TIP
To make this move harder, walk into a plank position and hold it for 10sec

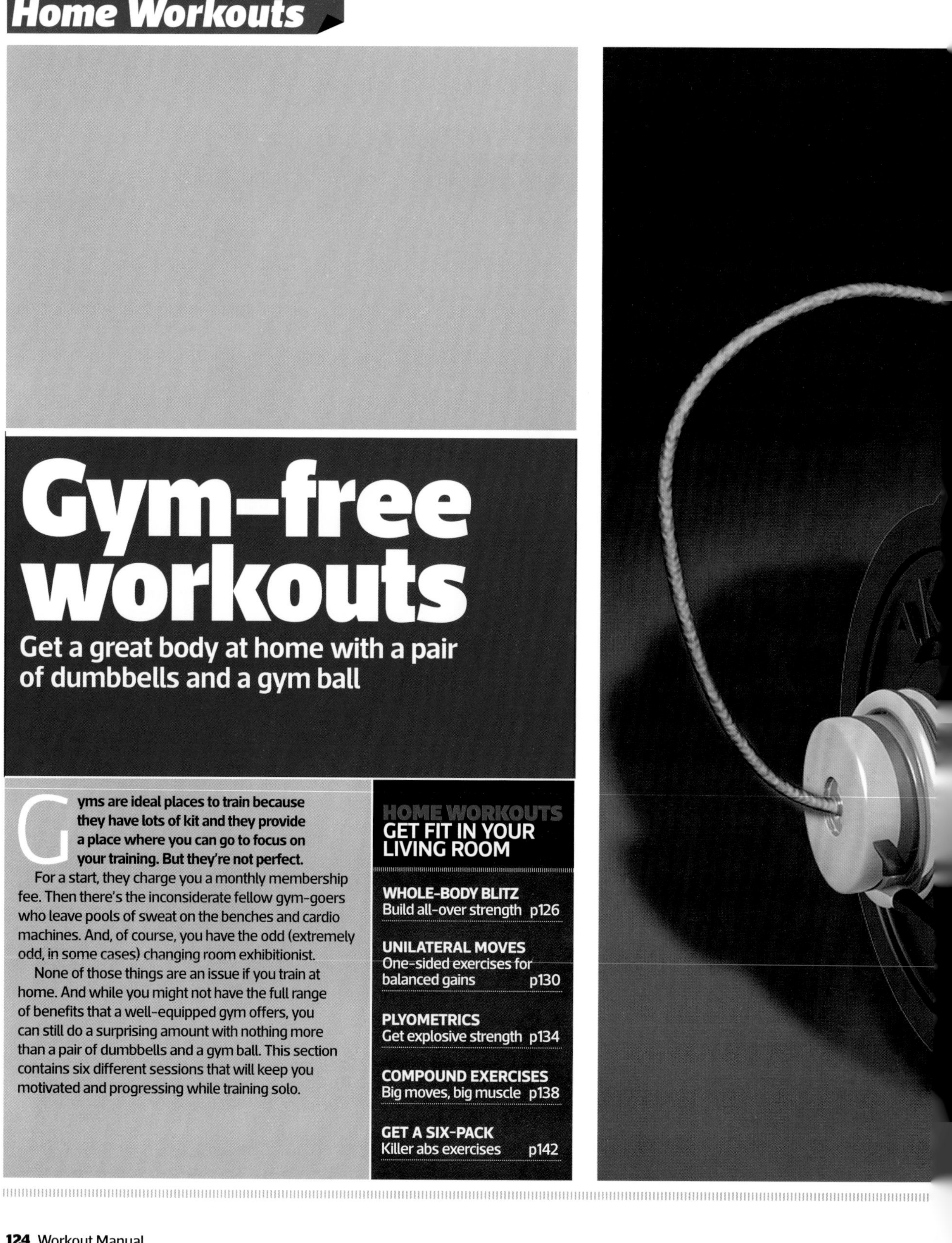

Gym-free workouts

Get a great body at home with a pair of dumbbells and a gym ball

Gyms are ideal places to train because they have lots of kit and they provide a place where you can go to focus on your training. But they're not perfect.

For a start, they charge you a monthly membership fee. Then there's the inconsiderate fellow gym-goers who leave pools of sweat on the benches and cardio machines. And, of course, you have the odd (extremely odd, in some cases) changing room exhibitionist.

None of those things are an issue if you train at home. And while you might not have the full range of benefits that a well-equipped gym offers, you can still do a surprising amount with nothing more than a pair of dumbbells and a gym ball. This section contains six different sessions that will keep you motivated and progressing while training solo.

HOME WORKOUTS

GET FIT IN YOUR LIVING ROOM

WHOLE-BODY BLITZ
Build all-over strength p126

UNILATERAL MOVES
One-sided exercises for balanced gains p130

PLYOMETRICS
Get explosive strength p134

COMPOUND EXERCISES
Big moves, big muscle p138

GET A SIX-PACK
Killer abs exercises p142

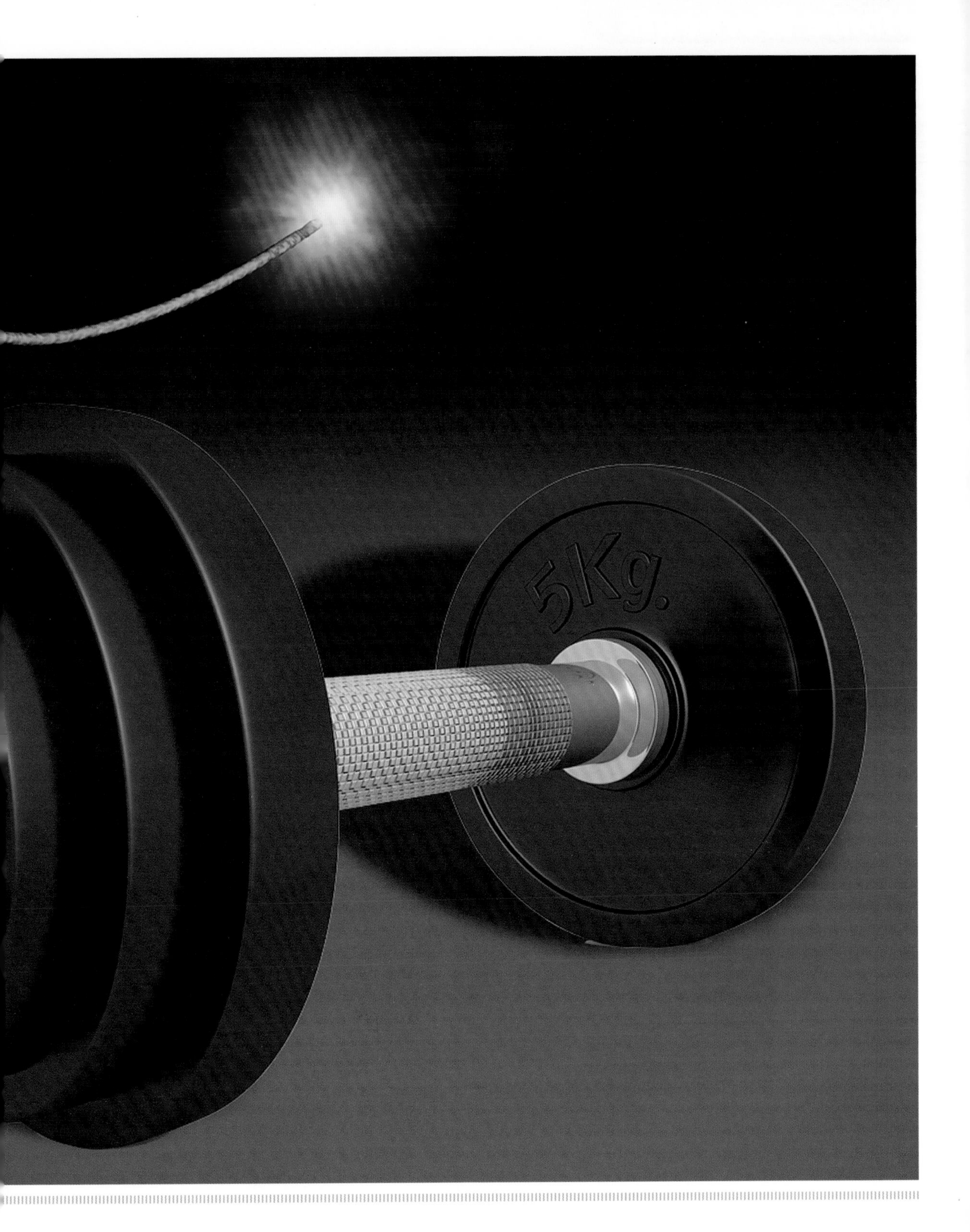
5Kg.

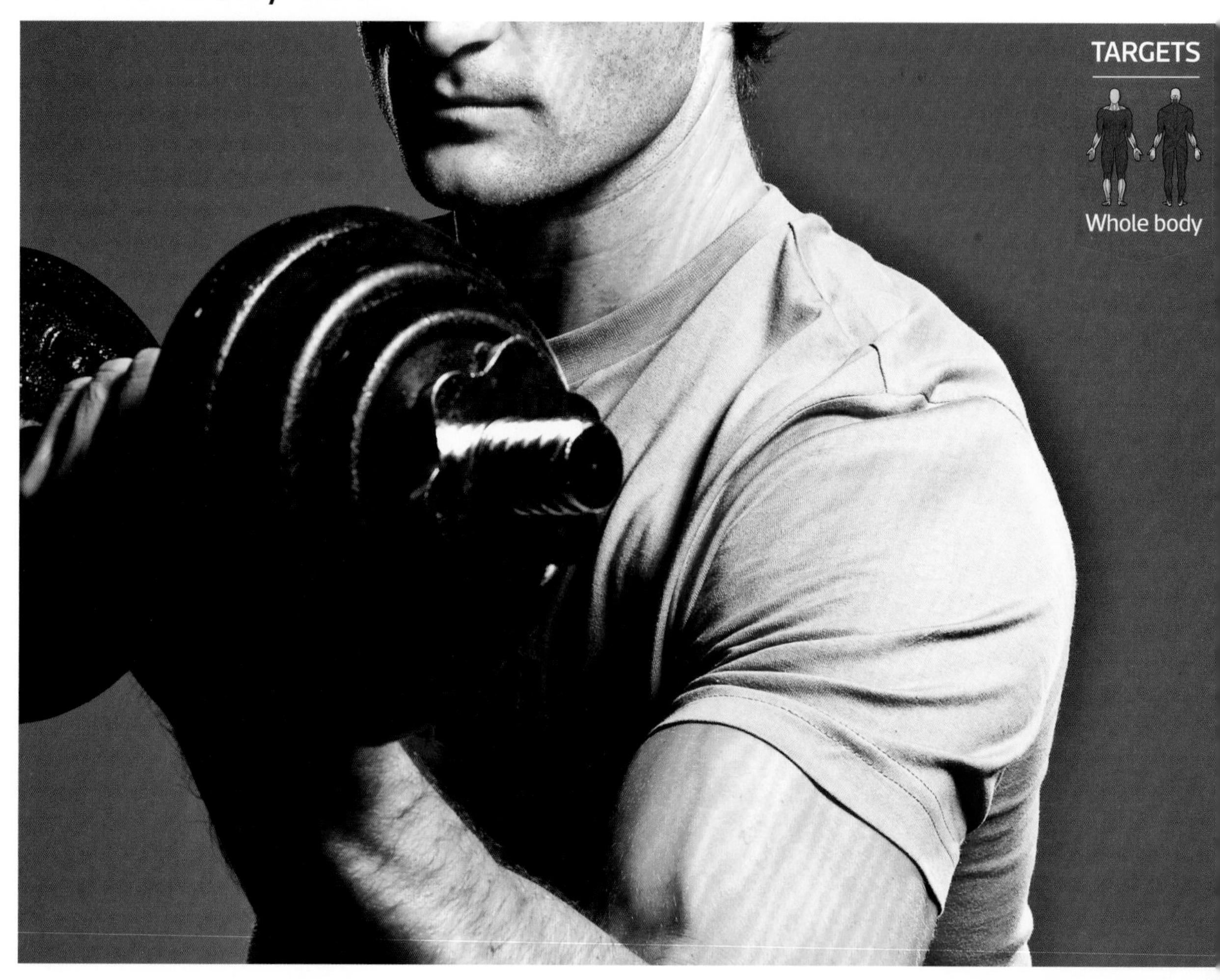

Strong all over

Do this total-body workout to get bigger and stronger without setting foot in the gym

The gym isn't always the best place to work out. Maybe your nearest one's a 40-minute drive away, or you can't manage the membership fees, or you're just not keen on exercising in front of dozens of other people. Fortunately, you don't need to go to the gym to get fitter and stronger. This half-hour workout doesn't involve any complicated kit, but its compound moves hit every body part. Alternating between the upper and lower body allows you to keep rest times short, getting your heart rate up and keeping your session time down. After four weeks of this you'll see serious muscle gains without having to go anywhere near a gym.

HOW TO DO IT

Days Do this workout three times a week for four weeks. For a new four-week home workout, get the next issue of *Men's Fitness*.

Timing It should take about 30 minutes, including the warm-up.

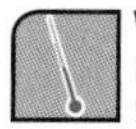

Warm-up Spend five minutes doing bodyweight moves such as press-ups, squats and lunges.

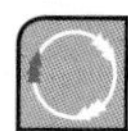

Sets and reps Follow the set and rep counts indicated for each exercise.

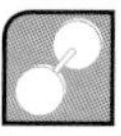

Weight Choose a weight that allows you to complete all your reps but no more.

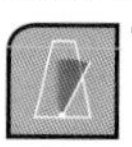

Tempo Take one second to lift the weight, pause, then take three seconds to lower it.

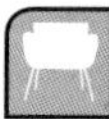

Rest Have a 30-45 secon rest between sets and on minute between exercise

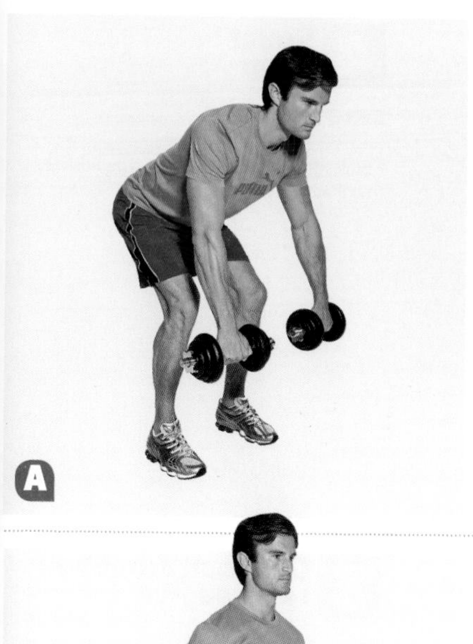

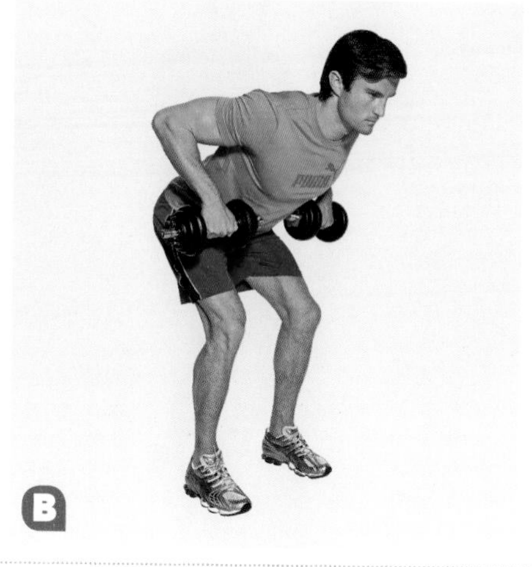

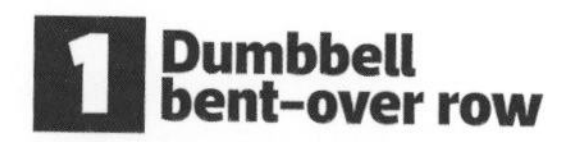

1 Dumbbell bent-over row

Sets 2 **Reps** 12

> Pull the dumbbells up to your chest, leading with your elbows.

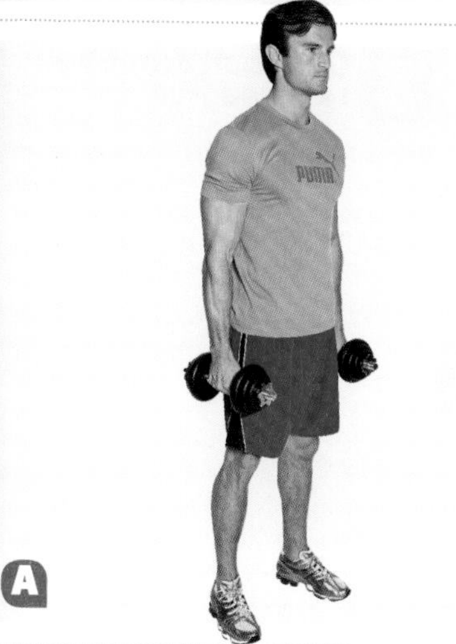

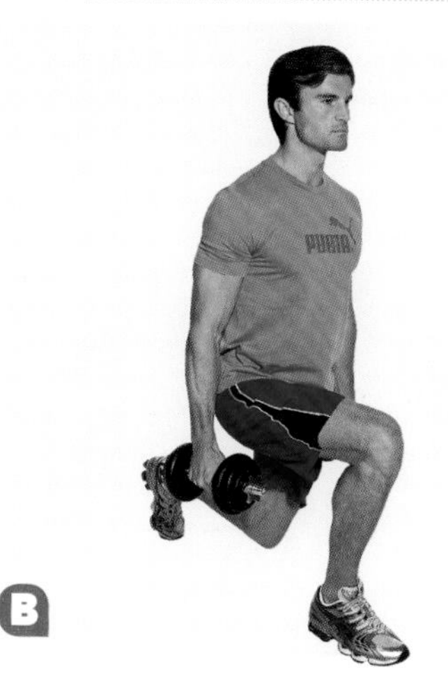

2 Dumbbell lunge

Sets 2 **Reps** 8 each side

> Step forward and, keeping your back upright, lower until your knees are bent at 90°.

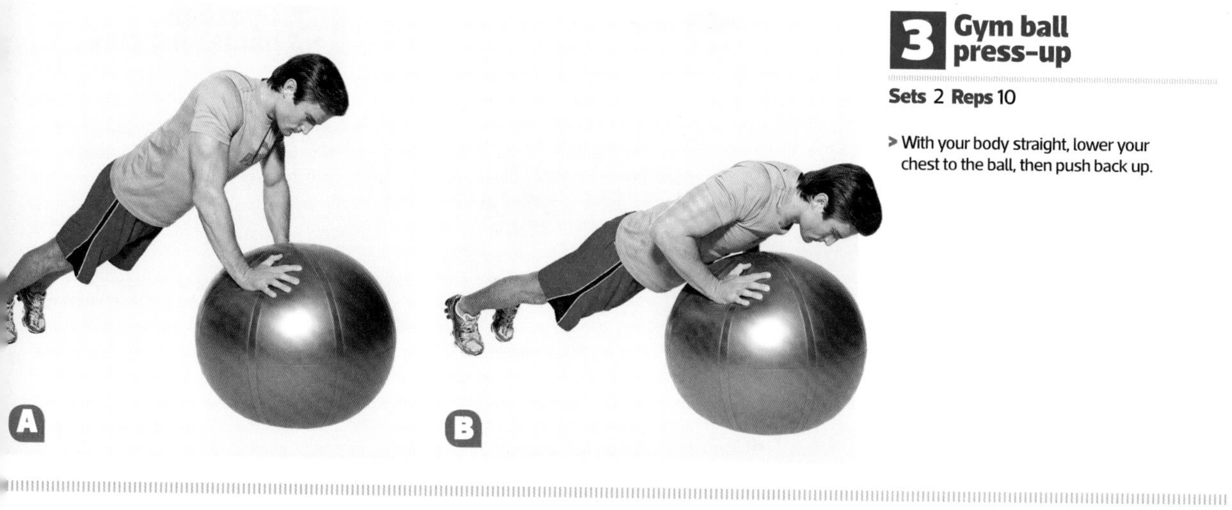

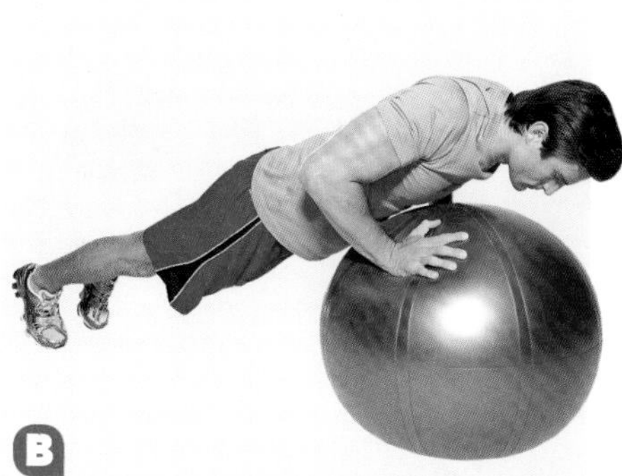

3 Gym ball press-up

Sets 2 **Reps** 10

> With your body straight, lower your chest to the ball, then push back up.

Whole-Body Blitz

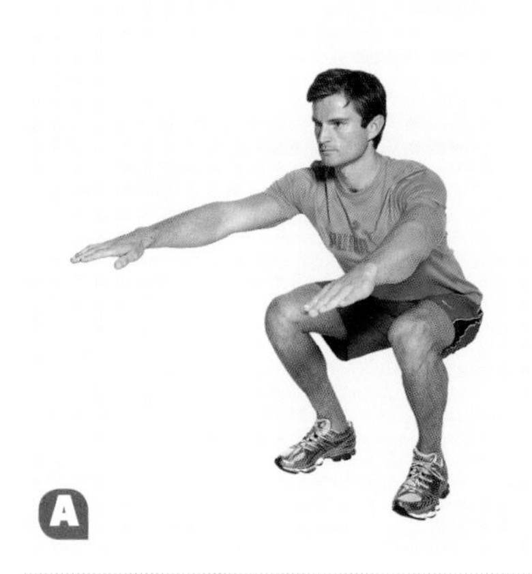

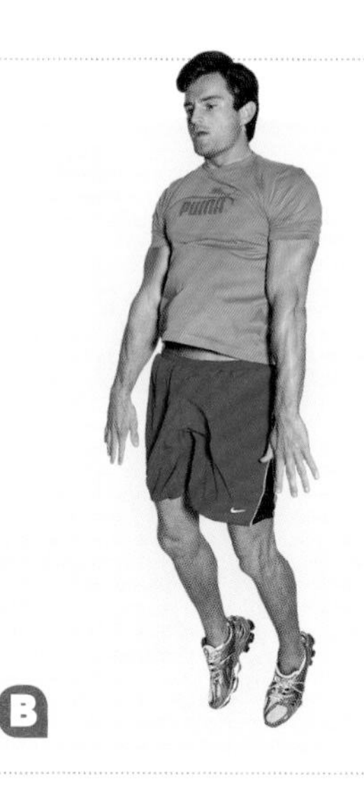

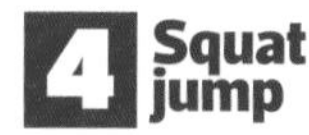

4 Squat jump

Sets 3 **Reps** 8

> Sink into a squat, then jump up explosively so that your feet leave the floor.

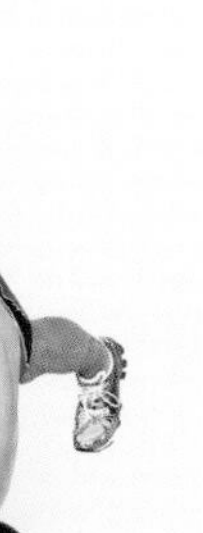

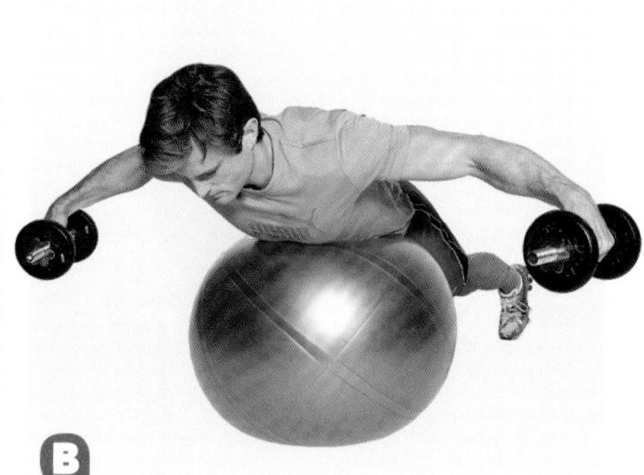

5 Gym ball dumbbell reverse flye

Sets 2 **Reps** 12

> Keep your body straight and your feet on the floor for balance. Raise the weights slowly out to the sides.

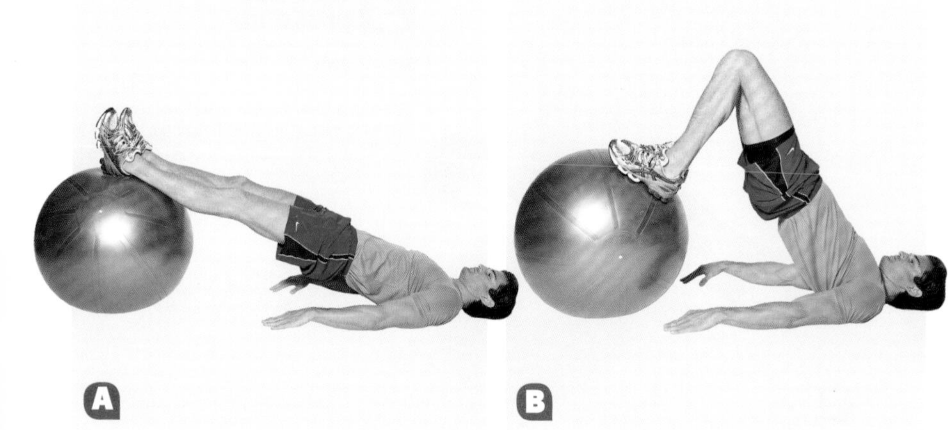

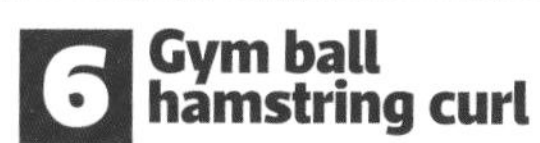

6 Gym ball hamstring curl

Sets 2 **Reps** 12

> Rest your calves on the ball and draw it in to your backside, keeping a straight line from knees to shoulders.

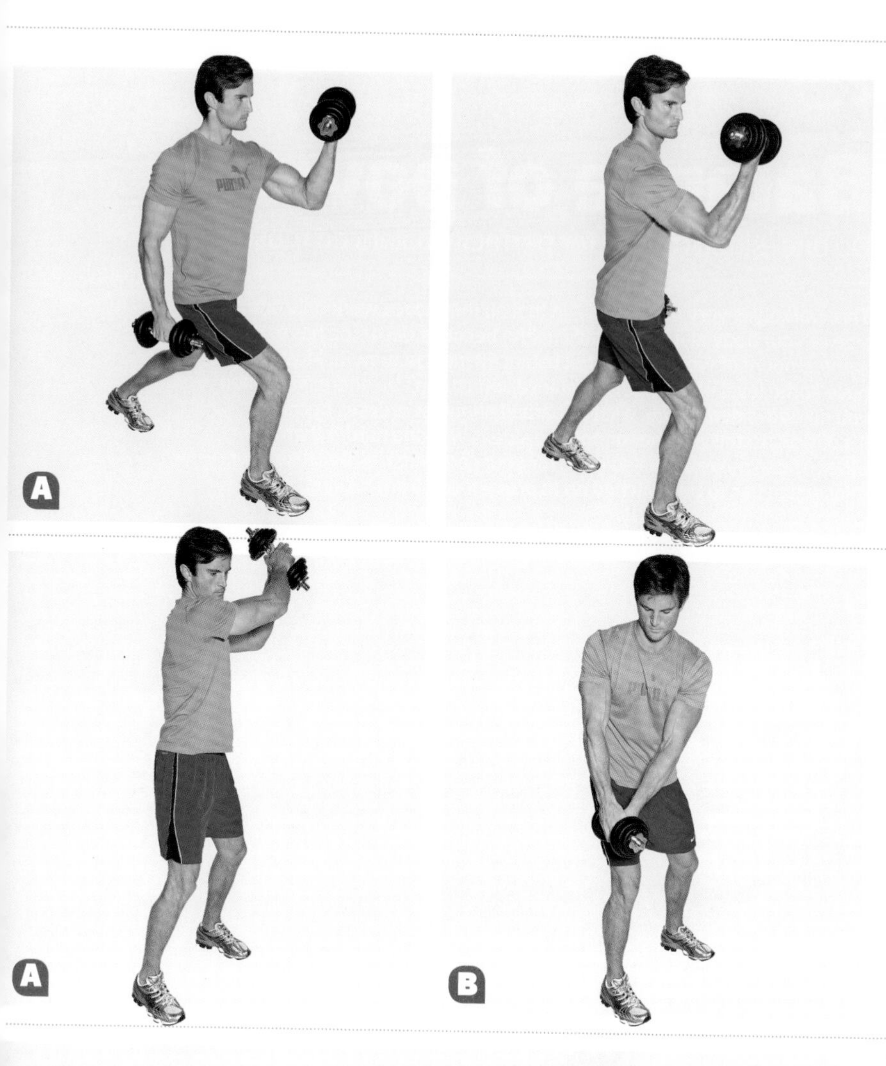

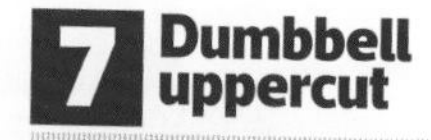

7 Dumbbell uppercut

Sets 2 **Reps** 8 each side

> Using a split stance, punch the weights up, alternating sides.

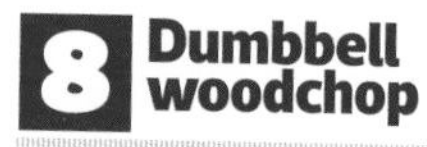

8 Dumbbell woodchop

Sets 2 **Reps** 8 each side

> Draw the dumbbell down and across your body.

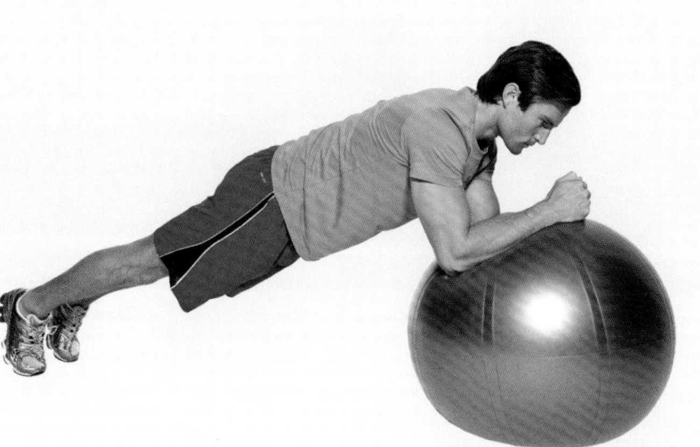

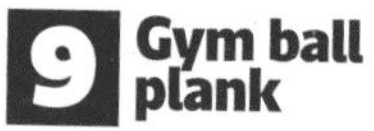

9 Gym ball plank

Sets 2 **Time** 30-45sec

> Rest your forearms on the gym ball and keep your body in a straight line from head to heels.

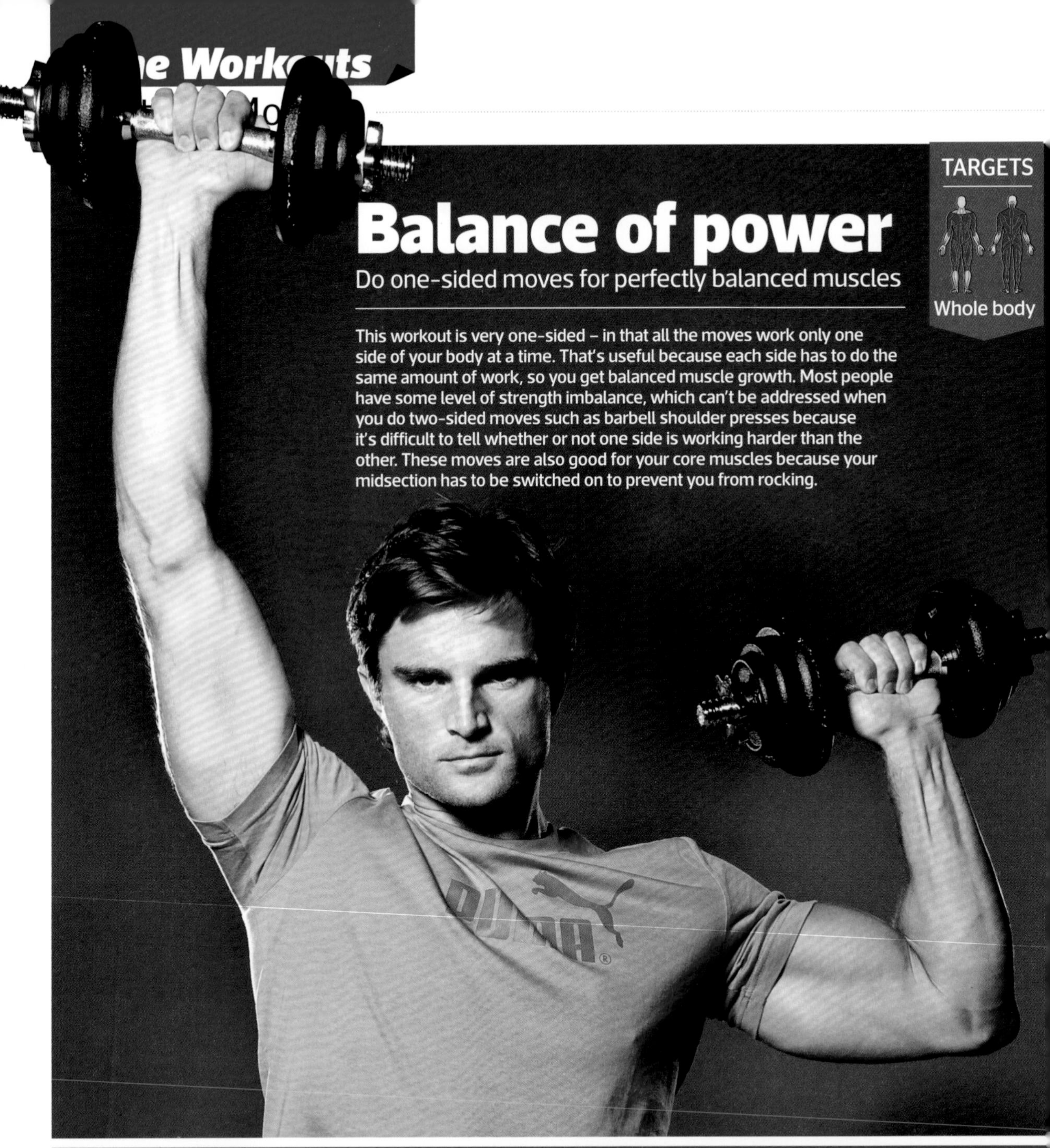

Balance of power

Do one-sided moves for perfectly balanced muscles

This workout is very one-sided – in that all the moves work only one side of your body at a time. That's useful because each side has to do the same amount of work, so you get balanced muscle growth. Most people have some level of strength imbalance, which can't be addressed when you do two-sided moves such as barbell shoulder presses because it's difficult to tell whether or not one side is working harder than the other. These moves are also good for your core muscles because your midsection has to be switched on to prevent you from rocking.

HOW TO DO IT

Days Do this workout three times a week for four weeks and then switch to a new home workout for the next four weeks.

Timing This workout should take about 30 minutes, including a quick warm-up.

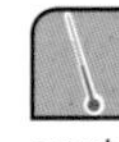

Warm-up Spend five minutes doing bodyweight moves such as press-ups, squats and lunges.

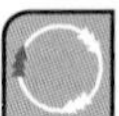

Sets and reps Follow the set and rep counts indicated for each exercise.

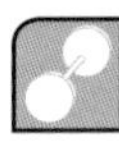

Weight Choose a weight that allows you to complete all your reps but no more.

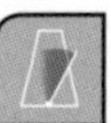

Tempo Take one second to lift the weight, pause then take three seconds to lower it.

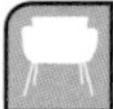

Rest Rest for 30-45 seconds between sets and for one minute between exercises.

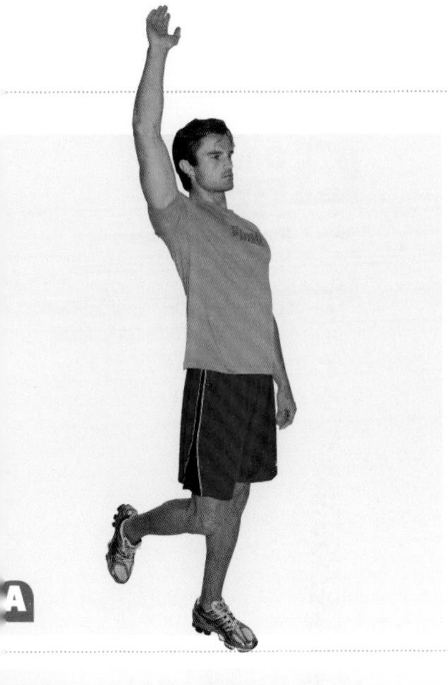

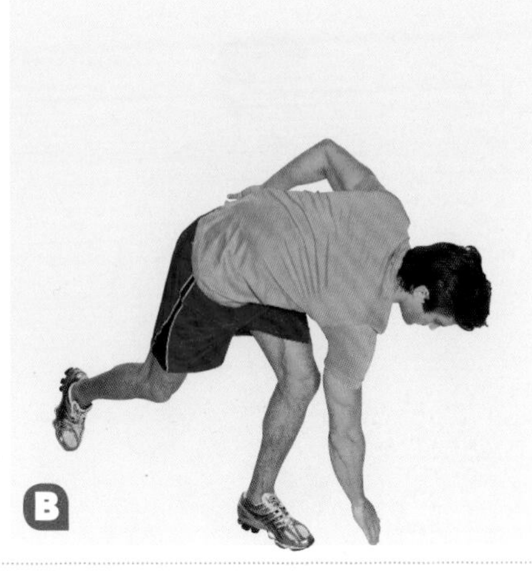

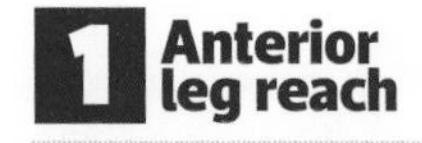

1 Anterior leg reach

Sets 2 **Reps** 10 each side

> Raise your arm and arch your back slightly, then bend at the hips to bring your hand down to your opposite foot.

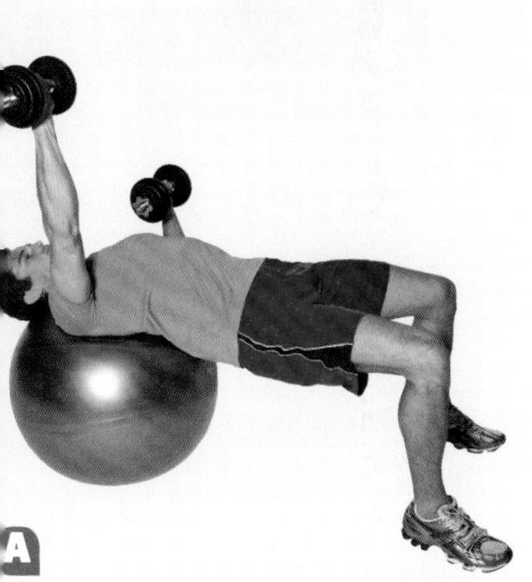

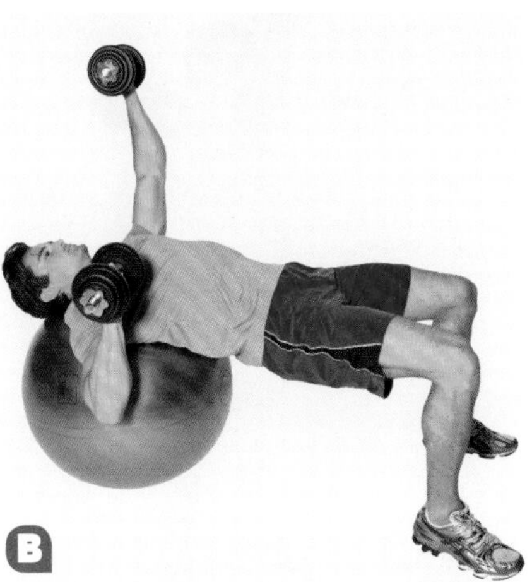

2 Gym ball dumbbell alternating chest press

Sets 2 **Reps** 10 each side

> Lie with your shoulders on the gym ball and press one dumbbell. As you lower the weight, start to press the other dumbbell.

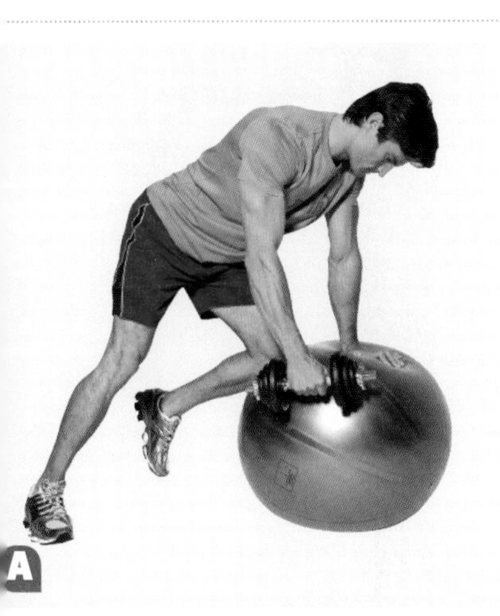

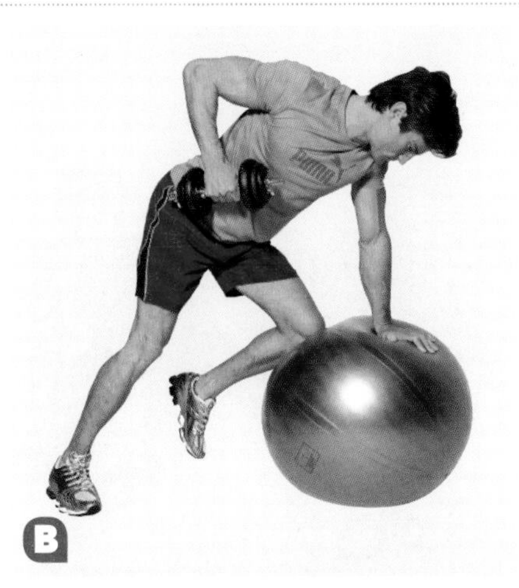

3 Gym ball dumbbell one-arm row

Sets 2 **Reps** 10 each side

> Kneel on a gym ball, supporting yourself on one hand with a dumbbell hanging down in the other.
> Pull the dumbbell up to your chest, keeping your elbow high.

Unilateral Moves

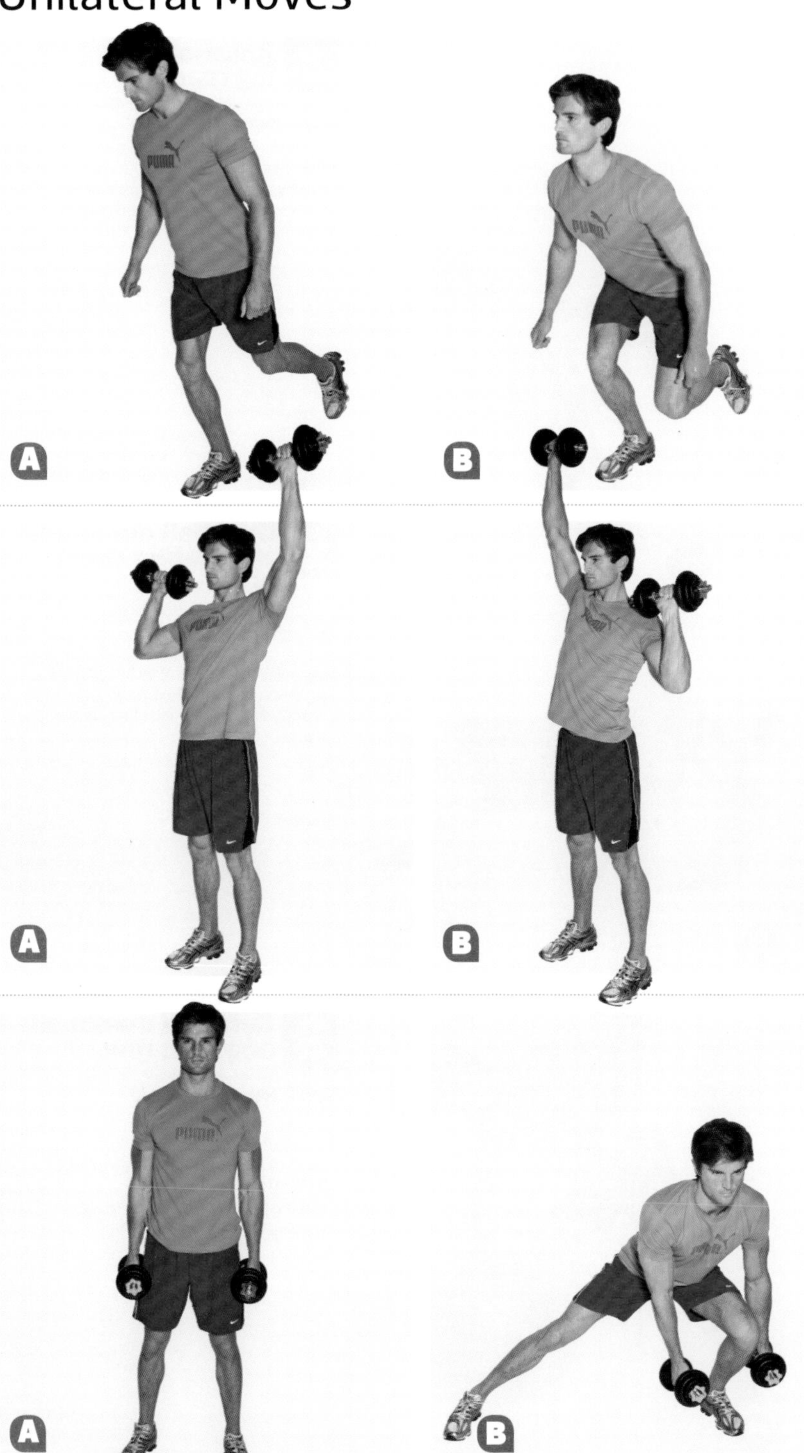

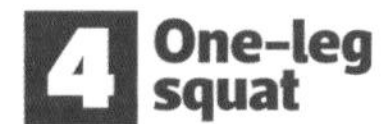

4 One-leg squat

Sets 3 **Reps** 8 each side

> Stand on one leg with your other foot off the ground. Sink down into a squat, keeping your torso upright and your knees in line with your toes.

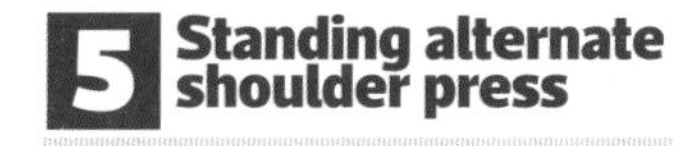

5 Standing alternate shoulder press

Sets 2 **Reps** 10 each side

> Press one dumbbell overhead. Then, as you lower it, press the other dumbbell overhead.

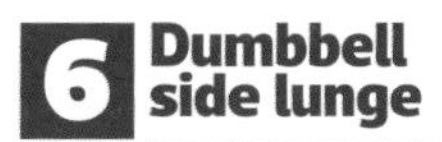

6 Dumbbell side lunge

Sets 2 **Reps** 10 each side

> Take a big side step, keeping your trailing leg straight and the knee of your leading leg over your toes.

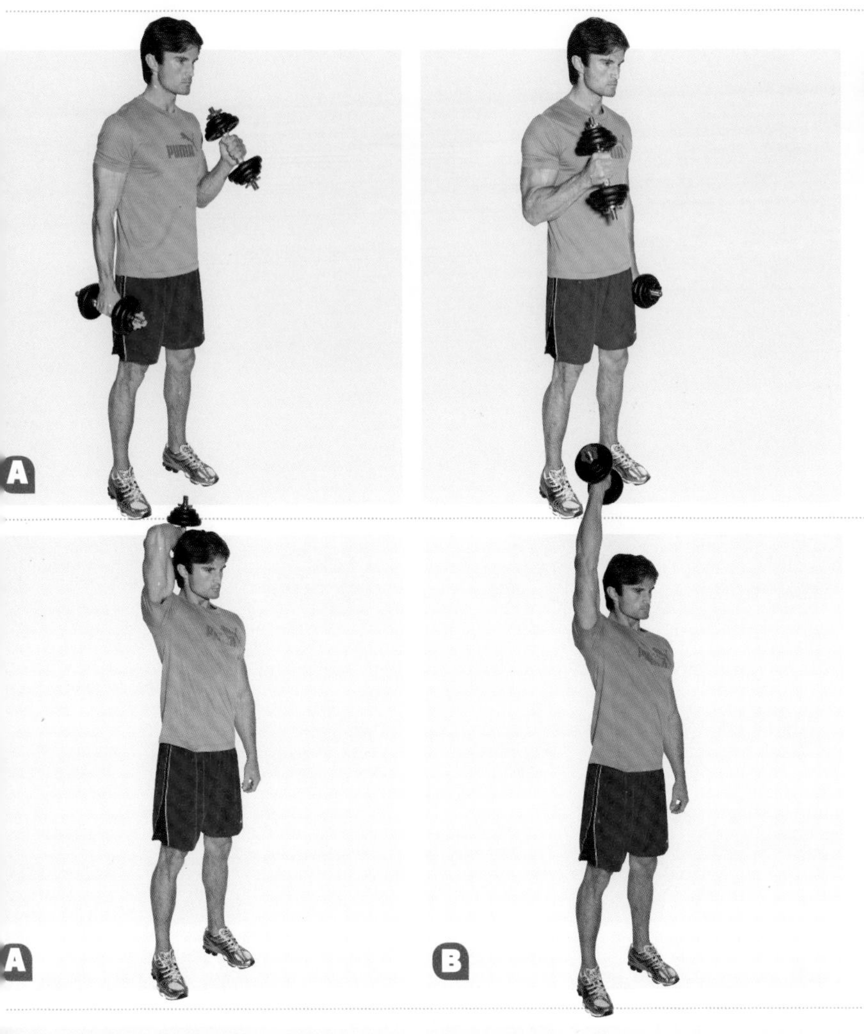

7 Hammer curl

Sets 2 **Reps** 10 each side

> Perform a biceps curl while holding the weights with a neutral grip. Alternate sides.

8 Standing overhead triceps press

Sets 2 **Reps** 10 each side

> With your upper arm vertical and the dumbbell behind your head, straighten at the elbow.

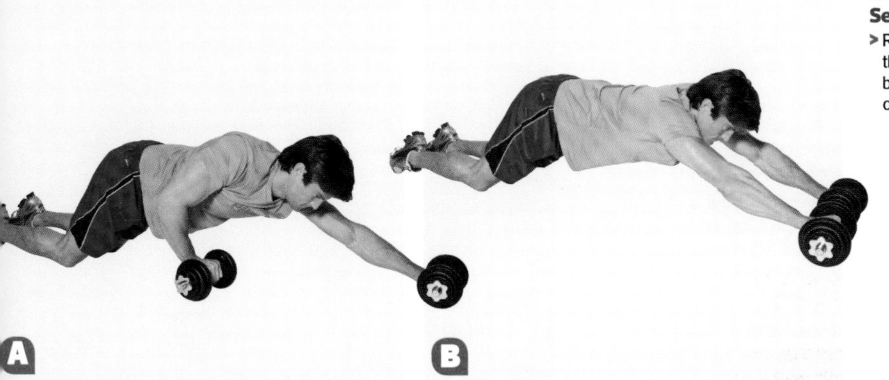

9 Alternate dumbbell rollout

Sets 1 **Time** 10

> Roll both dumbbells out together, then draw one back into your body and roll it out again. Repeat on the other side for one rep.

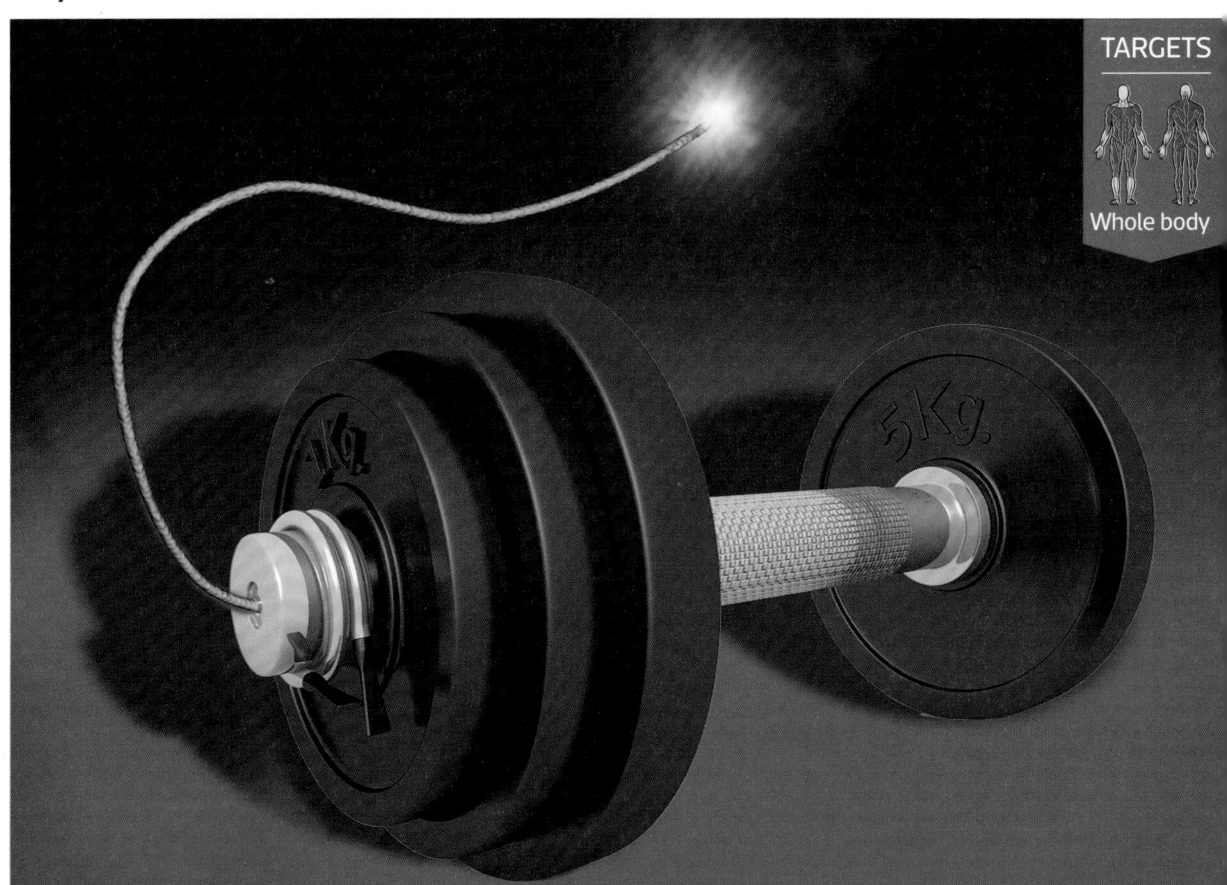

Explosive device

Use plyometric moves to fire up your training sessions and develop explosive power

If you're struggling to motivate yourself for a workout, doing a plyometric session – exercises that involve fast, explosive power movements – is a good way of ramping up your enthusiasm. That's because performing big movements at speed will engage your brain, as well as giving your muscles a new stimulus. They'll make you better at sporty, explosive moves and target your muscle fibres with most growth potential.

Before you perform each plyometric move, you'll warm up with an exercise that targets the same body part. This fires up the target muscle fibres so they're responsive when you do the plyometric move. Just make sure you don't exhaust the target area when you're doing the warm-up. You perform fewer plyometric reps than you would for normal sets because you're training for power rather than strength endurance.

How to do this workout	Beginner	Intermediate	Advanced
How many workouts should I do per week?	3	3-4	4
How long will each session take?	14min	26min	44mi
How many circuits per workout?	2	3	4
How many reps for non-plyometric moves?	8	10	12
How many reps for plyometric moves?	5	6	7
How much rest should I take between circuits?	1min	2min	2mi

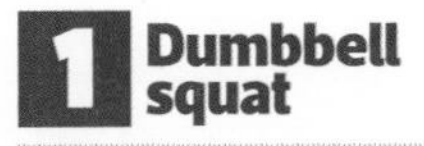

1 Dumbbell squat

> Keeping your back upright, lower until your thighs are parallel to the floor, making sure your knees stay in line with your toes.

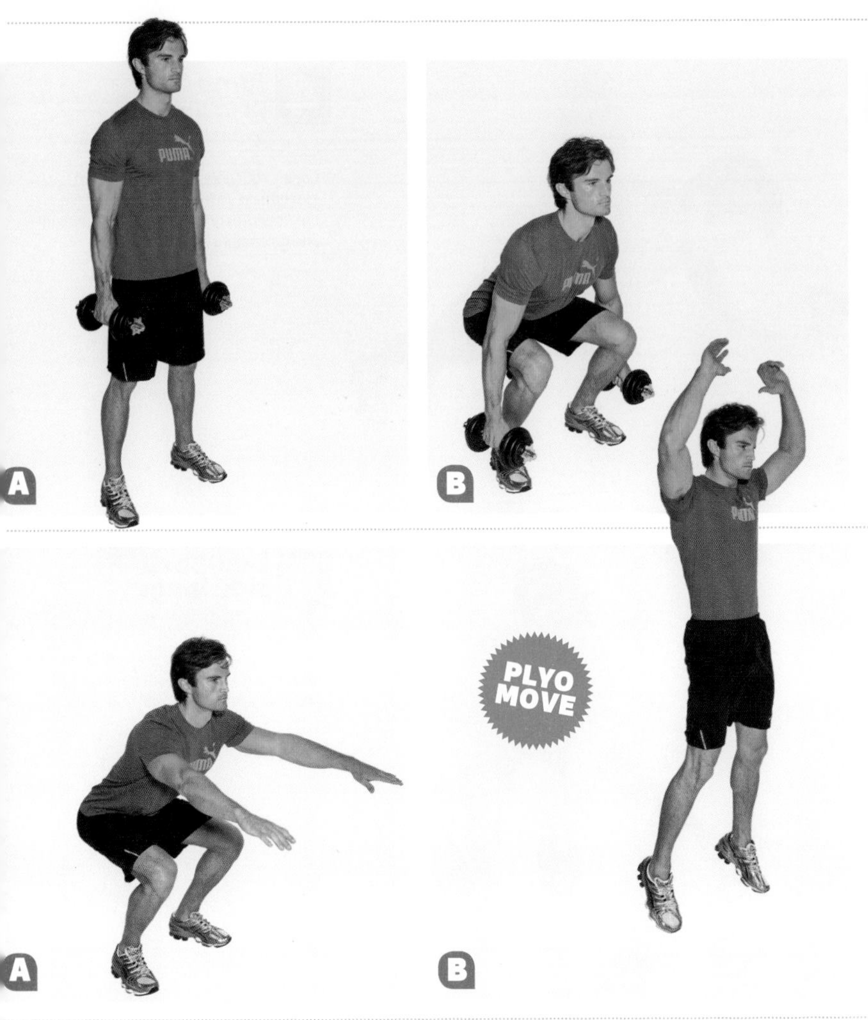

2 Jump squat

> Sink into a squat, then explode upwards. When you land, go straight into the next rep.

Fit tip
Once you've mastered the jump squat and jump lunge (see p136), boost the effect by doing them holding dumbbells.

3 Gym ball chest press

> Lie with your upper back on the ball and press the dumbbells directly up, then lower them under control.

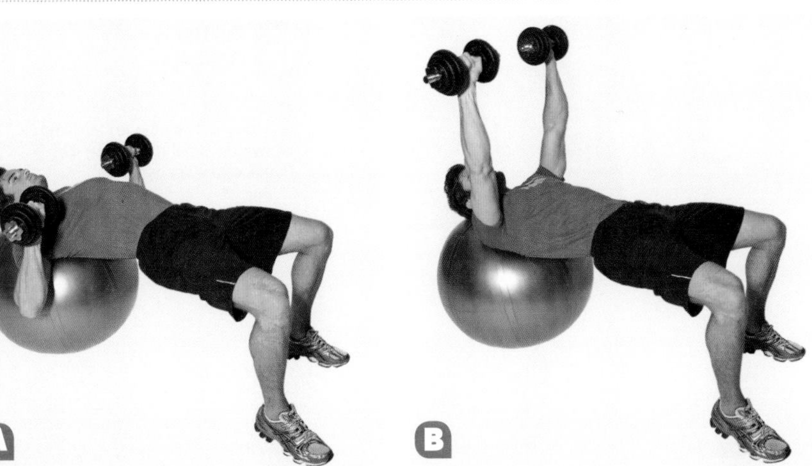

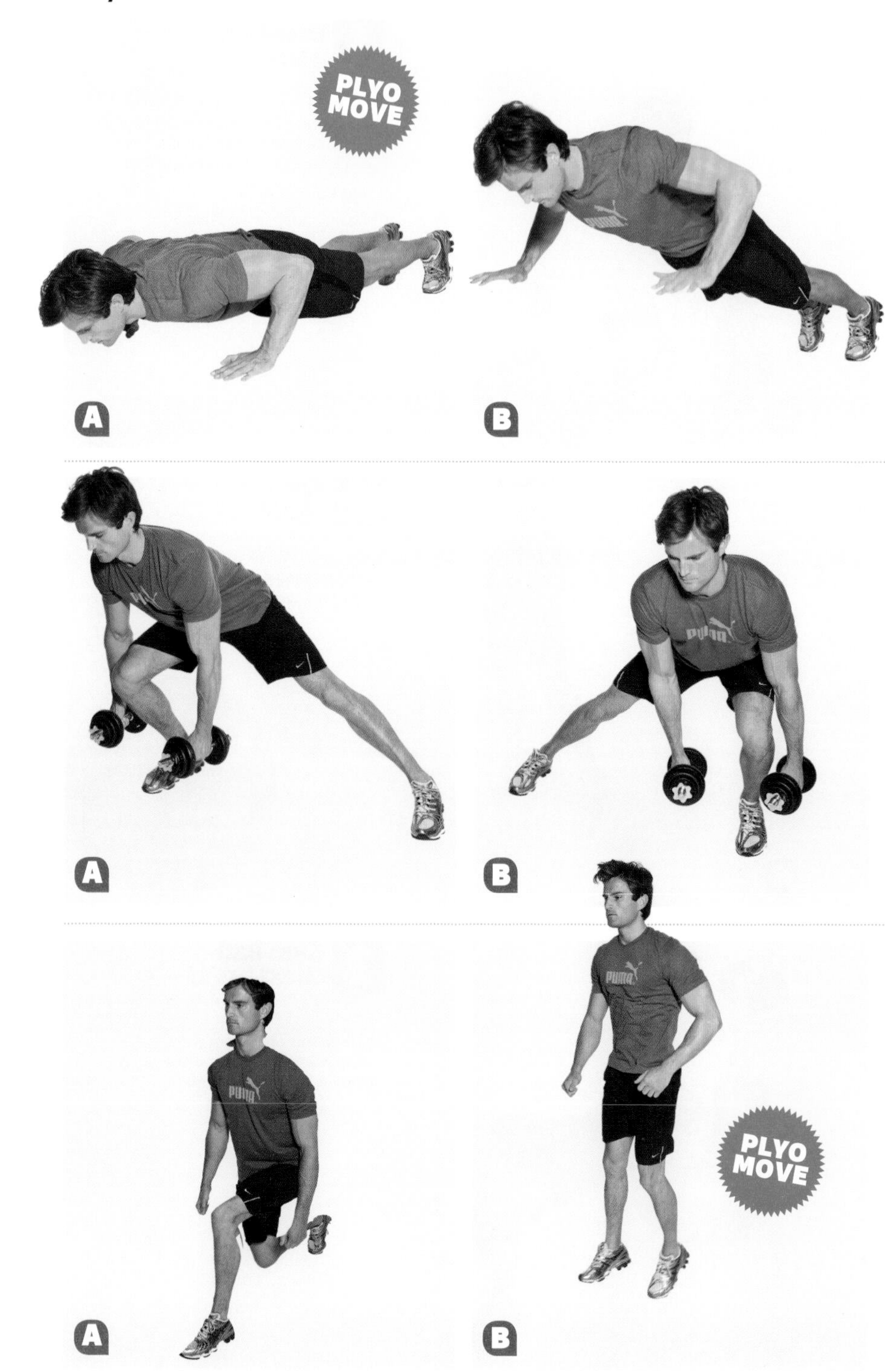

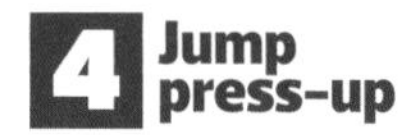

4 Jump press-up

> Lower your chest to the floor, then explode up so that your hands leave the floor. Absorb the impact on landing and go straight into the next rep.

5 Dumbbell side lunge

> Take a big step to one side and bend your leading leg, keeping your back upright and your knee in line with your toes.

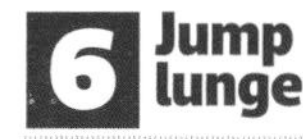

6 Jump lunge

> Step forward into a lunge then jump up, swap legs in the air and land in a lunge on the opposite side.

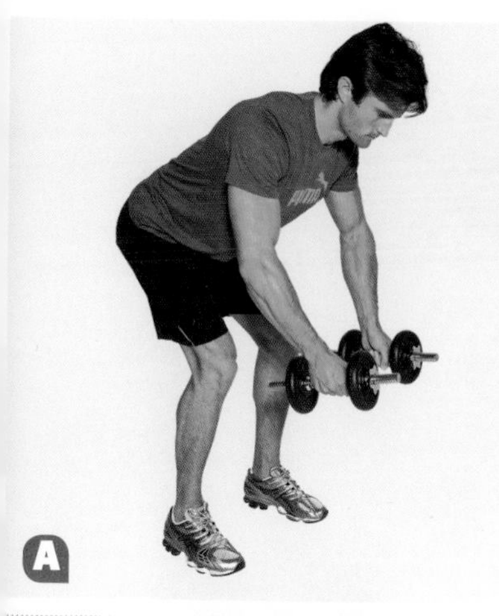

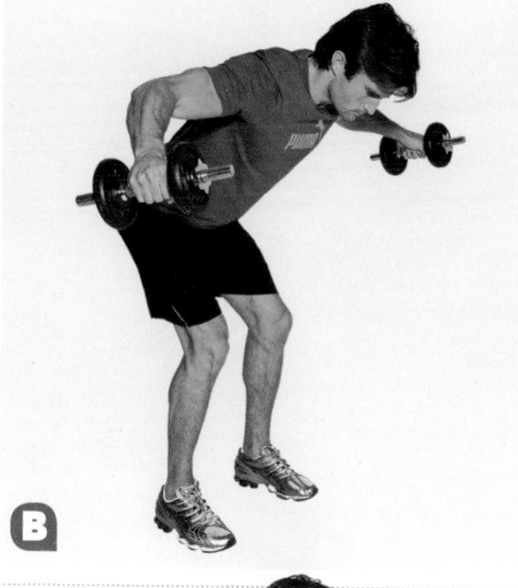

7 Dumbbell reverse flye

> Bend forward from the hips, not the waist, and raise the dumbbells out to the side, keeping a slight bend in your elbows.

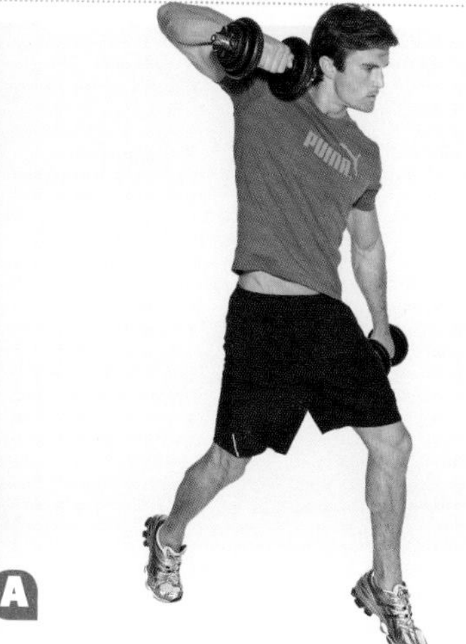

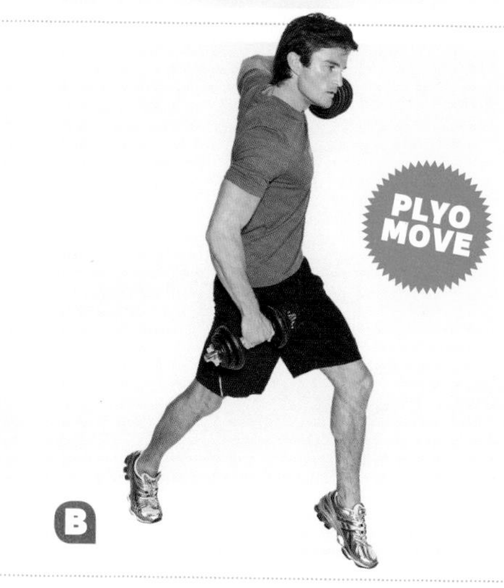

8 Dumbbell plyometric one-arm high pull

> Get into a split stance with the dumbbells hanging down. Explosively pull one up to your chest, then lower it back to the start. Alternate sides with each rep.

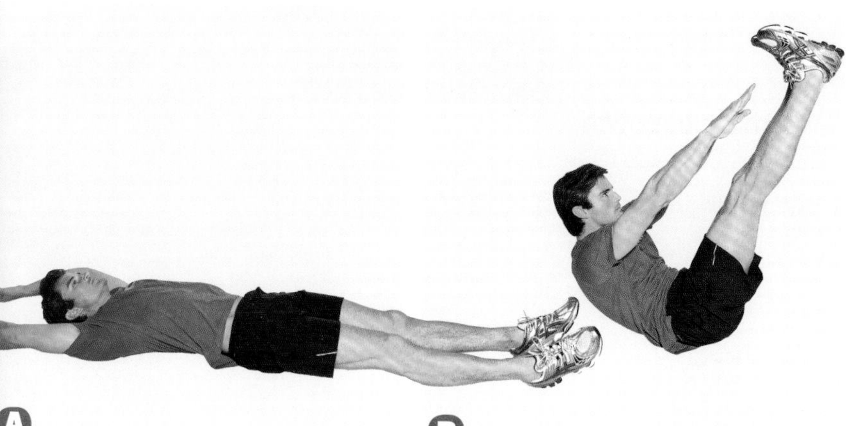

9 Jackknife

> Lie on your back with your legs and arms straight and raised slightly. Simultaneously raise your arms and legs until they meet in the middle.

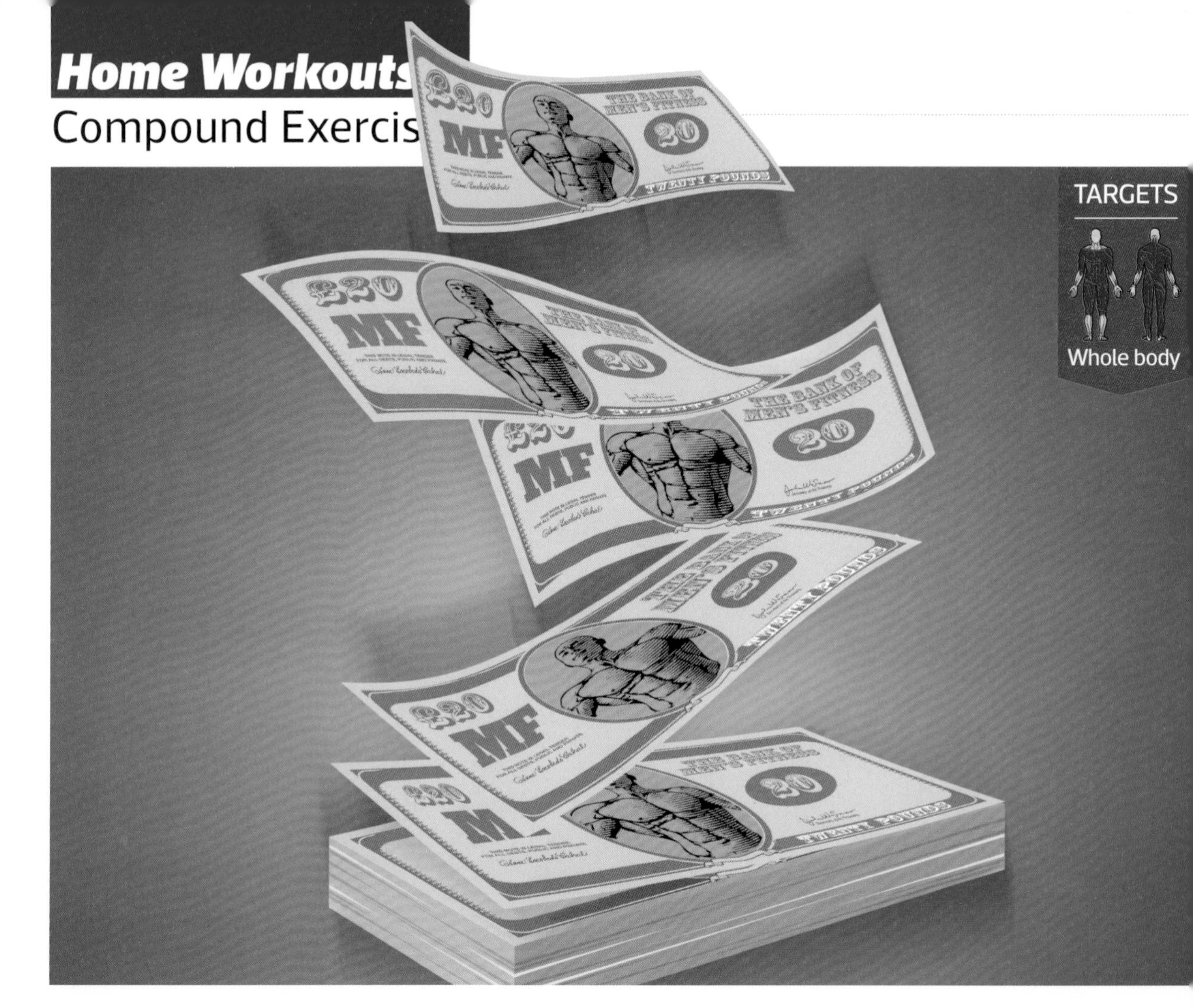

Bang for your buck

Use compound moves to cash in on muscle growth

You might think that to work every major muscle group in your body effectively you'd need to spend several hours training. But the truth is that you can perform an effective whole-body session in less than half an hour.

The key is to maximise your time and efforts. That's why this workout uses compound moves that target more than one muscle group at a time, so you work more muscles in less time. It also alternates between upper-body and lower-body exercises. That way your heart and lungs will be working constantly throughout the session – but each body part gets a chance to recover before it's targeted again.

How to do this workout	Beginner	Intermediate	Advanced
How many workouts should I do per week?	3	4	4
How long will each session take?	19min	26min	29mi
How many circuits per workout?	3	4	5
How many reps for per exercise?	10	12	12
How much rest should I take between circuits?	2min	2min	1min

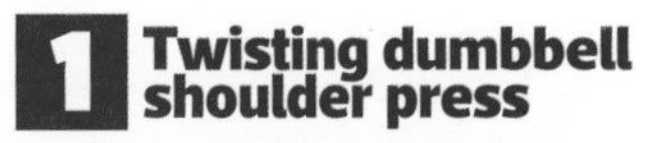

1 Twisting dumbbell shoulder press

> Press the weights directly overhead while rotating your torso. Alternate sides.

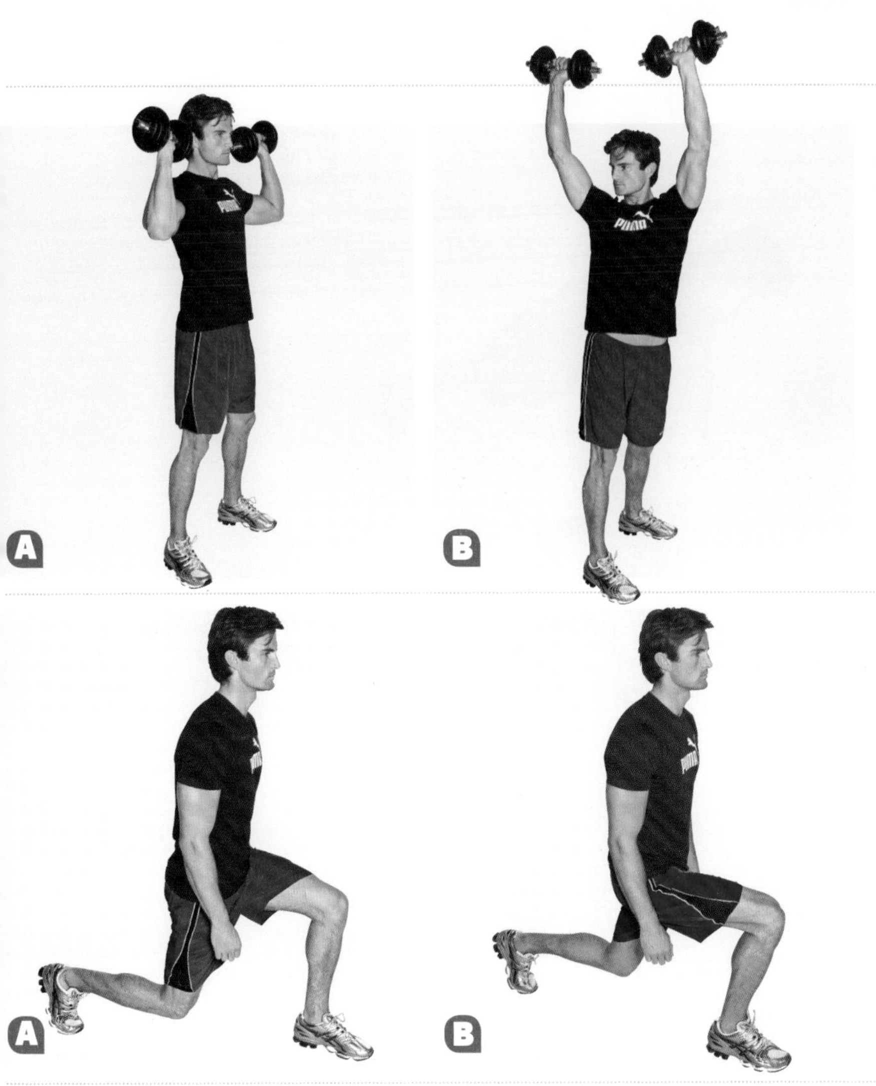

2 Lunge jump

> Start in the lunge position. Then jump up, swapping your legs over in mid-air. Land and go into the next rep.

3 Modified V-sit

> With your arms by your sides, crunch up to bring your knees to your chest.

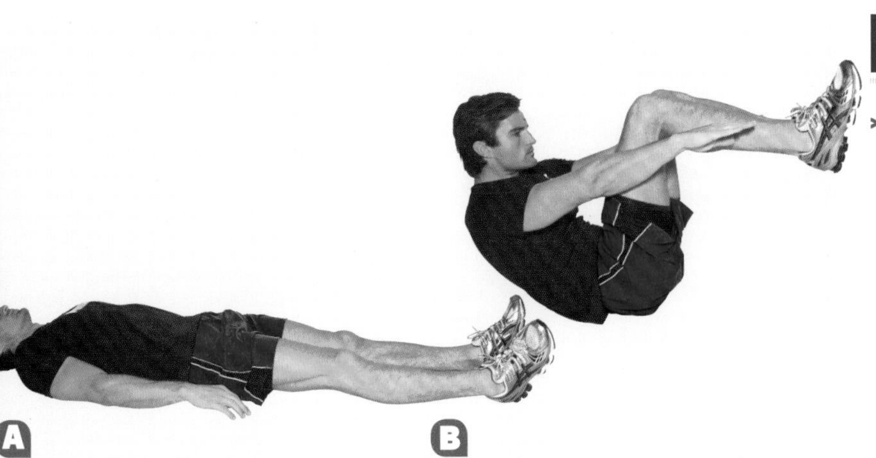

Compound Exercises

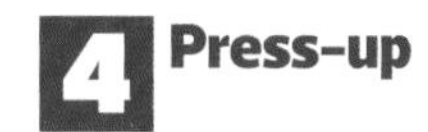

4 Press-up

> Lower your chest to the floor, keeping your elbows by your sides.

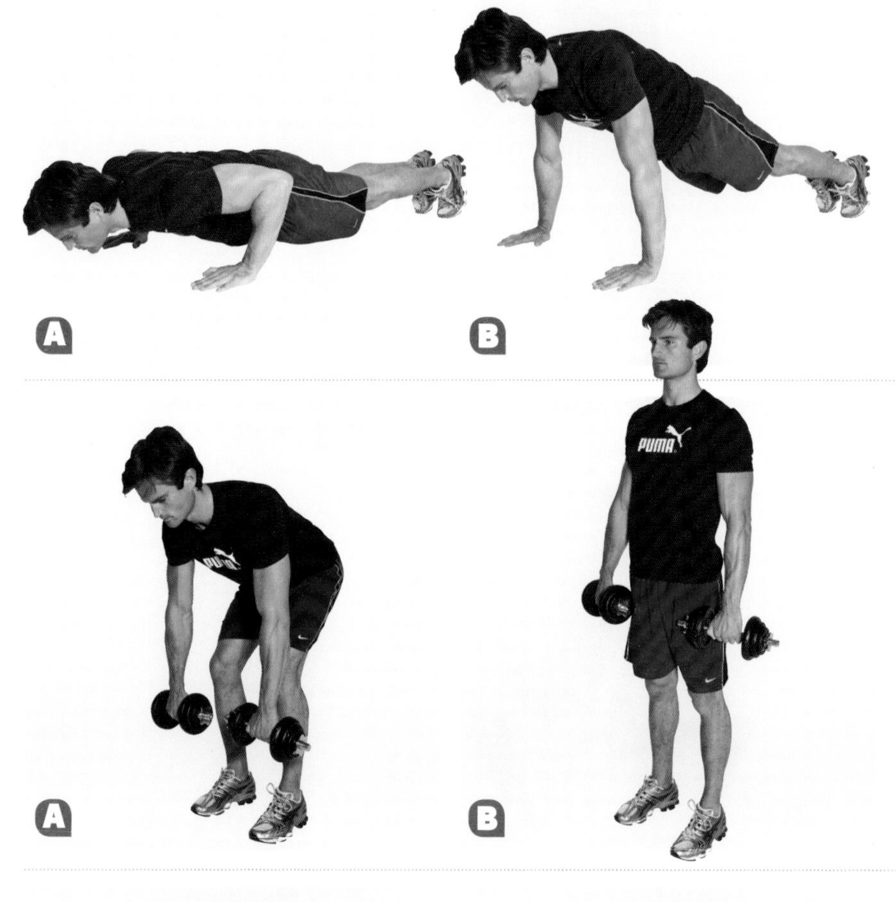

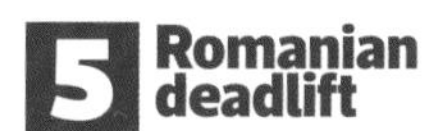

5 Romanian deadlift

> Bending from the hips, not the waist, lower the weight in front of your shins. Stand up smoothly.

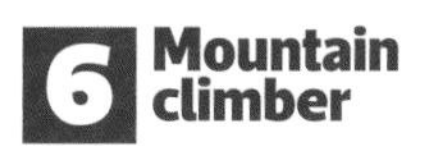

6 Mountain climber

> Jump one leg forwards while simultaneously jumping the other back. Alternate legs.

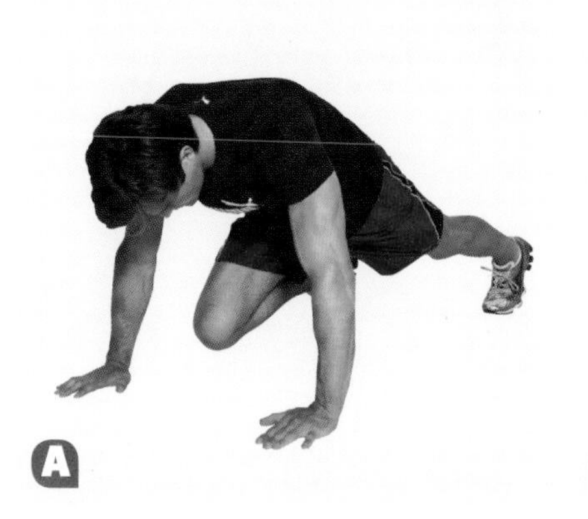

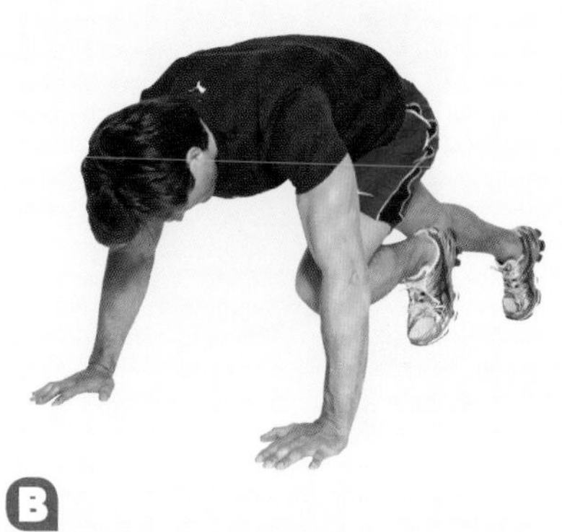

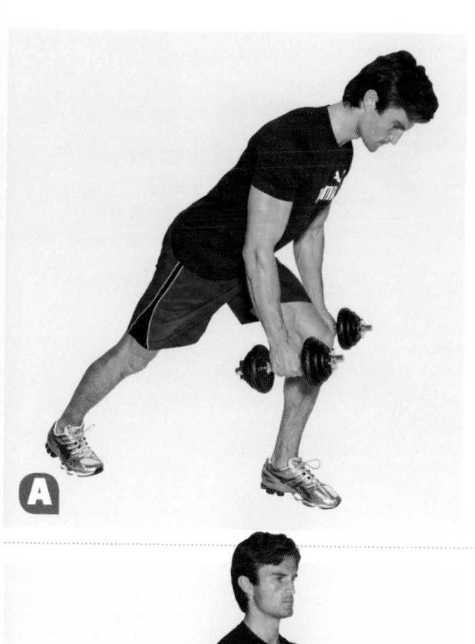

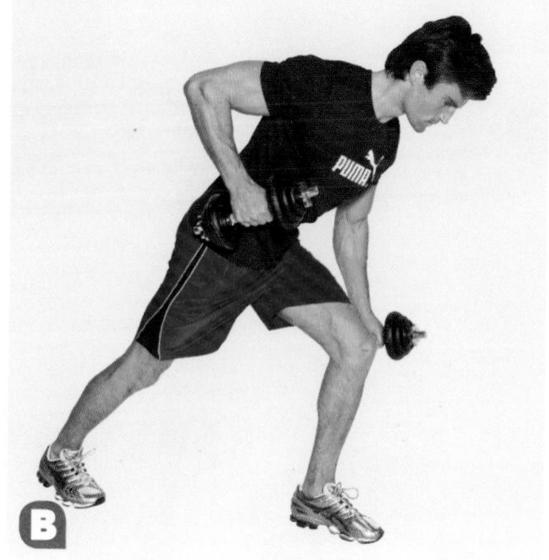

7 Split dumbbell row

> In a split stance, row one of the dumbbells up to your chest, keeping your elbows high at the top. Alternate sides.

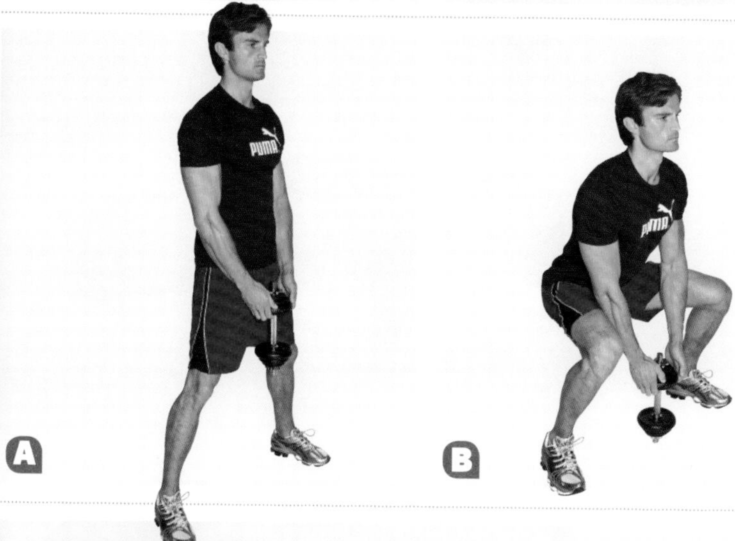

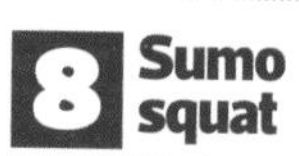

8 Sumo squat

> Adopt a wide stance, then lower until your thighs are parallel to the floor. Return smoothly to standing.

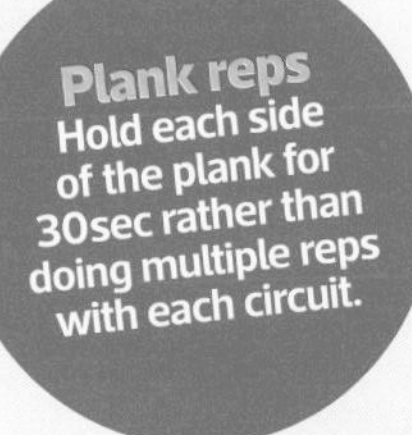

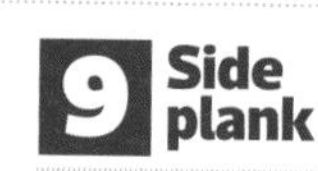

9 Side plank

> Your body should be straight from head to heels with your elbow below your shoulder. Alternate sides.

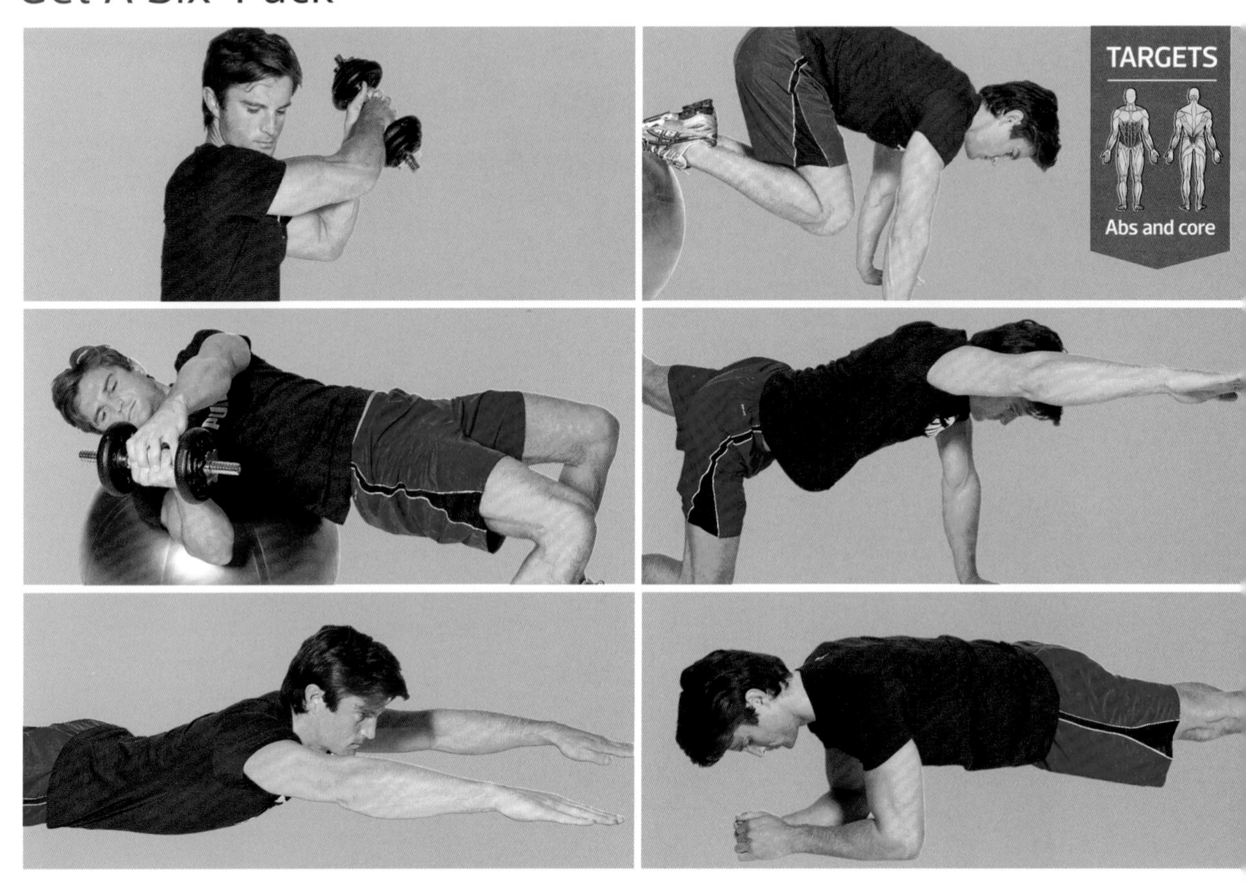

Six-pack in six moves

Build a rock-solid midsection with this balanced routine

Your abs are the perfect body part to train at home because you don't need heavy weights to give them a real test. But often, people don't include enough variety, meaning they don't develop strength and stability in all parts of their abs and core. It's also important to balance abs exercises with lower-back work – neglect this and you'll end up with a hunched posture as your abs pull your torso forwards.

This routine contains moves that work in all three planes of motion (side to side, forward and backward, and rotational) and will work your upper, lower and side abs, the deep-lying core muscles and the lower back. Your increased stability will have a positive effect for your other lifts and you'll be a step closer to getting that six-pack.

How to do this workout	Beginner	Intermediate	Advanced
How many workouts should I do per week?	3	4	5
How long will each session take?	16min	26min	30min
How many circuits per workout?	3	4	4
How many reps for per exercise?	12	12	15
How much rest should I take between circuits?	1min	2min	2min

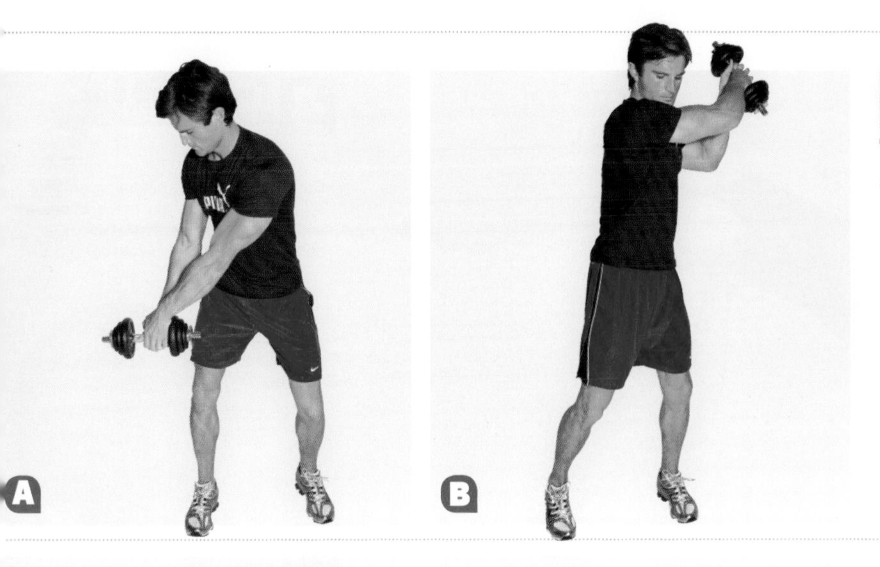

1 Woodchop

> Start with the dumbbell outside your knees and bring it across your body as you rise up.

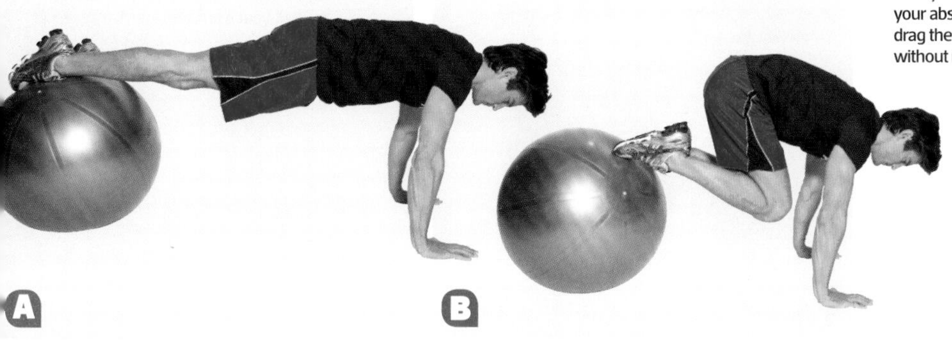

2 Gym ball jackknife

> Rest your feet on the ball, then contract your abs and bend your knees to drag the ball towards your chest without raising your backside.

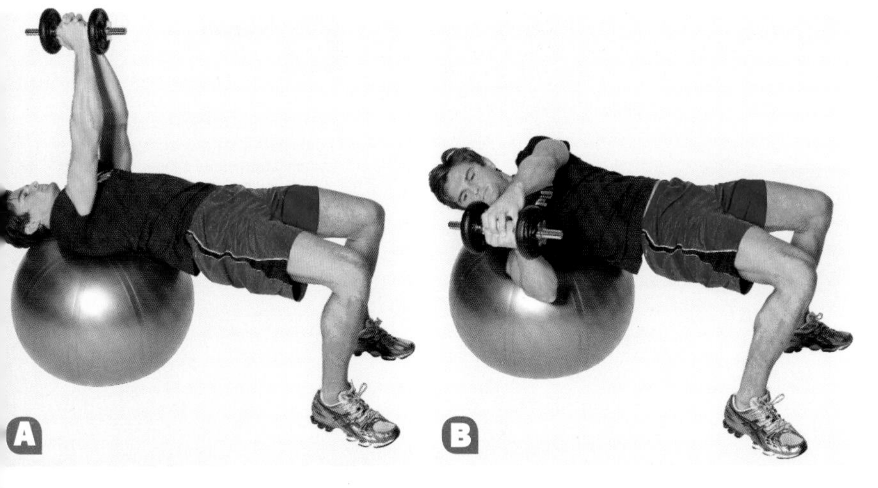

3 Gym ball Russian twist

> Rest your upper back on the ball and hold a weight above your face, then twist to one side. Return to the start and twist to the other side to complete one rep.

Get A Six-Pack

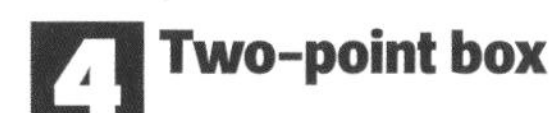

4 Two-point box

> Get on all fours with a neutral arch in your spine. Without tilting your pelvis, lift one arm and your opposite leg. Repeat the move on the other side to complete one rep.

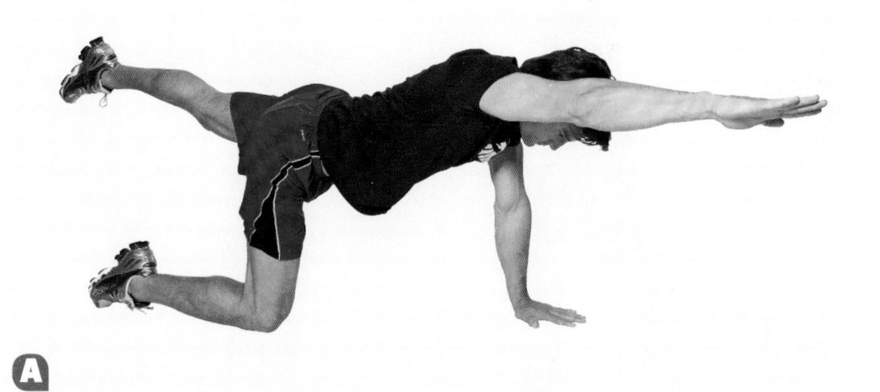

Hip hold
Make sure you don't tilt your hips as you extend your leg when performing the two-point box.

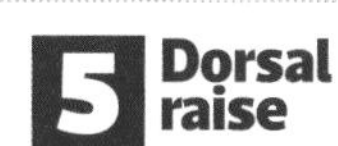

5 Dorsal raise

> Lie on your front with your arms out in front of your head. Engage your core and lower back to lift your torso off the floor.

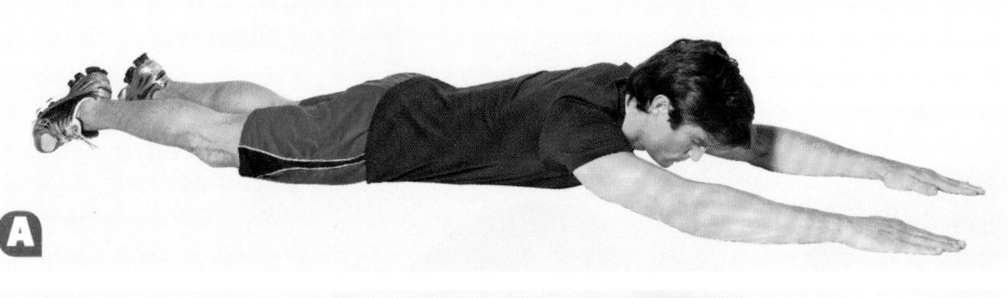

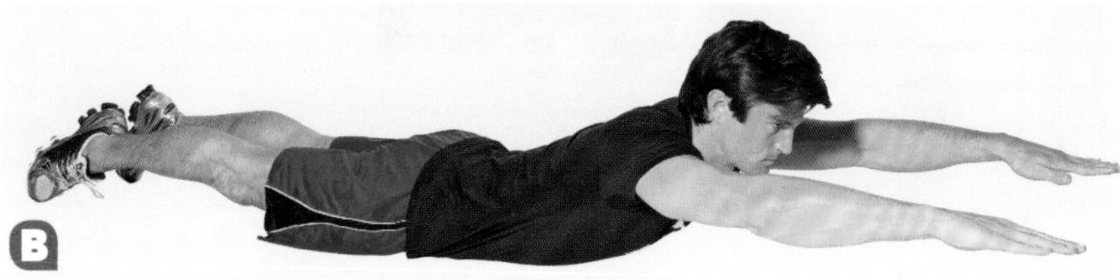

6 Plank

> Position your elbows below your shoulders and make sure your body is straight from head to heels. Don't sink your shoulders or let your hips sag.

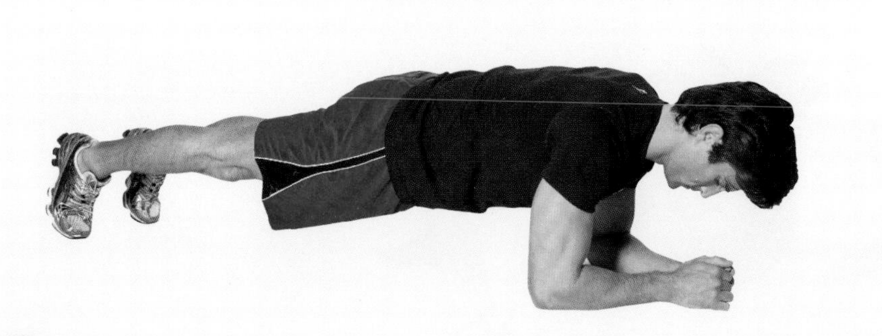

Plank time
Beginners should hold the plank for 30sec, intermediates 45sec and advanced exercisers 1min. Instead of the prescribed number of reps, do this three times.